"When I finally decided to turn my life around through exercise and better nutrition, one of the first things I did was give up eating refined, processed sugar. This well-researched book should be considered must-reading for anyone interested in the complex health discussion under way in America today!"

—Arkansas Governor Mike Huckabee

"This book is long overdue. Millions of people, including me, have been plagued by their relationship with sugar, and Connie Bennett has done a superb job bringing the topic into the public's eye."

—Film producer Harvey Weinstein

"Just about every American—or anyone who regularly eats sugar and processed carbs—needs to read this eye-opening, hard-hitting, and ultimately inspiring book."

—"Nutritionist to the Stars" Oz Garcia, Ph.D., author of *Look and Feel Fabulous Forever*

"I am sure that *SUGAR SHOCK!* will become the leading authority on this subject."

—Keith DeOrio, M.D., integrative physician (Connie's doctor who, back in 1998, "prescribed" that she kick sugar)

"This groundbreaking, hard-to-put-down book opens your eyes to little-known facts about how the typical American diet [high in sugar and refined carbs] could be wreaking havoc on your health, emotions, and relationships."

—Human relations expert Barbara DeAngelis, Ph.D., author of 14 bestsellers, including the #1 *New York Times* bestsellers *Secrets About Men Every Woman Should Know* and *Are You The One For Me?*

"Wish this book had been around when I was a teen—my whole life would have been better!"

—Naura Hayden, author of 8 books, including the #1 *New York Times* bestseller *How to Satisfy a Woman Every Time . . . and Have Her Beg for More!*

"*SUGAR SHOCK!* offers the best kind of 'sweet' that exists. This book is 'Brain Candy' for the smart consumer."

—Marilu Henner, actress and author of *Marilu Henner's Total Health Makeover*

"Follow Connie's powerful advice in *SUGAR SHOCK!* and finally break the sugar habit for good."

—Fitness expert Kathy Smith, author/creator of bestselling books and DVDs

"Through Connie's exhaustive research, interviews, and citations, she convinces us that, like drug addiction, sugar addiction is an environmental-biological disorder and a disease, not a moral weakness."
> —Marilyn E. Carroll, Ph.D., professor of psychiatry and neuroscience at the University of Minnesota, who has spent 30 years researching drug addiction and its interaction with feeding behavior

"A must-read!"
> —Dharma Singh Khalsa, M.D., author of the international bestseller *Brain Longevity*

"*SUGAR SHOCK!* tells the shocking truth about the devastating physical and mental effects of overconsumption of sugar and refined carbs."
> —Christiane Northrup, M.D., author of the bestsellers *Mother-Daughter Wisdom*, *The Wisdom of Menopause*, and *Women's Bodies, Women's Wisdom*

"Read this book. It could save your life."
> —Mark Hyman, M.D., *New York Times* bestselling author of *UltraMetabolism*

"Like *Fast Food Nation* and *Super Size Me*, *SUGAR SHOCK!* provides a much-needed wake-up call."
> —Donald I. Abrams, M.D., Director of Clinical Programs, OSHER Center for Integrative Medicine, University of California, San Francisco; and Chief, Hematology-Oncology, San Francisco General Hospital

"*SUGAR SHOCK!* is a must-read for anyone who cares about his or her health and well being!"
> —Jill R. Baron, M.D., integrative medicine physician and stress-management expert

"For years I've been warning my patients about the dangers of sugars and refined carbohydrates. At long last comes a book that tells the full story! I'll be recommending this to all of my patients."
> —Fred Pescatore, M.D., author of *The Hamptons Diet*

"A detailed, compelling, and scientific book that will become an instant classic."
> —Joshua Rosenthal, director of the Institute for Integrative Nutrition

"Everyone, whether hypoglycemic or not, will benefit from these provocative stories, powerful information, and health-healing messages."
> —Roberta Ruggiero, founder and president of The Hypoglycemia Support Foundation, Inc., and author of *The Do's and Don'ts of Hypoglycemia: An Everyday Guide to Low Blood Sugar*

"*SUGAR SHOCK!* is an engrossing, ultimately hopeful book that is brimming with fascinating, little-known facts and insights."
> —Nancy Appleton, Ph.D., author of *Lick the Sugar Habit*

"*SUGAR SHOCK!* is the ultimate antiaging, weight-loss, mood-management, optimal-health-and-detoxification book!"

—JJ Virgin, C.N.S., C.H.F.I., nutritionist for Dr. Phil's "Ultimate Weight Loss Challenge"

"Connie does a remarkable job in explaining in lay terms the plethora of research, myths, and associated health concerns of the sugar addict."

—Kenneth Blum, Ph.D., the first to associate the dopamine receptor gene with alcoholism and creator of the term "Reward Deficiency Syndrome"

"Connie Bennett delivers a potent 1-2-3 knockout punch to the sugar demons infiltrating our lives and threatening our health and well being."

—Ronald F. Feinberg, M.D., Ph.D., reproductive endocrinologist and author of *Healing Syndrome O: A Strategic Guide to Fertility, Polycystic Ovaries, and Insulin Imbalance*

"*SUGAR SHOCK!* contains powerful, cutting-edge, very accurate information that can help millions."

—Russ Bianchi, managing director, Adept Solutions, Inc., a global food and beverage product development firm

"Sugar is sweet. Tasty to eat. But, it mightily depletes. Read *SUGAR SHOCK!* your wisdom to complete."

—Mark Victor Hansen, coauthor of *One-Minute Millionaire* and coauthor of more than 65 titles in the bestselling Chicken Soup for the Soul series

"This is an important book done in a professional and meaningful way. Buy it to change your life."

—Liz Lipski, Ph.D., C.C.N., author of *Digestive Wellness* and *Digestive Wellness for Children*, and founder of Innovative Healing and Access to Health Experts

"Connie Bennett delivers a mind-blowing, provocative, easy-to-read book about how eating lots of sweets can throw you into SUGAR SHOCK!"

—Julia Havey, eDiets.com Master Motivator and author of *The Vice Busting Diet*

"*SUGAR SHOCK!* provides helpful, much-needed information."

—Dr. Eric Plasker, chiropractor; founder and CEO of The Family Practice, Inc.

"*SUGAR SHOCK!* . . . is an eye-opening book that should be in every home and doctor's office."

—Barbara Reed Stitt, Ph.D., president, Natural Ovens Bakery; author, *Food & Behavior* and *Roadmap for Healthy Foods in Schools*; and former Chief Probation Officer in Ohio, who helped probationers kick sugar and stay out of trouble with the courts

"Connie Bennett has written one of the most important health books of the twenty-first century in *SUGAR SHOCK!* Every single diabetic and obese person needs to read this book!"

    —Jimmy Moore, blogger and author of *Livin' La Vida Low-Carb: My Journey from Flabby Fat to Sensationally Skinny In One Year*

SUGAR SHOCK!

HOW SWEETS AND SIMPLE CARBS CAN DERAIL YOUR LIFE—AND HOW YOU CAN GET BACK ON TRACK

CONNIE BENNETT, C.H.H.C.,
with STEPHEN T. SINATRA, M.D.

Foreword by NICHOLAS PERRICONE, M.D.

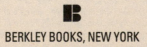

BERKLEY BOOKS, NEW YORK

THE BERKLEY PUBLISHING GROUP
Published by the Penguin Group
Penguin Group (USA) Inc.
375 Hudson Street, New York, New York 10014, USA
Penguin Group (Canada), 90 Eglinton Avenue East, Suite 700, Toronto, Ontario M4P 2Y3, Canada
(a division of Pearson Penguin Canada Inc.)
Penguin Books Ltd., 80 Strand, London WC2R 0RL, England
Penguin Group Ireland, 25 St. Stephen's Green, Dublin 2, Ireland (a division of Penguin Books Ltd.)
Penguin Group (Australia), 250 Camberwell Road, Camberwell, Victoria 3124, Australia
(a division of Pearson Australia Group Pty. Ltd.)
Penguin Books India Pvt. Ltd., 11 Community Centre, Panchsheel Park, New Delhi—110 017, India
Penguin Group (NZ), Cnr. Airborne and Rosedale Roads, Albany, Auckland 1310, New Zealand
(a division of Pearson New Zealand Ltd.)
Penguin Books (South Africa) (Pty.) Ltd., 24 Sturdee Avenue, Rosebank, Johannesburg 2196,
South Africa

Penguin Books Ltd., Registered Offices: 80 Strand, London WC2R 0RL, England

This book is an original publication of The Berkley Publishing Group.

Material from Dr. Stephen P. Gyland's 1957 study "Functional Hyperinsulinism in General Practice,"
published in the *Journal of the American Medical Association* 163; 507, reprinted with permission from
the American Medical Association. Copyright © 1957, American Medical Association. All rights reserved.

A listing of trademark information can be found on page 397.

Copyright © 2007 by Connie Bennett.
Cover design by axb group.
Text design by Tiffany Estreicher.

PRINTING HISTORY
Berkley trade paperback edition / January 2007

Library of Congress Cataloging-in-Publication Data

Bennett, Connie.
SUGAR SHOCK!: how sweets and simple carbs can derail your life, and how you can get back on
track / Connie Bennett and Stephen T. Sinatra ; foreword by Nicholas Perricone.
p. cm.
Includes bibliographical references and index.
ISBN: 978-0-425-21357-5
1. Sugar—Pathophysiology. 2. Carbohydrates, Refined—Pathophysiology. 3. Nutritionally
induced diseases. I. Sinatra, Stephen T. II. Title.
RC627.R43B46 2007
616.3'998—dc22

2006024574

PRINTED IN THE UNITED STATES OF AMERICA

10 9 8 7 6 5 4 3 2

SPECIAL DEDICATION

To the millions of mystified, anxious, panicked, depressed, moody, sluggish, wiped-out, fuzzy-headed, memory-impaired, libido-sapped, headache-ridden, lethargic, often–weight-challenged women and men, who are unknowingly trapped in SUGAR SHOCK! Your symptoms might not be "all in your head," as your doctors, friends, and loved ones may have been insisting. Rather, your habit of eating too many sweets and quickie carbs could be triggering your many mysterious ailments. Hope, health, and happiness await you.

DEDICATIONS FROM CONNIE

To my medical savior Keith DeOrio, M.D., who rescued me from a lifetime of horrific ailments and being doomed, branded, and shunned as an off-putting "Sugar Shrew," "Sugar Crybaby," "Sugar Zombie," and irrepressible "Sugar Junkie." I'm still marveling: All you did was give me a correct diagnosis ("reactive hypoglycemia") and accurate "prescription" (insisting that I renounce those sugary foods and processed carbs that I was overconsuming). Thank you always for my new lease on life!

To Roberta Ruggiero, founder of the nonprofit Hypoglycemia Support Foundation. Roberta, all I can say is "Wow!" You were my entire kick-sugar support network back in spring 1998, and I will always be tremendously grateful for your help. You are a selfless inspiration.

Last, but not least, to my ultra-extraordinary, talented, hardworking SUGAR SHOCK! research director and good friend Mary Kittel (1969–2004). You were simply amazing in your devotion and superhuman abilities to dig up all the latest scoops on the dark side of sugars and refined carbs. Because of you, I was able to piece together a complete picture of the devastating impact and far-reaching harm that could result from consuming all those sweets. Mary, I truly miss you and wish you'd seen this published book.

DEDICATION FROM DR. SINATRA

To all my patients, who've placed their trust and faith in me for the past 30 years to help heal them and improve the quality of their lives. You've touched my heart on multiple occasions as I hope I have yours.

CONTENTS

PART 3

WHERE WE ARE: ON A FAST TRACK
TO DANGER, DISEASE, AND LITIGATION

PART 4

HOW SUGARY FOODS COULD MESS WITH
YOUR MIND AND EMOTIONS

PART 5

HOW EXCESS SWEETS CAN SABOTAGE
YOUR HEALTH

PART 6

PULL THE PLUG ON SUGAR SHOCK! FOR A
HAPPIER, HEALTHIER LIFE

SUGAR SHOCK!

A mood-damaging, personality-bending, health-destroying, confusion-creating constellation of symptoms affecting millions of people worldwide, who often eat processed sweets and much-like-sugar carbs. "SUGAR SHOCK!" describes the often misdiagnosed and maligned condition of reactive hypoglycemia (low blood sugar), as well as other blood sugar disorders, from insulin resistance to diabetes. Research reveals that repeatedly overconsuming sweeteners, dessert foods, and quickie carbs (white rice, chips, etc.) wreaks havoc on your blood sugar levels, overstimulates insulin release, triggers inflammation, and could contribute to more than 150 health problems, including obesity, diabetes, heart disease, cancer, polycystic ovary syndrome, severe PMS, failing memory, mental confusion, *Candida*, sexual dysfunction, infertility, wrinkles, acne, and early aging. Victims of SUGAR SHOCK! also may experience depression, fatigue, headaches, dizziness, cold sweats, anxiety, irritability, tremors, crying spells, heart palpitations, forgetfulness, nightmares, blurred vision, muscle pains, temper outbursts, suicidal thoughts, and more. Ultimately, this insidious roller-coaster effect hampers sufferers' ability to function at full or even half throttle.

FOREWORD

Sugar and foods that convert rapidly to sugar in the bloodstream are toxic.

This highly charged statement might seem unduly harsh, especially as we gaze lovingly and longingly at that chocolate-chip cookie, Danish, or plate of rice cakes sitting on our desks. However, it is true. This very basic fact has been at the core of every book I have written, beginning with *The Wrinkle Cure* and continued in *The Perricone Prescription*, *The Perricone Promise*, *The Clear Skin Prescription*, and *The Perricone Weight Loss Diet*.

You may be asking yourself how something as American as apple pie could be regarded with both fear and loathing. The answer is simple. Sugar and high-glycemic carbohydrates are *proinflammatory*: that is, they create an inflammatory response in the body. My decades of research have shown that chronic, subclinical inflammation is the single greatest precipitator of aging and age-related diseases. These include diseases as diverse as heart disease, diabetes, Alzheimer's disease, arthritis, certain forms of cancer, obesity, unwanted weight gain, loss of muscle mass, and wrinkled, sagging skin.

This inflammation takes place on a cellular level and exists in all of our cells. It does its harm by triggering free radicals, which accelerate aging by damaging cells—leading to their eventual breakdown. Unfortunately, this inflammation is invisible to the naked eye: we can't see it or feel it until it is too late, and the damage is done. Many factors can trigger inflammation, including a proinflammatory diet, stress, environmental stressors (such as air pollution, pesticides, herbicides, etc.), weakened immune system, excess exposure to ultraviolet light, and hormonal changes. However, I believe the primary cause is diet—with stress running a close second.

Diet and Aging: The Sugar Connection

Foods that we eat can be either proinflammatory (i.e., they provoke an inflammatory response) or anti-inflammatory (i.e., they suppress the inflammatory response). The chief culprits in the proinflammatory arena are sugar and foods that quickly convert to sugar in the body (also known as high-glycemic carbohydrates). These include cakes, cookies, desserts, potatoes, most packaged breakfast cereals, breads, pastries, baked goods, juice, soda, chips, and rice cakes. Proinflammatory foods will exacerbate acne lesions, cause us to pack on the pounds, make us old before our time, and place us at serious risk for the many diseases and degenerative conditions listed above.

Understanding the Mechanism

Proinflammatory foods cause a sudden spike in blood sugar, triggering an insulin response from the pancreas in an effort to control the rising level of blood sugar. Diabetics do not have a properly functioning pancreas, and consequently they suffer from high blood sugar, which usually must be treated with insulin, diet, and exercise. Diabetics with poorly controlled blood sugar actually age one-third faster than do nondiabetics. Diabetics tend to have widespread, measurable inflammation in their bodies. Their constant high sugar levels cause kidney failure, blindness, heart attacks, and strokes. Studies have shown that when diabetics keep their blood sugar levels within normal range, they can cut their rate of health problems by 70 percent.

The bad news is that you don't have to be diabetic to experience the detrimental inflammatory response from sugar. Even a healthy body is damaged by sugar in a phenomenon known as glycation. Two decades in private dermatology practice and seeing thousands of patients, in conjunction with extensive study on the subject, has confirmed my belief that sugar is extremely damaging to the skin—in fact to all organ systems. I have used every platform available—from my books to my university lecture series on public television—to sound this alarm.

When we eat high-glycemic carbohydrates, they cause an immediate browning or glycating of the protein in our tissues. Glycation—a process long known to discolor and toughen food in storage—can occur in skin as well, creating detrimental age-related changes to collagen, and that means deep wrinkles. Glycation occurs when the sugar molecules permanently attach to collagen present in the skin and other parts of the body.

At the point of attachment, there is a small mechanism creating inflammation, which then becomes a source of inflammation in its own right. This inflammation produces enzymes that break down collagen, resulting in wrinkles. In addition to inflammation, glycation also causes cross-linking in our collagen, making it stiff and inflexible where it was once soft and supple.

This extensive cross-linking of collagen causes the loss of skin elasticity. Healthy collagen strands normally slide over one another, which keeps skin elastic. If a young person smiles or frowns, creating lines in the face, the skin will snap back and be smooth again when she stops smiling or frowning. But the skin does not snap back out in a person whose collagen has been cross-linked from years of eating sugar and the wrong carbs. Those deep grooves remain, because that is where the sugar molecules have attached to collagen, making the fibers stiff and inflexible.

The bond between the sugar and collagen generates a large number of free radicals leading to more inflammation. When glycation occurs in the skin, the ultimate effect is not unlike tanning a leather hide. Over time, skin begins to resemble a cross between beef jerky and an old boot, unevenly discolored and heavily striated with deep lines and grooves.

But it is not just the skin we have to worry about. These "sugar bonds" can occur throughout the body as we age. The sugar molecule attaches itself to the collagen, as well as our arteries, veins, bones, ligaments, even our brains, resulting in the breakdown of organ systems and the deterioration of the body. Glycation creates "free radical factories" known as advanced glycation end products (AGEs), which also increase cellular inflammation. These statements are based in solid scientific study. Glycation and advanced glycation end-products can be found in every medical textbook.

Although she is not a scientist, Connie Bennett is living proof of the havoc these proinflammatory foods can and do wreak. *SUGAR SHOCK!* is both a cautionary tale and one of hope. Connie shows us that, like her, we *can* beat the addiction and reclaim our health and well-being. I applaud her choice of Stephen Sinatra, M.D., F.A.C.C., as medical consultant.

Dr. Sinatra and I are colleagues of long standing and like minds. It is heartening to see more and more people—both physicians and scientists of Dr. Sinatra's caliber and laypeople such as Connie, with valuable firsthand experience—use their voices to raise awareness of the debilitating dangers of proinflammatory foods, with sugar leading the pack.

Nicholas Perricone, M.D.,
Madison, CT, April 2006

PART 1

OUR TALES: FROM SUGAR SEDUCTION TO SUGAR AWARENESS

1

Connie's Story: Confessions of the "Sugar Shrew No More!" and How I Changed upon the Scary Sugar Truth

My boyfriend, Mark, and I were dining at a trendy Malibu restaurant overlooking the Pacific Ocean. The crashing waves, caressing summer breeze, and flickering candles invited romance. Mark affectionately tousled my hair, then lifted his glass of zinfandel and toasted, "Here's to our first year together and to the sweet hereafter." I blushed.

Happy as I was to be in this idyllic setting with my beau, my thoughts were straying.

I confess: They were skipping ahead—to dessert. In fact, I was just about salivating at the thought of the establishment's famed, delectable chocolate mousse.

All evening, the enticing chocolate aroma had been wafting throughout the hip restaurant. Already, I could taste the velvety, creamy, delectable confection gliding down my throat. As if reading my mind, our waiter waltzed up, balancing a huge tray covered with sweet, dazzling, artfully prepared, mouthwatering presentations.

When my moist chocolate mousse and Mark's fluffy chocolate soufflé arrived, we shared, as always. First, we slowly, sensuously slipped dollops of our tantalizing treats into each other's mouths. Then, we sampled the plateful of complimentary miniature macaroons, chocolate truffles, lemon pinwheels, pecan pies, chocolate coconut stacks, and mints. Finally, we topped off dessert with a tasty amaretto liqueur. We were high on love, I thought.

After supper, we headed north to his house on the picturesque Pacific Ocean coastal route. We acted like a couple of giddy teens. We rolled with laughter and exchanged witty repartee. I, especially, was a fountain of clever remarks—so much so that Mark exclaimed, "Honey, you're so fun and funny."

In my mind, we were on cloud nine. Life felt sweet.

But, about 45 minutes into our drive, my mood shifted abruptly. My euphoria and elation moved out. Instead, panic and anxiety consumed me. The jitters struck. A brutal headache hit me. My innards shook. Dizziness overtook me. Edginess seized me. Even worse, I felt as if a monstrous force beyond my control had bubbled up inside me.

The calm, charismatic Connie had totally vanished. In her place, a crabby, cantankerous shrew had taken over. I felt as if this chilling creature was in control, holding my sweet personality hostage.

Then, the traffic light turned red. As Mark hit the brakes, "she"—certainly not I!—nastily snarled, "So why were you so late picking me up? You could have called. That was so rude!"

Startled, my boyfriend quickly turned toward me. Crestfallen, he asked, "Hey, Connie, we've been having such a great time. Why are you bringing this up now?"

Against my will, my demonic double irrationally bombarded him with a torrent of angry words. All logic had disappeared: I couldn't stop this bestial imposter from hurling a barrage of nonsensical criticism at him.

Mark's jaw muscles tightened. He gripped the steering wheel so tightly that his knuckles turned white.

He turned toward me. In Mark's eyes, I saw horrifying shock and complete befuddlement as more irrational words spewed out of me.

Time seemed to slow down as his gaze grew distant and his heart seemed to shut down. We drove in silence for several minutes until he couldn't contain his fury any longer. He finally demanded, "Why are you being so bitchy?"

I was dumbstruck. Flabbergasted, no reply came out. I had no rational answer.

Curling up against the car door, I wept and wailed uncontrollably. Suddenly, Mark made a quick U-turn and started driving south.

"Look, I can't handle this," he abruptly announced. "Let's cut the evening short. I'm taking you back to your place."

His chilled finality landed like a punch to my stomach. He opened the window, and it seemed that all the warmth we shared was sucked out into the night air.

Alone at my place, I collapsed on my couch and bawled. I was inconsolable. Worse yet, the charming, composed Connie—*the real me*—was nowhere to be found.

Later that night, after I'd hungrily devoured a small piece of leftover salmon, a handful of almonds, and some celery sticks, my tears subsided, and a sense of serenity enveloped me.

Then, the full impact of my intolerable behavior hit me like a sledgehammer. Much to my horror, I'd acted appallingly—probably way worse than the horrific "Wild Kate" in William Shakespeare's *The Taming of the Shrew*.

Remorse and shame flooded me. I was simply aghast at my transformation from loving sweetie to ranting bitch.

Indeed, I was forced to admit that I'd almost behaved as if I had a split personality: A cheerful, good-natured Connie had gone out to dinner. In her place, a distraught, ill-tempered Connie returned home.

That night, I crashed like an inflatable doll with the air squeezed out. Sleep came to claim me for a full 11 hours.

The next morning, I awoke with a ferocious "hangover" and overpowering malaise. Dragging myself out of bed took tremendous effort.

Overnight, I'd become a limp, lifeless zombie trapped in a depressed daze. It was fruitless to even *try* to research and write the magazine article whose deadline was looming. (At the time, I was a freelance entertainment and lifestyle reporter, which meant—thank goodness—that I had a flexible work schedule, leaving me free to try to make sense of the muck I'd landed in.)

In the days that followed, I laid low and agonized. Although downcast and demoralized, I tried to pinpoint the cause of my volatile outburst.

My bizarre behavior deeply disturbed me. I was scared and alarmed. A blue mood gnawed at me without abatement. What's more, despite my sincere, profuse apologies, Mark wouldn't see me. Sadly, I couldn't blame him.

Amidst my torment, I asked myself searing questions over and over again: *Why* had I, for no apparent reason, become unreasonable, argumentative, and irrational? *Why* had I become so overly emotional? *Who* was this woman who spewed odious, unloving remarks? And more importantly, I wondered, *What* the heck is wrong with me?

Alas, no answers came. Without much else to do, I continued to beat up on myself.

From Mortification to Revelation!

Scenes like the one I've just described—I'm horribly embarrassed to admit—used to be periodic, if not frequent, occurrences in my life. But that was before my stunning, life-changing revelation.

In spring 1998, after years of surviving way too many mortifying situations and freaking out more loved ones than I care to admit, I finally realized and accepted that I quickly transform from an easygoing Dr. Jekyll to a monstrous Ms. Hyde *whenever* I overindulge in sweet foods such as candies, cookies, cakes, cereals, sodas, ice cream, and waffles smothered with powdered sugar.

Likewise, I become outright irrational and illogical after filling up on refined, fiber-stripped breads, rolls, crackers, spaghetti, chips, or white rice—in short, any processed, devitalized baked goods or what I call "much-like-sugar carbs" or "quickie carbs."

Even one little glass of wine or a shot of sake, which, like all alcohol, turns to sugar in your bloodstream, wallops me with a horrific hangover, excessive exhaustion, and a blast of irritability.

There's simply no escaping the terrifying change that occurs against my will. After eating or drinking a lot—or a polite portion—of sweets or refined carbs, I turn into my own worst nightmare, uncontrollable and unstoppable.

After eating quickie carbs, I become an untamable, irascible "Sugar Shrew"; a fuming, disagreeable "Sugar Monster"; a sobbing, pitiful "Sugar Crybaby"; and finally, a listless, lethargic "Sugar Zombie"—never intentionally evil—but really, really difficult to be around.

Would that I could stop my switch from sweetie to shrew, from good to bad—believe me, I've tried hard and often. Doesn't work.

Alas, my dreadful, dramatic sugar-induced transformation is inevitable.

As predictable as the moon rising.

As sure as the swallows coming home to Capistrano at the same time every year.

As expected as the crowds flocking to Macy's or Bloomingdale's for an annual blowout sale.

Perhaps, to you, my reaction seems over the top or quite out of the ordinary. Certainly, I can comprehend that point of view.

But, lest you think I'm unique in my Sugar Shrew scenario, you'll hear later from other sensitive "sugar sufferers," who talk about similar volatile outbursts, quarrelsome behaviors, and illogical reactions after eating sweets or refined carbs.

Actually, I hope that my "coming out of the closet" about my sugar addiction will pave the way for millions of others to do so as well.

In fact, difficult as it may be to accept the fact that *both* emotional reactions and physical problems may be linked to your habit of eating too many desserts and quickie carbs, compelling research buttresses this theory.

Bewitched, Bewildered, Beleaguered

For *more* than a decade—*before* I learned about the dire consequences of my over-the-top sugar habit—I and a steady stream of medical specialists had been consistently stumped by the swarm of seemingly unconnected physical and emotional ailments that besieged and waylaid me. (You'll soon learn that there were medical reasons for my emotional ups and downs and for my plethora of perplexing ailments.)

To this day, I marvel in disbelief when reminiscing about my many strange, seemingly unconnected, disparate symptoms.

For starters, I was socked by "brain fog" so my thoughts wouldn't coalesce properly. This meant I often had to reread sections of documents and newspapers so they'd make sense. Meanwhile, my nagging forgetfulness occasionally got me into trouble, like the time it simply slipped my mind to meet my friend Helen for dinner. (Furious, she ended our friendship.)

My dazed mental state also made me accident prone. On one embarrassing occasion, I actually sprained my ankle merely walking down a ramp while covering a film premiere for a national magazine.

QUICK GUIDE TO THE WORDS "SUGAR," "SUGARS," ETC.

Throughout this book, we interchangeably use the words "sugar," "sweets," "sugars," and "sugary" to mean ALL caloric sweeteners, sugars, or desserts. These terms also apply to ALL processed, fast-acting carbs such as refined pasta, chips, white breads, and bagels. We call these foods "much-like-sugar carbs" or "quickie carbs." Furthermore, sugar signifies all alcoholic beverages, because they turn to sugar in your bloodstream. Please see chapter 4, "Clearing the Carb Confusion," for further explanations and clarification.

Moreover, much of the time I felt dizzy, woozy, and light-headed. The room often swirled around me. My hands and insides shook when hunger hit, and I was besieged by sudden, overpowering feelings of "I've got to have food now!" And my sleep was haunted by vivid, unsettling nightmares.

Other strange, inexplicable symptoms hit me, too. Much of the time my eyes burned and ached. Light blinded me whenever I went outside, even if the sun wasn't shining. My skin itched and crawled, and my hands and feet frequently felt cold. Even worse—and perhaps one of my most troubling symptoms—I was often plagued by a crippling, crushing, unrelenting exhaustion, where eight hours of sleep didn't even help. (Sure sounds like chronic fatigue syndrome, doesn't it?)

Then, all too frequently, I was beset by throbbing, unbearable, migrainelike headaches, which made it almost impossible to get anything accomplished—that is, other than lying down. Even more scary—every few weeks, loud, frightening palpitations would strike, making me feel as if my heart were about to jump right out of my chest and onto the floor in front of me.

What's more, every month, without fail, horrific PMS turned me into hell on heels, complete with mood aberrations and unbridled anger. And my period always entailed horrible, must-lie-me-down cramps, nagging backaches, and more.

Besides being a physical mess, I was an emotional volcano, as you "witnessed" earlier. Much to my mortification, for no good or logical reason, I'd flip from euphoric and enthusiastic to depressed and dejected within any one hour.

For example, I'd surrender to tears or be overcome by mercurial moods, troubling anxiety, and even—I'm embarrassed to admit—occasional thoughts of suicide. Worse still, this volatile, overly emotional, undignified Connie would appear—against my will, of course—at the most inopportune moments. (Yeah, I know, "she" sounds like one unsavory chick and a basket case! Thank God, we're not talking about me anymore.)

Even more frustrating and infuriating is that none of the doctors I saw over the years were able to explain my myriad of perplexing symptoms. They certainly didn't think my turbulent, on-again, off-again love/hate affair with sweet snacks was to blame.

Depending upon when you caught me, I'd have quickie-carb favorites. Toward "the end" (as I call it), before my "eureka" moment, I'd become overly attached to red licorice, which first seductively beckoned to me at a screening for us film reporters. Without realizing what was happening, I let one piece lead to a fistful, and soon I was scouting them out at grocery stores so I could devour 10 to 15 at a time. Chocolate-covered peanuts, small wheat crackers, and low-calorie hard candies in several flavors also played starring roles in my life at one time or another.

"You were hoarding them like a closet alcoholic," revealed my friend Devo, who once opened a drawer at my place looking for paper clips, but instead discovered my secret stash of chocolate, cinnamon, cherry, and butterscotch candies.

As memory serves me, I reached for those "treats" for a turbo-charged burst of concentration, a much-needed pick-me-up, and sometimes for solace or comfort.

Although I ate way too many quickie carbs, you wouldn't have known it by looking at me. My weight was normal other than the fact that I occasionally battled (at least in my mind) five lingering, unwanted pounds. My "crime" is a common one among weight-conscious females: I counted calories, all the while shortchanging myself by only minimally eating high-quality, healthier foods.

Actually, years previously—I'm saddened to admit—my sugar-and-carb-filled binges had played a pivotal part in a hard-to-break eating disorder. Even though I'd finally overcome my bulimia and anorexia (thanks to determination, positive thinking, therapy, and belief in the divine), my sugar addiction was, nevertheless, still raging unabated.

Years and Years of Misdiagnosis

Perplexed and frustrated, I made the rounds of medical practitioners—one after another, year after year.

"Chronic fatigue syndrome," pronounced one physician.

"Epstein-Barr virus," proclaimed another.

"Too much coffee," insisted a third. "Cut it out." (I did.)

"Absolutely nothing wrong with you," yet another declared.

"It's the diet soda. Quit it," suggested one more. (Again, I followed the advice.)

"It's all in your head. Get into therapy," maintained another M.D. (I obliged.)

"Take Prozac," one psychiatrist urged repeatedly. (I adamantly refused.)

You get the idea. Sure, the mystified physicians had "answers," but *none* was ever totally correct.

So, much to my dismay, I remained a pooped-out, fuzzy-headed, confusion-laden, anxiety-ridden, depression-plagued, sugar-obsessed woman with the energy and life force of an immobile, inert slug.

My Turning Point

After that last mortifying flip-out with my boyfriend, Mark, I sought yet another doctor, hoping to unlock the key to my woes.

Luckily, after years of puzzled agony, I found Dr. Keith DeOrio, an integrative physician, who was well versed in nutrition, vitamins, homeopathy, and acupuncture, and who had an amiable, caring bedside manner. This M.D., who had a thriving practice in Santa Monica, quickly pieced the clues together—something his ignorant medical colleagues had been unable to do for years.

Soon after learning of my excruciating symptoms, running a battery of tests, and grilling me about my chronic consumption of candies and refined crackers, Dr. DeOrio delivered an *accurate* medical diagnosis—one that had eluded me for years:

"You have severe reactive hypoglycemia or low blood sugar," he pronounced.

Then, he issued a unique, if not shocking, "prescription"—if you want to call it that—which didn't involve medications of any sort:

- "Cut out all sugary foods and all processed carbohydrates, and, mark my words, you'll feel better."

- "Eat ample protein, plenty of fresh vegetables, low-sugar fruits, nuts, seeds, legumes, some whole grains, and healthy fats."

- "Take these herbs, vitamins, and supplements."

Sure enough, my doctor's prediction came true within weeks.

After following his advice to shun sweets and quickie carbs and enjoy nourishing foods, my life miraculously changed. *All* 44 of my dreaded symptoms *totally* disappeared!

Quite remarkably, soon after kicking sugar, I became full of zest, verve, spunk, vitality, enthusiasm, optimism, and joie de vivre.

Imagine how delighted I was to discover a new, improved, happier, sweeter, more coherent Connie! At the risk of sounding trite, I truly felt *reborn*.

It was mind boggling to me that simply quitting dessert foods and fast-acting carb favorites such as bagels, chips, popcorn, and French bread could trigger such dramatic, drastic, far-reaching improvements in my health, moods, energy levels, frame of mind, and, as a result, relationships.

My transformation was extraordinary to fathom, especially given the fact that I'm a skeptical, prove-it, give-me-all-the-facts journalist.

My Sugar Education and the Hypoglycemia Connection

Restored to good health and humor, I became *driven* to dig up more information about reactive hypoglycemia and what part sugar plays in it. After devouring the few books I could find and talking to fellow sufferers, I learned that hypoglycemia is a baffling, misunderstood, much-maligned medical condition that can produce more than 100 debilitating ailments, including manic depression, migraines, crying sprees, and even suicidal impulses. (I would have learned about low blood sugar on the Internet, but this was 1998, and the Web didn't have nearly as much information as it does now.)

Much to my relief, I also found *every single one* of my ailments described

CONNIE, THE "SUGAR SHREW" OF 1998: MY SYMPTOMS

Get ready to be amazed, as I am now, by my extensive list of ailments—**all of which** my books told me are symptoms of low blood sugar. Much to my surprise, every single one disappeared within weeks of kicking sweets and quickie carbs!

1. Mood Swings
2. Temper tantrums
3. Crying spells
4. Drowsiness
5. Overwhelming fatigue (or the reverse—being wired)
6. Insomnia or sleeping difficulties
7. Waking up exhausted
8. Craving for sweets
9. Sleeping too much
10. Headaches
11. Difficulty concentrating
12. Mental confusion
13. Restlessness
14. Anxiety
15. Depression
16. Irritability
17. Heart palpitations (tachycardia)
18. Dizziness and vertigo
19. Forgetfulness
20. Fainting
21. Light-headedness
22. Nightmares
23. Aching eye sockets
24. Ravenous hunger between meals
25. Severe PMS
26. Unnecessary worrying
27. Feel best after 7 p.m.
28. Digestive problems
29. Muscle pains
30. Joint pains
31. Cold hands and feet
32. Internal trembling
33. Indecisiveness
34. Nervousness
35. Sensitivity to light and noise
36. Peculiar breath/perspiration odor
37. Lack of coordination
38. Suicidal thoughts or tendencies
39. Anorexia and bulimia (at one point)
40. Muscular twitching or cramps
41. Antisocial or unsocial behavior
42. Itching or crawling sensations on the skin
43. Sighing and yawning
44. The shakes when hungry

with uncanny accuracy! In fact, all my symptoms were listed in the literature—and I counted a whopping 44 in all!

The Experts' Startling Supposition

The more research I conducted, the more astounded and intrigued I became, because all experts arrived at the same conclusion: Eating too many sweets or processed carbs is almost always to blame for hypoglycemia's many mysterious symptoms. This discovery was enlightening but unsettling.

Questions began to stick to me like Krazy Glue:

- How could eating yummy chocolate, beautifully decorated cakes, delicious pasta, and freshly baked dinner rolls lead to emotional and physical ailments as wide ranging as forgetfulness, fainting, and fatigue?

- Why would a devastating, perplexing, far-reaching medical condition such as hypoglycemia be so consistently ignored, overlooked, and underplayed?

- Why weren't our nation's newspapers, magazines, and TV talk shows brimming with stories containing hard-hitting warnings about the potential for problems that often plague dessert delighters?

Since my startling sugar discovery in 1998, I've learned that I have a lot of company. Millions of Americans suffer similar fates at the hands of sweets or much-like-sugar carbs.

But emotional turmoil is only *part* of the story. Your reaction to eating quickie carbs might be less obvious and quite different from my overly emotional Sugar Shrew, hypoglycemic meltdown.

For many, over time, a heavy-duty dessert routine or quickie-carb overload can erode energy levels, corrode powers of concentration, or even sap their sex drive. For many more, blood sugar disorders such as insulin resistance or prediabetes set in. For still others, the effects of their excessive, long-term sugar or carb habit might not emerge until years later, when they're ambushed by severe physical problems such as diabetes, cancer, or heart disease.

Are You Suffering, Too, and Don't Know Why?

At this point, I invite you to explore the possibility that some of your baffling, unexplained maladies might be related to your eating patterns, too.

- Are you buffeted about by wildly fluctuating mood swings, panic attacks, angry outbursts, and sobbing spells that make your sweetheart throw his or her hands up in puzzlement and eventual disgust?

- Are you bewildered by overpowering exhaustion, fuzzy thinking, incapacitating blues, aching eyeballs, rapid heartbeat, unbearable migraines, and severe PMS?

- Are you engaged in a seemingly endless battle of the bulge—but nonetheless always make room for dessert foods or quickie-carb snacks?

- Are you "hooked" on chocolate, chips, or pasta—even identifying with people who can't go a single day without cigarettes, booze, or drugs?

If you answered yes to any of the above questions, then you *might* be among the estimated 74 million to 147 million Americans—or from one-quarter to one-half of the U.S. population—who have difficulty processing sweets and refined carbs. Perhaps you, too, are a victim of this terrifying, menacing epidemic that I call SUGAR SHOCK!

From Sugar Shame to Sugar-Free Success

To be honest, I have tremendous, overpowering "Sugar Shame." I'm quite humiliated and horrified by moments such as the one I recounted earlier.

Frankly, I was initially very reluctant to tell the world how my sugar and quickie-carbs habit twisted my personality, nearly destroyed my health, and wreaked havoc on my love life and relationships.

Worse still, I'm disappointed in myself that I didn't take action or heed

SUGAR SHOCK! DEFINED

A mood-altering, emotionally devastating, mentally damaging, physically destructive constellation of symptoms affecting millions of people worldwide, who are caught in a cycle of overindulging in refined sweets and much-like-sugar carbs like white bread, pasta, and chips. "SUGAR SHOCK!" describes the often-misdiagnosed condition of reactive hypoglycemia (low blood sugar) and other blood sugar disorders, from insulin resistance to diabetes. Mounds of research reveal that repeatedly overconsuming these nutrient-deprived quickie carbs and caloric sweeteners wreaks havoc on your blood sugar levels, overstimulates insulin release, triggers inflammation, and could contribute to 150-plus health concerns, including obesity, diabetes, heart disease, cancer, polycystic ovary syndrome, failing memory, sexual dysfunction, and infertility. Victims of SUGAR SHOCK! may also experience depression, fatigue, headaches, dizziness, cold sweats, anxiety, irritability, tremors, crying spells, severe PMS, nightmares, heart palpitations, mental confusion, muscle pains, blurred vision, temper outbursts, suicidal thoughts, and more. Ultimately, this insidious roller-coaster effect, which occurs whenever you eat lots of sweets and quickie carbs, hampers sufferers' ability to function at full or even half throttle.

warnings I'd heard years earlier when I first learned about hypoglycemia and the "sugar blues," as author William Dufty calls it.

Let's face it: naturally, it would be far easier to hide my living sugar-induced nightmares, pretend they never happened, close that chapter of my life, and move on.

But now that I've had nine wonderful years to distance myself from this distasteful, despicable Sugar Shrew, Sugar Crybaby, and Sugar Monster, I realize that millions of you out there could greatly benefit from my dreadful, almost unbelievable tales and needless health woes, as well as my insights, research, and conclusions.

You, too, might be able to leave behind your moody, nasty demeanor simply by kicking all sugars and fast-acting carbs.

You, too, might be able to bid adieu to innumerable, inexplicable symptoms such as debilitating depression, horrible headaches, and awful PMS.

You, too, might be able to finally find the peace of mind that has continually eluded you. It's my greatest hope that this book will help you do just that.

2

Dr. Sinatra's Story: From Witnessing My Mom's Dangerous, Diabetic Blood Sugar Swings to Unmasking the Cholesterol and Low-Fat Myths

By Stephen Sinatra, M.D., C.N.S.

For two decades, I've been warning my patients and those who hear me speak that the more sugar and refined carbohydrates they consume, the more quickly they will age. Therefore, when Connie first approached me to come on board as medical consultant for her book, I jumped at the opportunity to get the truth out—that overconsuming sugar and your resulting high blood sugar levels can be highly toxic.

Furthermore, I'm eager to correct the misconception about the dangers of high cholesterol that's been so widely accepted by an unsuspecting public. As a board-certified cardiologist, certified nutrition specialist, and antiaging specialist, I can tell you this: there are far more significant and devastating causes of coronary artery disease than cholesterol, and too much sugar and high blood sugar levels are at the top of the list.

It's unfortunate that Americans, who are, at least by and large, somewhat savvy about cholesterol's dangers, are almost completely ignorant about the many perils of eating too much sugar.

The truth is that, over time, consuming too many sweets and refined carbohydrates could cause even more profound clogging of your heart vessels than high cholesterol levels ever could. Too much sugar can give you heart disease. What's more, it can get you there much faster than cholesterol.

To be sure, cholesterol does play a role in developing heart disease, but in my opinion, it's only a minor player. And unfortunately, its role has been overexaggerated by the scientific community, as well as the media. In fact, millions of people in this country are on cholesterol-lowering drugs, but frankly, I don't think they need it.

A look at my youth and medical training will help you to understand how I arrived at my conclusions about sugar's role in heart disease and other illnesses.

My Awareness of Sugar's Dangers and Diabetes Began in Childhood

As a young child, I first began to witness the dangers of too much sugar and wide blood sugar fluctuations. From age 10 to 17, I was exposed to frequent blood sugar nightmares and scares because my mom was a type 1, insulin-dependent, brittle diabetic (with wide blood sugar swings), who was often in and out of the hospital. A few times, I even found her passed out on the floor.

Eventually, in 1998, my mother tragically died from diabetic complications. It was awful: She developed cardiac arrhythmias, severe osteoporosis and bone fractures, and blindness. Even worse, it was painful to stand by helplessly when physicians were unable to help her. In fact, because of that horrible experience during my teenage years, I was inspired to become a doctor so I could help heal people.

You'd expect that, growing up with a diabetic mom, I would learn how to moderate sugar intake and properly manage blood sugar levels. But that didn't happen.

Instead, given the bad advice diabetics were being given in those days, we didn't learn about the value and health benefits of limiting sugar intake. Doctors were wrongly teaching diabetics to eat a lot of sugary foods such as orange juice, cereal, breads, and flour. So that's what my mom ate.

Today, of course, it's obvious why, after eating high-sugar, low- or no-protein meals, my mom would frequently swing from episodes of low blood sugar, where she'd get shaky, sweaty, or faint, to high blood sugar, where she'd have ketosis, with blurred vision, the shakes, difficulty concentrating, weakness, and a strong acetone breath.

Once I'd begun practicing as a cardiologist, I realized how inappropriate my mother's dietary recommendations had been. For years she had eaten poorly, yet she was simply following standard teachings of the day!

In fact, you'll learn here, in this book, about the considerable research that flat-out refutes this advice.

My Hypoglycemic High School Moments and My Sugar Sensitivity

While watching my mother sink further and further into her disease, I also unknowingly had my own strange sugar experiences. For example, in high school, I would often fall asleep in my honors English class, which took place right after lunch.

In those days, we'd eat a lot of carbohydrates at the midday meal— sandwiches on white bread, macaroni and cheese, and then ice cream for dessert. Even though the course was interesting, I'd take naps all the time.

I sat in the front row, and the teacher was constantly waking me up. I remember thinking, "What's this all about?"

Years later, when I became a doctor, I realized that each time I had snoozed like that in class, I was having a hypoglycemic reaction in response to my sugary lunch. Those carbs had triggered a blood sugar high and then an insulin reaction, which brought my blood sugar down too low.

Actually, I was having similar reactions to the ones my mom had experienced years earlier. My mother would occasionally pass out, but I would just fall asleep.

In high school, I also learned that sugar gives you a fake "high." I used to wrestle, and the coaches would tell us to drink honey and orange juice right after the weigh-in to give us energy during the bout. Afterward, I would feel very jittery and wired—what I realize now to be a maladaptive, energized state.

As time went on, I came to realize that whenever I ate sugar, my body gave me a strong message. For example, if I had a dessert and some wine with my dinner, I'd get a rapid heart rate for hours and then horrible insomnia. Knowing my family history of diabetes, I came to realize that I'm sensitive to sugar and that if I'm not careful, I'm a likely candidate for diabetes. That's why I work hard to keep my weight down and watch my sugar intake like a hawk.

Although most of the time I stay away from sweets, I'm not perfect. I do allow myself tastes of sweets from time to time. For example, I'll have an occasional piece of dark chocolate—the darker the better, because it contains antioxidant properties similar to those found in green tea.

Or, sometimes, to be social, I'll taste one forkful of dessert when I'm out with friends. But if I do plan to eat a little sugar, I'll always add protein to my meal to counteract the insulin surge, because our bodies metabolize sugar and insulin more slowly if we ingest protein at the same time.

While, in an ideal world, it's, of course, better and more healthy to eliminate sweets entirely, I'm also realistic. For example, over the years, in my practice, I've found that my patients find it extremely difficult to be a "purist" 100 percent of the time. Rather, they have the most success when they eat healthily at least 80 percent of the time and allow themselves less-ideal foods the other 20 percent.

In short, by permitting themselves small portions of planned "treats" or "indulgences," they find it much easier and doable to eat right most of the time. Otherwise, I've found, they might fail entirely. But I certainly don't recommend this 80/20 approach if you have an urgent reason to avoid sweets such as a metabolic disorder, diabetes, or hypoglycemia.

However, as Connie will explain later, many people just can't have any sweets at all. They react to sugars the way alcoholics react to alcohol. They just cannot take even one small bite of a dessert: if they do, it leads to another bite and eventually to a binge or a sugar overload. Or they have overpowering, horrible reactions to sugary foods, such as those Connie so colorfully and eloquently shared in chapter 1.

While you're deciding if you're one of millions in SUGAR SHOCK!, here are some facts about sugar, aging, and heart disease you should know.

How I Witnessed Firsthand That Sugar Ages You More Quickly

Already, in my first year of medical school in 1968, it dawned on me that people with diabetes and poor blood-sugar-control age more quickly. One day, as part of our training, a radiologist put up a woman's abdominal X-ray and asked us to guess the systemic disease it indicated. What it showed was a calcified femoral artery (calcium deposits inside a blood vessel) that looked like it belonged to a 60-year-old. None if us could figure out what disease this person had.

I'll never forget this X-ray. It turned out she had diabetes—and she was only in her early 40s. I remember thinking, "Yeah, that's just like my mom. My mom is aging too quickly. This is such a rotten illness!" So this early med-school lesson showed me without a doubt that diabetes ages you about 15 years more quickly than the general population.

Then, in the late 1970s, as a busy, young cardiologist, I started seeing the evil side of sugar on a day-to-day basis. I would work long hours in a hospital, doing cardiac catheterizations and angiograms and take care of hundreds of people stricken by heart attacks.

Sadly, the sickest people I saw were elderly diabetics—just like my mom. Working with these diabetics made me realize how vulnerable they were and how important it was to maintain proper blood sugar control.

Around this time, I also began reading books by nutritionist Carlton Fredericks such as *New Low Blood Sugar and You*, and my mind was opened.

Here I was, a relatively new cardiologist treating elderly diabetics' hearts, and my diabetic mother was rapidly getting worse, and it all came together for me: I saw that sugar, not cholesterol, was the real evil. In 1982, I included vital information on how excess sugar can harm your heart in my first book, *All about Me: Hercules, the Heart*, which was for children.

Over the years, the relationship between sugar and aging kept coming up time and time again, including about 20 years later, when I was getting certified as a nutrition specialist.

Simply put, high blood sugar and high insulin are a lethal combination. Later in *SUGAR SHOCK!* you'll learn more about advanced glycation end products, or AGEs, which—as my colleague Dr. Nicholas Perricone mentioned in the foreword—occur when insulin levels are consistently elevated as a result of consuming too much sugar. What you need to know now is that inflammation causes AGEs to be formed, which fatigues the vital mitochondria, your cells' source of energy.

Essentially, if you eat an excess of sugar, you diminish your cells' life force, but if you cut back on sugar, you delay the aging of your cells as inflammation is diminished.

The majority of both conventional and alternative doctors now believe that chronic silent inflammation is the root cause of disease—whether it's cancer, coronary artery disease, Alzheimer's disease, Parkinson's disease, or diabetes.

What causes this silent inflammation? The hormone insulin is at the top of the list. What releases insulin? Sugar. Surges of sugar trigger surges of insulin.

What happens is this: As you digest sugar, dessert snacks, or fast-acting carbohydrates, your body converts these foods into glucose. When glucose enters your bloodstream, it triggers your pancreas to produce insulin, which helps to convert the excess glucose into glycogen for storage in your liver and muscles, and the unmetabolized calories are stored as fat. That is why you gain weight.

So the more sugar you consume, the higher your insulin levels will be and the more inflammation you will have. In short, sugar affects not only the tiny mitochondria but also the skin, heart, and all the cells in your body. And that's why excess sugar ages you prematurely.

How I Found Out That Low-Fat Diets Don't Work, But Cutting Carbs Does

Back in the early 1990s, I, like most of my medical colleagues across the country, wrongly bought into the low-fat craze. We thought that the best way to lose weight was to go on a high-carb diet and to avoid fats like the plague. It made sense to take fat out of the diet because fats are nine calories per gram, and carbohydrates are four calories per gram.

At the time, I was eating lots of pasta, salad, and bread, and I stayed away from all fats. Then, I made the worst error of all—even eliminating the good omega-3 essential fatty acids. And over the years, I started to gain weight—and so did my patients. My pants size started to increase, and when I checked my blood lipids, my HDL (the "good" cholesterol) was going down, my triglycerides were going up, and I was developing early insulin resistance.

That's when I realized that my high-carb diet was contributing to early insulin resistance syndrome. And it dawned on me that this was why my patients also were getting heavier and developing the same syndrome.

After years of mistakes, I learned that I'd been wrong. I literally had to rewrite my book *Optimum Health* because my opinion had changed, and I had to tell the truth about the evils of a high-carb diet.

Actually, my patients were my best messengers. They helped teach me that the best diet of all is one that includes a little protein at every meal, along with some healthy fats and low-glycemic-load carbohydrates such as vegetables, fruits, and whole grains. I became a broccoli addict overnight. It's also best to really restrict foods made with white flours such as bread, bagels, crackers, and pasta.

When my patients ate this way, their triglyceride levels fell, their HDL (the "good" cholesterol) increased, their blood pressure went down, and they began losing weight. This way of eating works because moderate amounts of protein and healthy fats do not trigger the production of insulin, but carbohydrates, especially sugar, require an enormous insulin response.

The Fallacy That Cholesterol Causes Heart Disease

As I've already mentioned, in the early 1980s, after taking care of hundreds of diabetics who were having heart attacks, helplessly watching my ailing diabetic mom, and getting further nutrition education, I realized that the American public—and even doctors—were being improperly educated. They'd all been led to believe that you need to take medications to lower your cholesterol, and that if you do, you'll lessen your risk of heart disease or even prevent a heart attack.

But taking meds isn't necessarily the best way to prevent heart problems. Too much sugar, not cholesterol, is the real evil. Cutting out sweets and refined carbohydrates—or at least eating a lot less of them—is perhaps the best way to protect your heart.

The reason more cardiologists haven't focused on the evils of sugars and simple carbs rather than cholesterol is because there is no patent on blood sugar. Basically, I'm saddened to admit, most doctors are indoctrinated or educated by the pharmaceutical industry. Drug representatives often come to doctors' offices with briefcases full of samples of cholesterol-lowering medications. These drug reps are there to talk about how the meds work, and they're armed with all kinds of literature—periodicals and copies of research studies—that "prove" the meds work.

Of course, these drug reps aren't talking about studies that show the relationship between excess sugar consumption and heart disease, despite the fact that so much information is out there. As you'll soon learn in *SUGAR SHOCK!*, we seek to fill in these many, many educational gaps.

In the last 25 years, many cardiologists have come to believe that high ("bad") LDL cholesterol (greater than 160) causes heart disease. I, however, see cholesterol as only a small part of the disease process. It's a minor player, but it's been built up to be the major player. Thankfully, a number of open-minded, nutrition-oriented physicians and cardiologists have now arrived at my point of view.

Actually, you may be surprised to learn that cholesterol is very important to our bodies. It lubricates our skin. It forms the basis for our sex hormones—testosterone, estrogen, and progesterone. It's vital for our brain function. And cholesterol's release into our bloodstream provides our bodies' natural defense against toxicity, particularly from heavy metals. LDL cholesterol also carries the coenzyme Q10, a naturally produced antioxidant that is vital for sustaining life.

We tend to hear a lot about the dangers of high cholesterol, but I daresay most Americans don't know that very low cholesterol is unsafe, too. When people's LDL cholesterol falls too low—less than 70mg/dL—they may develop transient global amnesia, meaning that they forget who they are.

Years ago, in the early 1980s, when cholesterol-lowering drugs first hit the mass market, studies found an increase in suicides, homicides, and automobile accidents. But those results were somehow overlooked in the rush to prescribe these "wonder" meds.

At the 2005 American College for Advancement in Medicine (ACAM), I attended a lecture by a prominent cardiologist, Dr. Thomas Levy, who theorized that when people took these medications to lower their cholesterol, their bodies' normal protective mechanism against heavy metal toxicity was diminished and they got depressed, hostile, and angry—hence the increase in homicides and suicides. They also lost their agility and ability to react in technical situations—hence more car accidents.

That is not to say that lowering cholesterol does not have advantages for some. It does, especially in middle-aged men (50–70) with coronary heart disease. The newer cholesterol-lowering drugs (i.e., statins) not only lower cholesterol but also lower inflammatory mediators in the body.

And since we know that chronic relentless inflammation causes arteries to be on fire, controlling cholesterol by either lowering oxidized LDL or raising HDL will be advantageous. I still recommend statins as part of my plaque reversal plan in patients with documented coronary artery disease.

My grievance is when we aggressively treat high cholesterol numbers and not patients, and when we overprescribe these drugs for healthy people, especially women. Statins should be prescribed and chosen with great care and scrutiny. They may have many side effects, including changes in liver function; muscle pain or weakness; memory problems; depression; shortness of breath; and, on rare occasions, even death.

Tragically, despite the studies showing the downside of cholesterol-lowering drugs, the medical community, including cardiologists nationwide, have concentrated on the alleged wonders of lowering cholesterol and continue to ignore the relationship between high blood sugar, insulin surges, and heart disease.

Excess Insulin Hurts Your Heart

Today, cardiovascular disease is the number one killer of both men and women in the United States. But did you know that 60 percent or more of those people with type 2 diabetes or insulin resistance develop some form of heart disease?

When our blood sugar levels get too high, we have higher insulin. And I believe that the number-one cause of the hardening of the blood vessels is excess insulin. The most important way to prevent coronary disease is to keep your insulin levels down, and that means eating fewer refined carbs and sweets. And yet this valuable piece of information is largely overlooked by members of the medical community.

A bit of history is in order. Before the Agricultural Revolution some 10,000 years ago, we followed the caveman diet—meat we hunted, fish we caught, and fruits and vegetables we plucked or picked. But now most Americans regularly load up their systems with more sugar and refined carbohydrates than they can easily metabolize. And millions of people are unknowingly diabetic or prediabetic. They consume sweets, gain weight, and literally wear out their insulin-producing cells, which simply can't keep up.

As a cardiologist, I treat a lot of diabetics. That's right. I am a heart specialist, yet I help a lot of patients with a disease that involves high blood sugar. Sounds strange, doesn't it?

Even more curious—many of my heart patients don't even know they have insulin resistance or diabetes before I diagnose them. Many of these patients come to me with a big belly, low levels of HDL (the "good" cholesterol), high triglycerides, and high blood pressure. We now call this scenario metabolic syndrome.

Too many physicians send these people away with four or five different prescriptions to treat each problem separately when what they really need is to exercise regularly and change their diets—cut out the very foods that are causing their high blood sugar levels and insulin surges.

With any luck, I've been catching these patients early in the disease process. Over the years, the ones who followed my advice did really well. They lost weight, exercised, and quit or drastically curtailed their intake of simple carbohydrates. Those who continued to gain weight and eat a lot of refined carbs inevitably developed full-blown diabetes and lots of complications, including heart disease.

Unfortunately, many patients with diabetes take their disease lightly and don't follow their doctors' advice. By not making drastic dietary and exercise changes and properly monitoring their blood sugar levels, they are at risk for heart attacks and stroke, kidney disease, blindness, nerve damage, and diabetic neuropathy, which can lead to amputation, impotence (if they're male), loss of libido (if they're female), skin disorders, and depression. And, ultimately, some of them will die at an early age.

What saddens me is that many people with high blood sugar, insulin resistance, metabolic syndrome, or full-blown diabetes could be spared from many complications with the right diet and a regular exercise program.

We can stop the toxic cycle of excess sugar/excess insulin that is inflaming our arteries, endangering our hearts, and aging us quickly. We can protect our cells and slow down the aging process. Now you know why I don't condone sugar. Trust me, sugar is not your friend but rather your foe.

Americans need to know that not only will sugar make you fat, but it will also make you age faster because of the havoc it wreaks on your blood sugar and insulin levels. Keeping both these levels under control is the best way to slow down the aging process and stay trim. Trying to stay sugarfree and steering clear of processed carbohydrates brings you closer to the fountain of youth.

PART 2

YOUR STORIES: FROM SUGAR IGNORANCE TO SUGAR EDUCATION

3

FROM ENTICEMENT TO ENTRAPMENT:

HERE'S THE SHOCKING SUGAR NEWS!

If you speed walk two to six miles along the sidewalks of New York City, as I like to do, you'll be struck by the fantastic "landscape"—a kaleidoscopic collage of sweet-smelling bakeries, trendy ice cream parlors, and neon-lit candy stores, as well as pizza joints, bagel shops, pretzel stands, hot-dog and soda carts, delis, and much more, all of which provocatively offer an array of enticing fiber-stripped fare.

In this 40- to 120-block area, you'll find drugstores displaying mounds of colorful candy pegged to the next holiday (even if it's months away), supermarkets pushing the latest processed cookies, crackers, or breads from some major food manufacturer, fast-food outlets promoting French fries, apple-pie pockets, and bulging burgers on mammoth white-flour buns.

Inevitably, you'll also catch folks chowing down on discount or gourmet chocolate, gooey pastries, frozen yogurt, and piles of processed pasta. And you'll undoubtedly see them swigging sodas, sugary sports beverages, or sweet, caffeinated drinks. And, more often than not, these same people are loaded down with excess weight.

Manhattan is not unique in this almost unstoppable sugar-and-quickie-carb reality. Indeed, what occurs in this East Coast metropolis is replicated elsewhere. More to the point, New York City simply offers a microcosm and an amplification of what occurs in industrialized nations around the world.

Inevitably, wherever you go, wherever you live, in pharmacies, minimarts, malls, movie theaters, gas stations, ballparks, office buildings, street fairs, even hospital cafeterias and gift shops, and, of course, grocery stores, diners, and restaurants, tantalizing sugary or quickie-carb "treats" are conniving or conspiring—it seems—to land in our stomachs.

Enticed and Seduced Since Almost Before Birth

Our love affair with sugar starts early. We're born with an innate preference for sweets—the natural kinds found in vegetables, fruits, and nuts. But by the time we're toddlers learning about the world around us, most of us have become inducted into the world of soft drinks, candies, cookies, chips, cake, and ice cream.

Yale University psychology professor Kelly D. Brownell, Ph.D., one of the world's foremost experts on obesity and eating disorders, suggests that this gloomy, sugary predicament confronts and bombards us as soon as we leave our mother's womb.

"We're born into a preordained, toxic environment that grabs our children and won't let them go," maintains Dr. Brownell, director of the Yale Center for Eating and Weight Disorders and author of the book, *Food Fight: The Inside Story of the Food Industry, America's Obesity Crisis, and What We Can Do about It.*

"It's a perfect recipe for making a nation obese," he observes.

This contaminated atmosphere is teeming with calorie-dense, easily accessible, convenient, oversized, supersweet snacks and vitamin-bereft fast foods, as well as laborsaving appliances that would make our lean, fit, active Cro-Magnon ancestors gawk in disbelief. Small wonder, then, that so many hectic, time-strapped, sedentary Americans overload on simple-carb junk food and while away hours in front of their TVs, computers, or video games.

Almost from the get-go, we're groomed, programmed, and conditioned to become the next wave of brand-loyal consumers of particular breakfast cereals, candy bars, sodas, and largely non-nutritious snacks.

Although it's an inadvertent move on the part of unsuspecting parents, it's a deliberate, planned corporate strategy included in far-reaching marketing plans.

"Everything conspires to make us eat cheap food, which happens to be sugar, fat, and salt," observes Adam Drewnowski, Ph.D., professor of epidemiology and director of the Center for Public Health Nutrition at the University of Washington.

"The major factors that make people choose or buy a given food are taste, cost, and convenience," Dr. Drewnowski continues. "So that gives us a triple whammy. Taste? Sugar, fat, and salt. Cost? Sugar, fat, and salt. Convenience? Sugar, fat, and salt. How are you going to win?"

Indeed, "winning" is virtually impossible when we "learn" our love of sweet, refined, nutrient-poor foods from one or both parents. That was the case for "Sugar Kickers" Charletta P. and Leila A., both of whom I met in my free, online, international KickSugar support group (on Yahoo!).

Take Charletta, 49, who grew up in Benton, Kentucky. "I was raised on lots of simple carbs, sugar, and fat," she says. "My mother thought a healthy meal was fried meat, high-starch veggies, and dessert. So when I grew up I ate the same way."

And Leila, 23, of Belmont, California, is convinced that she was "born hooked on sugar. While I was a fetus, my mom drank Coca-Cola and wine daily and often ate chocolate and pastries. Then, when I was a toddler, my relatives tell me, I would get fussy when I was denied sweets, but happy when I got them. And when I was a child, my father would show his love by bringing home pastries." By the time Leila hit puberty, she was, as she put it, "so dependent on sugar and hitting the school vending machines every day for a midday pick-me-up."

Leila's experiences are typical. "Caring" parents, doting relatives, frustrated teachers, and other well-meaning adults often dole out sweet "treats" to reward or manipulate growing children. Then, as they grow up, many kids develop lifelong attachments to "comfort" foods such as pancakes slathered in maple syrup and butter, chocolate fudge ice cream, and mashed potatoes drowned in creamy gravy.

By the time we reach elementary school, many of us have experiences akin to those of Stacie S., 32, of New York City.

"I would save up pennies to buy little 'pucker ups' in the candy machines. It was so exciting to put the coin in, turn the handle, and hit the jackpot: candy, candy, candy," recalls Stacie, whose habit eventually triggered hypoglycemia and forced her to start eating healthily.

Then, every holiday celebration calls for something sugary. You have chocolate eggs and malted milk balls for Easter, pumpkin pie and candied marshmallow yams for Thanksgiving, green-glittered cookies and candy canes for Christmas, and foil-covered chocolate "gelt" and applesauce-covered potato latkes for Hanukkah.

Naturally, for Valentine's Day, it's deemed fitting (except in our sugar-free circles) to give chocolates to your beloved—the richer and creamier, the better. And, of course, frosted cakes are inextricably linked to every rite of passage, from birthdays to graduations to weddings.

Even popular books, songs, games, and movies are littered with references that indicate our society's sugar fixation. Just think of "The Good Ship Lollipop," *The Chocolate Touch*, "A Spoonful of Sugar" (from the film *Mary Poppins*), and the book *Charlie and the Chocolate Factory*.

And let's not forget the nursery rhyme reminding us that little girls are made of "sugar and spice and everything nice."

"Last night I stopped dead in my tracks while reading that to my little boy," marvels Cheryl N., 38, of Lake Zurich, Illinois. "I'm noticing just how pervasive sugar is in our society, starting at a young age," adds Cheryl, who suffers from diabetes.

Certainly, the outcome is inevitable and predictable. There's simply no hiding. We are being led into temptation. Would that only enticing, succulent apples were beckoning us—as in the Garden of Eden.

Indeed, not only have we become a "fast-food nation," as author Eric Schlosser so eloquently describes in his book of the same name, but Dr. Sinatra and I maintain that we've also become a nation trapped in a state of SUGAR SHOCK!—as have industrialized countries the world over.

Studies Show an Upswing in Sugar Intake and Junk Food

Americans are ingesting so many empty calories that three nutrient-poor groups—sweets and desserts, soft drinks, and alcoholic beverages—now contribute almost 25 percent of the calories we consume, recent data shows. If you then add such items as pizza, potato chips, and hamburgers, junk food makes up nearly one-third of the calories the average adult American consumes daily.

"We knew people are eating a lot of junk food, but to have *almost one-third* of their calories coming from those categories is appalling," bemoans Gladys Block, Ph.D., a professor of epidemiology and public health nutrition at the University of California at Berkeley's School of Public Health.

Soft drinks alone contributed 7.1 percent of the average American's total calories, and salty snacks and fruit-flavored drinks comprised another

5 percent, explains Dr. Block, who studied data from two governmental surveys, which together looked at the food habits of more than 38,000 people nationwide.

"What I worry about is that we're getting one-third of our calories from foods that contribute *no* vitamins and minerals. Because people are eating all that junk, a large proportion of Americans are undernourished," adds Dr. Block, whose findings were published in the *Journal of Food Composition and Analysis*.

"Yes, you can actually be obese and undernourished," explains Dr. Block, noting that taking in nutrient-lacking foods contributes to the development of most chronic diseases. Here's what folks surveyed consumed, listed in order of popularity:

1. Regular soft drinks
2. Cakes, sweet rolls, donuts, pastries
3. Hamburgers, cheeseburgers, meat loaf
4. Pizza
5. Potato chips, corn chips, popcorn
6. Rice
7. Rolls, buns, English muffins, bagels
8. Cheese or cheese spread
9. Beer
10. French fries, fried potatoes

These findings, Dr. Block concludes, were simply "shocking."

We're appalled, as are nutritionists, by this typical American diet.

A number of other recent studies also point to the alarming escalation in our consumption of soft drinks and other processed, sugary foods around the globe.

One study, published in *Obesity Research*, aptly titled "The Sweetening of the World's Diet," showed that "80 percent of this sweet increase comes from soft drinks and sugar-sweetened beverages," according to the study's coauthor Barry M. Popkin, Ph.D., nutrition professor and economist at the University of North Carolina at Chapel Hill.

Curiously, urbanization and increased income accounted for 82 percent of the rise in caloric sweetener consumption worldwide. In other words, sugar intake increased as people earned more money and more folks moved into cities in developing countries, both of which gave them greater access to processed foods, which are higher in sweeteners.

"If both urbanization and the processing of the food supply continue unabated, this trend in the worldwide diet will persist," Dr. Popkin's study asserts.

"Thus, we will inexorably move away from foods that are potentially important sources of calcium and other key nutrients and toward foods that provide fewer nutrients."

Sweetener Consumption Is Going > Going > Going—Higher > Higher > Higher

Another way to grasp the magnitude of the sweet tooth problem is by looking at America's astronomical sugar-intake figures. The United States is the world's largest consumer of sweeteners, including sucrose and high-fructose corn syrup, as well as one of the largest global sugar importers, according to the U.S. Department of Agriculture (USDA). Just look at how our intake of sweeteners has soared over the past two centuries:

- In 1801, historians estimate, each person consumed about 8.4 pounds of sugar, which comes to less than one tablespoon or 2.2 teaspoons a day.

- In 1909, when the first official U.S. statistics were released by the USDA, the typical American consumed less than 6 pounds of corn sweeteners and less than 80 pounds of cane and beet sugar. Overall, Americans were consuming close to 85 pounds of caloric sweeteners that year.

- By 1999, Americans' consumption of added sugars hit its all-time high, according to the USDA. Americans consumed a total of 151.4 pounds of added caloric sweeteners per person. The consumption of corn sweeteners alone skyrocketed to 83.5 pounds per person.

- By 2005, consumption reportedly dropped slightly, but the average person in the United States was still eating or drinking nearly 142.6 pounds of added caloric sweeteners per person, or a little more than three-quarters of a cup a day, according to the USDA's Economic

Research Service. That figure includes refined sugar from cane and beets (about 63.4 pounds); corn-based sweeteners such as high-fructose corn syrup, glucose syrup, and dextrose (about 77.7 pounds); pure honey (1.1 pounds); and edible syrups (1.4 pounds).*

While that 142.6-pound USDA figure might already seem high, some experts believe that the government's delivery estimates are *grossly underestimated* and that, in point of fact, Americans consume much more per person per year in food and drinks.

"The average American consumes more like 170 pounds per year, or just shy of a cup a day," estimates Russ Bianchi, an experienced food scientist who serves as managing director of Adept Solutions, Inc., a global food and beverage product development firm.

The reason the USDA figures fall short is that they neglect to include certain sugars. "The government's figures don't include high-intensity sweeteners; concentrated fruit juices; sugar alcohol or polyol sweeteners; or other corn-based, highly chemically refined sweetener components like maltodextrin or modified corn starches," Bianchi says.

That's not all. So-called "hidden sugars"—which are pervasive in the food supply today—have been ignored, too.

"These USDA numbers also don't include unlabeled sugars, which are injected or added to processed meats and prepared foods," Bianchi explains. "For example, about 63 percent of Americans are unknowingly consuming more sugar-infused foods at restaurants, fast-food places, colleges, military bases, rest homes, and even hospitals that are supposed to make you well but feed you sugary junk instead."

Furthermore, Americans are taking in added sugars not only from obvious foods such as candy, soda, cakes, and cookies, but from packaged, frozen, and canned foods, including cereals, crackers, yogurt, salad dressings, bagels, and peanut butter.

Whether Americans are taking in a cup of sugar a day or more, *any* amount is way too much, some experts insist.

"*Even three teaspoons* of refined sugars work to throw the body out

---

*Note: These USDA figures are for per capita estimated deliveries of caloric sweeteners to food and beverage companies, so actual human consumption may be lower because food is uneaten, spoiled, or lost in other ways.

of balance and compromise its health," explains Nancy Appleton, Ph.D., author of *Lick the Sugar Habit* and *Lick the Sugar Habit Sugar Counter*.

"All simple sugars—concentrated fruit juice, honey, maple syrup, rice syrup, agave, et cetera—suppress your immune system and attack your body like a foreign invader. If we were to eat no sugar at all, our bodies would still have plenty of glucose, which we need to live," explains Dr. Appleton, who has been studying sugar's dangers since the 1980s.

You Don't Eat That Many Sweets or Quickie Carbs, Right? Wait! Are You in Denial?

Perhaps the above statistics and conclusions don't convince you that *you've* boosted your intake of sugar and fast-acting carbs. In fact, if you're like most Americans—as I once was—you just know that you eat hardly any sweets or quickie carbs. You certainly don't have a problem, right? Well, before you rush to conclusions, I invite you to find out if you're in what I call SUGAR SHOCK! denial.

Jennifer C., 32, of Chicago, Illinois, witnessed this kind of denial behavior in an ex-boyfriend. "He told me my whole sugar-addiction problem was in my head—this from a guy who drinks at least a six-pack of Coke a day and whose favorite food is Pixy Stix [brightly colored straws filled with flavored sugar]."

I encourage you to find out if you, too, are in denial. Assess your quickie-carb consumption patterns. To begin, check out the sugar content for the following products, all of which have fanatical followers. Are you perhaps one?

- A half cup portion of Ben & Jerry's Chunky Monkey: contains 28 grams, or roughly 7 teaspoons of sugar. (A more likely portion size—a full cup—has some 14 teaspoons of sugar.)

- An 8-ounce Minute Maid Strawberry Slurpee from 7-Eleven: packs in 33 grams, or around 8.25 teaspoons of sugar. (Many folks buy Slurpees *twice* that size—which have about 16.5 teaspoons of sugar.)

- And a 16-ounce grande Starbucks Strawberries & Crème Frappuccino Blended Crème: includes 85 grams (with whipped cream) or some 21.25 teaspoons of sugar!

Still not convinced that you overindulge in sweets or much-like-sugar carbs? Then see if any of this rings a bell:

- ■ 7 a.m.: "Ugh, I feel groggy. Gotta have coffee now." (2 cups, with 4 teaspoons total sugar)

- ■ 8 a.m.: "Oh no, I'm late for work. I hardly have time for two Slim Fast peanut-butter bars, but at least I'll lose weight." (5 teaspoons of sugar for the bars, according to Dr. Appleton's *Lick the Sugar Habit Sugar Counter*)

- ■ 10 a.m.: "I need a pick-me-up now, because this report is due in an hour! Maybe this Krispy Kreme glazed devil's food donut will give me the energy boost I need." (7.5 teaspoons for the donut)

- ■ Noon: "I'm wiped out, hungry, and I have such a headache. Think I'll get a cream soda and Snickers bar with my tuna sandwich. (About 12.25 teaspoons of sugar for the soda, 7.5 teaspoons for the candy, and another 2 to 4 teaspoons for two slices of white bread. Even the mayonnaise mixed in the tuna has some sugar.)

- ■ 3 p.m.: "I just can't concentrate. I need pep—and now! Maybe these peanut M&M's and a Coke will give me that zap of energy." (6.25 teaspoons for the candy and another 10.25 teaspoons for the soda)

- ■ 6 p.m.: "What a rough day! I need to relax. Think I'll chill out with a couple of screwdrivers before dinner. They do, after all, contain orange juice, which has vitamin C." (9 teaspoons for two 7-ounce glasses)

- ■ 7 p.m.: "That pizza really hit the spot. I'm stuffed, but my sweetie will be hurt if I don't try her (or his) home-baked (or store-bought) carrot cake." (Two slices of Domino's pizza yields about 3 to 4 teaspoons of sugar and another 6.25 teaspoons or so for the dessert)

- ■ 10 p.m.: "Wonder why I'm so hungry and so wiped out. Maybe this fruit yogurt will help. It's healthy." (10 to 11.25 teaspoons for a Dannon 8-ounce low-fat yogurt with fruit on the bottom)

Sound familiar? All day long, as you'll learn in the next chapter, you've been continually exhausting your poor pancreas, overstimulating insulin production, and doing other damage just to keep your body functioning from hour to hour. Indeed, relying on sweets and quickie carbs when you're run down, headachy, or wiped out quickly shoots up your blood sugar levels, which ultimately rapidly plunge and hurl you into an insidious, perpetually repeating, almost continual state of SUGAR SHOCK!

Watch Out for Those Processed Carbs, Too

Even if you don't indulge in dessert foods, the carbohydrates from heavily processed, nutrient-deficient breads, crackers, and chips of all kinds will have exactly the same effect on your blood sugar, as we'll explain shortly.

And, as if that's not enough, "hidden sugars" lurk in just about any frozen or packaged food you can buy in a can, jar, or box. In addition, as food scientist Bianchi just warned you, while eating out at diners, making bagel pit stops, and grabbing takeout from fast-food places, you're likely to consume even more sweeteners, which have been surreptitiously slipped into your meals. You won't ever know about them unless you ask, and even then you might not get the full facts.

Your Body Can't Handle All That Sweetness

The bottom line is that in the last 200 years, sugar consumption has risen more than 1,500 percent, cautions nutritionist Ann Louise Gittleman, Ph.D., C.N.S., author of *Get the Sugar Out: 501 Simple Ways to Cut the Sugar Out of Any Diet.*

"Our bodies simply haven't had time to respond and adapt to this nutrient-poor source of calories—and it appears that our bodies are rebelling with a multitude of physical ailments, telling us loudly and clearly that they don't like what they're being fed," explains Dr. Gittleman, the author of the *New York Times* bestsellers *The Fat Flush Plan*, *The Fat Flush Fitness Plan*, and *The FastTrack, One-Day Detox Diet.*

"Saying 'sugar is bad for you' is the ultimate understatement," she insists. "The far-reaching problems sugar can cause are well documented in medical journals throughout the world, and new sugar-disease connections are made each year."

4

CLEARING THE CARB CONFUSION: THE PITFALLS OF PROCESSED CARBS AND THE BENEFITS OF QUALITY CARBS

If you're like many Americans, you're probably confused when it comes to the subject of carbohydrates. It's time to give you the skinny on these much-talked-about but often-misunderstood foods so you'll understand why and how to pick "smart" carbs.

Most important, you need to know that carbohydrates fall into two categories. You can select inferior, nutrient-poor, empty-calorie, fiber-stripped quickie carbs. Or you can pick superior, nutrient-dense, fiber-filled quality carbs—or "qual carbs."

"It's not that all carbohydrates are bad; it's the overabundance of the simple, processed carbohydrates and sugars—that's where we're going wrong," explains renowned obesity expert and pediatrics professor James O. Hill, Ph.D., director of the Center for Human Nutrition at the University of Colorado Health Sciences Center. "Americans need to eat the right kind of carbohydrates."

The best kinds of carbs to eat, experts say, are nutritious, flavorful, rainbow-colored, "Mother Nature's Carb Gifts." By this, I mean, for instance, cruciferous vegetables like broccoli, cabbage, brussels sprouts, cauliflower, kohlrabi, and kale; fruits such as strawberries, raspberries, blueberries, melons, and oranges; and legumes, nuts, and seeds. Better carbs also include whole grains like brown rice, quinoa, and steel-cut oats.

On the other hand, the worst kind of carbs are those nutrient-deficient sweet desserts and other processed "treats" that so many Americans crave—candies, cookies, cakes, ice cream, and soda. Of course, inferior carbohydrates also include a hundred-plus kinds of caloric sweeteners such as high-fructose corn syrup, sucrose, brown sugar, dextrose, fruit-juice concentrates, raw sugar, and crystalline fructose. Other low-caliber carbs, which I dub "much-like-sugar carbs," include processed (mostly white) foods such as white rice, white flour, and breads like bagels and French bread, most types of pasta, crackers, chips, rice cakes, puffed rice cereals, and pretzels.

Before delving into the benefits or pitfalls of the various health-promoting or health-damaging carbs, you need to know why this food group is of such critical importance to us all.

Basically, our bodies and brains *need* to fill up regularly on foods that convert to glucose in our bloodstream. That all-important glucose—a simple sugar or monosaccharide—gives us the energy to wake up in the morning, perform well at our job, score high grades in school, take care of our kids, hang out with friends, make love with our beloved, and have the stamina to exercise religiously. In short, having adequate glucose in our bloodstream allows us to go about our daily lives.

Or, to put it another way, just as our car needs gasoline to pull out of the parking lot and pick up speed on the highway, our body requires glucose to kick-start our engine and function at full steam so that we can survive—and preferably thrive. Deprived of this necessary glucose, we could develop a plethora of symptoms from headaches to crankiness. At worst, without glucose we could even go into a coma and die.

In particular, our brains—sometimes called the "crown jewel" of our bodies—are simply *desperate* for glucose. Indeed, although the brain represents only about 2 percent of our total body weight, "it uses a significant amount of our body's glucose supply from the bloodstream, with the rest going to our muscles and tissues," according to Antonio Convit, M.D., associate professor of psychiatry, medical director of the Center for Brain Health at New York University School of Medicine, and researcher at the NYU-affiliated Nathan Kline Institute.

"In fact, the brain is a virtual glucose hog, gobbling more than two-thirds of the circulating carbohydrates in the bloodstream while you are at rest," points out biotechnology pioneer Barry Sears, Ph.D., in his bestselling book *Enter the Zone*.

Where do we get this necessary glucose? We get it from carbohydrates. They provide our main and most easily accessible source of glucose, although it also can be manufactured, though not as easily, from proteins and fats.

The Complicated Processing Complex Carbs Undergo to Become Quickie Carbs

Before I explain how foods become fuel to keep us going, you need to know how a fiber-and-vitamin-rich, generally brownish whole grain is transformed through state-of-the-art technology into pristine-looking white flour. To help you understand how whole grains are ultimately robbed of their nutrients, world-renowned researcher and nutrition expert Walter Willett, M.D., chairman of the nutrition department at the Harvard School of Public Health and a professor of medicine, outlines the various steps that transform wheat berries into white flour.

"The milling process first cracks the wheat grains, then pulverizes them with a series of rollers. In this way the starchy, carbohydrate-rich center, called the endosperm, is separated from both the dark, fibrous bran and the wheat embryo, called the wheat germ," writes Dr. Willett in his book *Eat, Drink, and Be Healthy: The Harvard Medical School Guide to Healthy Eating*.

"At each stage of milling, something is lost. Removing the wheat germ pulls out vitamins and unsaturated fats. Whacking away the branny outer layer removes fiber, magnesium, and more vitamins. By the time whole-wheat grains have been turned into white flour, the final product is a pale shadow of the original, literally and nutritionally."

So why did this "pale shadow of the original" become all the rage in industrial societies? The shift from high-quality whole grains to low-quality refined grains came about because of perception, Dr. Willett explains.

"Once it became possible to refine wheat, it was marketed as being purer than whole-grain flour," Dr. Willett points out, noting that initially the upper classes found the white flour a novelty and that, in time, it became a status symbol.

The popularity of processed grains, Dr. Willett observes, was also "driven by the reality of storage—white flour, with almost none of the healthy oils found in whole-grain flour, keeps longer. Whole-grain flours must be used more quickly and/or refrigerated."

But what it comes down to is that when "whole grains are processed or refined, they're stripped of much of their nutritional value," points out fitness trainer and exercise physiologist Bob Greene, who is Oprah Winfrey's personal fitness coach. These fiber-deprived grains then "become, more or less, empty calories, which we want to avoid," Greene writes in his number one *New York Times* bestseller, *Get with the Program.*

Indeed, a growing number of medical studies are demonstrating that, over time, eating too much of that innocent-looking, processed white flour used in breads, pasta, and desserts, as well as white rice, which is similarly stripped of nutrients and fiber, could lead to a host of blood sugar disorders and debilitating diseases.

The Protective Features of Whole Grains

If you regularly relish white bread that you can easily smush in your hands and mold into a putty-type wad, you've been going for the refined carbs I've been discussing. Just think about it: If you can transform this food into an almost-sticky paste, how do you think it impacts your body?

YOUR HANDY CLEARING-THE-CARB-CONFUSION GLOSSARY

Here is a list of phrases, words, and terms Dr. Sinatra and I use throughout *SUGAR SHOCK!* These are their definitions for our purposes:

Quickie Carbs (Also Much-Like-Sugar Carbs, Inferior Carbs, Wrong Carbs, Fast-Acting Carbs, Refined Carbs, Low-Caliber Carbs, Simple Carbs, Processed Carbs or Starches, or Sugar Act-Alikes): Inferior, processed carbohydrates such as refined, nutrient-deprived, fiber-stripped breads, cereals, crackers, potato chips, bagels, pretzels, rice cakes, white rice, and alcoholic beverages. In your body, these refined grains and alcohol work much like sugar, because almost immediately after eating them, your blood sugar levels spike and you get a "sugar high" or "sugar rush."

These sudden sugar spikes can trigger SUGAR SHOCK!, which can lead to hunger, and ultimately to weight gain and many diseases.

Quality Carbs (Also Right Carbs, Superior Carbs, Smart Carbs, Better Carbs, Slow-Acting Carbs, Complex Carbs, Slow-Release Carbs, Mother Nature's Carb Gifts, and Nutrient-Dense Carbs): Vegetables, legumes, nuts, and seeds. These wholesome carbs contain "natural sugars" and provide beneficial vitamins, minerals, fiber, and antioxidants and are metabolized more slowly in our bodies than processed carbs so that they don't cause blood sugar spikes and a huge insulin overload. Many also tout the benefits of whole grains if you don't have gluten sensitivity. Better carbs also include fiber-filled fruits, which contain all kinds of nutrients and phytochemicals.

Sweets or Sugary Foods: All calorically sweetened desserts and snack foods such as chocolates, cookies, candies, cakes, donuts, ice cream, sweet rolls, pancakes, pies, soft drinks, fruit-juice blends, sweetened iced teas, and other sweet drinks, as well as chewing gum and breath mints.

Hidden Sugars: Sweeteners (often several kinds in one product) added to thousands of prepared products—including those where you'd never expect them. For instance, you'll find hidden sugars in most salad dressings, packaged meats, catsup, cocktail sauce, tomato sauce, and frozen dinners. (To get a free list of more "Foods with Sly Hidden Sugars," just visit my website, www.SugarShock.com, and sign up for my free report and e-zine.)

Sugars and Sweeteners: More than 100 varieties of sugars and sweeteners now used by food manufacturers, including beet sugar, brown sugar, brown rice syrup, evaporated cane juice, fruit-juice concentrate, and turbinado sugar. In addition, "sugars" applies to so-called natural sweeteners such as honey, barley malt, maple syrup, molasses, and raw organic cane sugar, which also raise your blood sugar levels. For the sake of simplicity, Dr. Sinatra and I, along with most nutrition experts, also use the word "sugar" and "sugars" to signify chemically created corn-based fructose and high-fructose corn syrup. Finally, I often use the term "sugar" or "sugars" to mean quickie carbs or much-like-sugar carbs. (Get your list of "Sugars by Any Other Name" at www.SugarShock.com.)

On the other hand, superior types of breads using whole grains are firmer to the touch, and whole-grain products, such as bulgur wheat, millet, kamut, and amaranth are often crunchy and chewy, and always flavorful when cooked.

For more than a decade, Dr. Willett and his colleagues have been examining the health effects of refined versus unrefined grains on thousands of people. Their studies offer compelling, convincing data indicating that whole-grain foods are clearly better for sustained good health than their refined counterparts. Not only that, but whole grains could protect you against a variety of chronic diseases, including type 2 diabetes, heart disease, many types of cancer, and more.

Although it may be impossible to isolate the exact ingredients that make whole grains so protective, a number of "contenders" have been identified, Dr. Willett notes. For starters, "the fiber in whole grains delays absorption of glucose and eases the workload for the insulin-making cells in the pancreas. Fiber [which is also found in vegetables, fruits, and legumes] also helps lower cholesterol levels in the blood," Dr. Willett believes. "Fiber may also rev up some of the body's natural anticoagulants and help prevent the formation of small blood clots that may trigger heart attacks or strokes.

"Antioxidants like vitamin E [found in whole grains] prevent cholesterol-containing low-density lipids from reacting with oxygen, a key early step toward the formation of cholesterol-clogged arteries. Phytoestrogens, or plant estrogens, may protect against some cancers."

What's more, Dr. Willett adds, "the bran layer of many grains contains essential minerals, such as magnesium, selenium, copper, and manganese that may be important in reducing the risk of heart disease and diabetes."

SHOULD WE TRUST NEW WHOLE-GRAIN CEREALS FROM FOOD COMPANIES?

Enter a grocery store today, and you'll see cereals galore trumpeting—usually in big, bold lettering—that they contain "whole grains." Often, they even feature the American Heart Association seal of approval. This begs the question: Are they healthy?

"This is one of the biggest labeling scams out there," charges Michele Simon, author of *Appetite for Profit* and founder/director of the Center for

Informed Food Choice (CIFC). "The federal government said to eat more whole grains but these processed-food companies are just adding a little whole grain and then slapping big labels on the box. And they're spinning these new cereals . . . as healthier when they're not." Indeed, many cereals contain lots of added sugars and processed carbs despite the whole-grain claim.

Here are some tips I compiled to help you identify the low-caliber carbs from the quality carbs:

- Before purchasing whole-grain products, read the label carefully. The word "whole" on the ingredient list ("whole wheat," "whole rye," or "whole oats") should be listed first. For example, "wheat flour" doesn't mean "whole-wheat flour." It probably contains primarily refined flour.
- Make sure no white flour has been added to the supposedly whole-grain product.
- Try brown rice, bulgur, wheat berries, millet, or hulled barley.
- Choose grains with at least three grams of dietary fiber per serving.
- Make sure the whole-grain product doesn't contain artificial or caloric sweeteners.
- To ensure freshness and quality, don't buy grains past their expiration date.
- Buy whole grains in sealed packages, which protect them from air, moisture, and spoilage, and store them in airtight containers in a cool, dry place. To extend their storage life, keep grains in the fridge or freeze them for long-term storage.
- Cook most grains in water, preferably purified. Add grains to boiling water and simmer until the food absorbs most of the liquid. Generally, use one part grain to two or three parts water. Then cook until tender.
- If you're on a diet, keep quick-to-grab grain foods—even if they're whole grain—out of the house.
- If you want to have cereal for breakfast, try old-fashioned steel-cut oats, quinoa, or a whole-grain combination such as Kashi, the Breakfast Pilaf.

Those Quickie Carbs Turn to Fuel Too Fast

To better understand why experts consider some carbs virtuous and others villainous, you need to understand what happens after you drink or eat them. Whenever you consume caloric carbs—whether they're superior or inferior—they, as we've noted, ultimately convert to glucose in your bloodstream. (The one exception, according to research, is chemically refined fructose or high-fructose corn syrup, which studies show takes a different pathway, as we'll discuss in the following chapter.) At that point they become "blood sugar," which Merriam-Webster defines as "the glucose in the blood."

So if all carbs end up as glucose anyway, why would some be good for us while others contribute to our widening waistlines and declining health? You get these negative results from processed or refined carbs and starches not only because they're lacking in nutrients and fiber and generally high in calories, but also because of the rapidity with which they're metabolized (processed or broken down in your body).

Again, think of your body as a car. "When you consume refined sugars and processed foods, it's like running your car on low-octane gas instead of high-octane gas and neglecting to recharge the battery and add oil to the engine," explains integrative physician Keith DeOrio, M.D., who has helped thousands of folks kick sugar and refined grains. "Or, to put it another way, your body's metabolism gets ramped up on refined carbs because you're putting in a bunch of low-quality fuel that has no vitamins, nutrients, minerals, and antioxidants."

How are processed grains similar to low-grade fuel? Well, those refined carbs are turned into glucose more quickly, meaning that your body doesn't need to work so hard to break down and digest them, because, as Dr. Willett has explained, machinery has already done the work for you during processing.

To put it as simply as possible, let's say you gulp down the contents of a 20-ounce bottle of soda and chomp on a handful of frosted cookies. Your blood sugar will rise rapidly. In fact, whenever you eat a carb, the "rise in the level of blood glucose is commensurate with the type and amount of carbohydrate ingested (i.e., higher for sugar, lower for fresh fruit)," explain the four authors of *The New SUGAR BUSTERS! Cut Sugar to Trim Fat*.

You might suspect that sugary foods would make your blood sugar skyrocket the most. But, according to Dr. Willett that's not necessarily true. "In fact, your digestive system turns white bread, a baked potato, or white rice into glucose and pumps this sugar into the bloodstream almost twice as fast as it delivers the sugar in a cocktail of pure glucose," he observes.

Indeed, all processed, refined carbohydrates end up being metabolically similar to sweets (which is why Dr. Sinatra and I call them "much-like-sugar carbs"). In short, both sweets and quickie carbs cause a surge in your blood sugar level.

The Glycemic Index and Glycemic Load: Boon or Bane for Carb Watcher?

Now that you know it's preferable to monitor your food intake by picking quality carbs that convert to sugar gradually, you also should know something about the glycemic index (GI), a much-ballyhooed or much-criticized tool (depending upon the source) for identifying how much a particular food will raise your blood glucose.

The glycemic index measures the effect that a 50-gram serving of a particular food (eaten by itself) will have on your circulating blood glucose about two hours after you eat it. The GI is a mathematical system developed in the late 1970s and introduced in the early 1980s by researchers from the University of Toronto, including nutritional science professors David Jenkins, M.D., Ph.D., and Thomas Wolever, M.D., Ph.D., to aid in statistical analysis for research projects. Since 2002, the GI has been heavily promoted for consumer use by the University of Sydney in Australia.

For years, people with diabetes also have been using the GI to plan meals and snacks that generate the smallest possible increases in blood sugar, and more recently, the GI has been touted by experts as a valuable dieting tool as well.

Nowadays, a number of nutritionists and experts recommend that their carb-cutting clients watch out for white bread, white rice, and other sweets or starchy foods because "they rank high on the glycemic index." What this means is that they trigger a dramatic rise in blood sugar levels.

Essentially, the premise of the glycemic index is to encourage people to be cautious or shy away from foods with a GI of 70 or higher because they provide the biggest blood sugar blast. The ideal is to gravitate toward foods with a GI of 55 or less—these include most vegetables, legumes, whole grains, and low-sugar fruits—because they trigger a small, steady rise in blood sugar. You also may wish to cautiously select foods with a medium GI of between 56 and 69, which cause a moderately higher glycemic response.

(It should be noted, however, that GI numbers will differ because one glycemic index uses glucose as the value and another uses white bread.)

Although glycemic-index advocates note that eating foods with a low GI means you'll get a smaller rise in blood glucose after meals, improve your sensitivity to insulin, and get help losing weight, some insiders lament that consumers find the glycemic index confusing. What's more, they say, it's very easy to misuse and misinterpret it.

For example, as Dr. Willett explains, the GI number doesn't always accurately reflect the real effect of eating a food. Vitamin-rich carrots, for example, have a glycemic index of 131, which could cause many people to avoid them. But to get 50 grams of carbohydrates from carrots, you'd have to eat roughly an entire pound's worth in one sitting, which most people are unlikely to do. (Since then, however, other studies have shown carrots to rank medium or even low on the GI.)

Critics claim other flaws exist as well. "The glycemic index is scientifically and metabolically flawed, as well as misleading and potentially dangerous," charges food scientist and formulator Russ Bianchi, head of Adept Solutions, Inc.

"One of the biggest problems with the measure," he contends, "is that foods containing corn-derived fructose, specifically, high-fructose corn syrup (HFCS) rank low—anywhere from 10 to 32—on the glycemic index, although medical studies are showing us that they're being converted to fat and triglycerides. Thus, the glycemic index provides information that could be very harmful to people such as diabetics who specifically choose low-GI foods containing HFCS. And polyols such as malitol and sorbitol also are low on the glycemic index, because they're not absorbed, but they could cause additional adverse health consequences such as diarrhea."

Another dilemma presented by the glycemic index is that some carbohydrates, including medium- or high-glycemic plant foods such as pineapples, bananas, mangoes, papayas, parsnips, cantaloupes, watermelons, and, of course, carrots, have been vilified, points out Cynthia Geyer, M.D., director of women's health at Canyon Ranch health resort in Lenox, Massachusetts. "I think, in balance, that these foods can be part of a healthy diet," Dr. Geyer maintains.

The glycemic index offers other misleading numbers, too. For example, some fruits—which contain more natural sugars—rank higher on the GI than particular fatty, sugary, processed foods like ice cream. But, let's face it, nutritive, high-fiber fruits are clearly healthier by a landslide than these heavily refined sweets.

Other experts believe that another, more recently developed tool, the glycemic load (GL), which was pioneered by Dr. Willett and his associates, offers more valuable information, because it takes into account the *amount* of carbs in your portion size rather than testing a standardized amount of 50 grams (as in the GI). For that system, 10 or less is considered low, 11 to 19 is medium, and 20 and up is high.

Neither the glycemic load nor the glycemic index gives you the true blood sugar impact of a meal, points out nutritionist Jonny Bowden, Ph.D., C.N.S., resident nutrition and weight-loss expert on www.ivillage.com and author of *Living the Low Carb Life* and *The 150 Healthiest Foods on Earth*.

"Any time you add different foods together, you get another response that would be different from the glycemic load or glycemic index of a food by itself," Dr. Bowden explains. "The glycemic impact of any meal is a product of the interaction of the different macronutrients—carbs, fats, and protein, and, of course, fiber. Usually the glycemic index alone is not a good way to choose foods. I like the glycemic load, but it's still not perfect, because it still only talks about foods in isolation."

Furthermore, some experts argue, for the average health-minded American, both of these measures may be superfluous.

"I challenge the fundamental concept of the glycemic index," says Jack Challem, writer/editor of the monthly *Nutrition Reporter* and author of *Syndrome X* and *The Inflammation Syndrome*.

"In some ways, the whole glycemic index is a rationalization for processed foods," contends Challem, noting the irony that refined foods full of fat and sugar may rank much lower on the GI than superior, wholesome, nutrient-loaded foods.

Indeed, Challem and others argue that you simply don't need either the glycemic index or the glycemic load if you're choosing high-fiber, high-quality carbs.

In the end, some experts contend that while the glycemic index and the glycemic load may be invaluable to scientists conducting research studies or to sophisticated carb-watching consumers, these measures may be too complicated for many Americans.

So, while Dr. Sinatra and I recognize that some people may wish to learn the GI of certain fruits and vegetables, we believe that your best bet is to simply stay away from fiber-stripped, nutrient-deficient, processed carbs, particularly ones containing high-fructose corn syrup.

In short, we recommend that you shun prepared foods that come in plastic packages, boxes, or jars. Instead, opt for superior, high-fiber, nutrient-dense, slow-release vegetables, legumes, nuts, and seeds, limited amounts of whole grains (if you can have them), and low-sugar fruits. As you'll learn next, you can moderate your blood sugar levels further by consuming the above along with some lean protein, fiber, and healthy fat.

The Power of Protein, Fat, and Fiber to Curb Hunger and Stall Carb Absorption

If you can learn one lesson here, it's that you don't ever want to eat carbohydrates all by themselves, whether they're low-caliber or quality carbs.

"If you regularly eat carbs alone, your blood sugar will be harmfully spiking in response," warns nutritionist and exercise physiologist Jill Vollmuth, C.N.C., a consultant who helps physicians implement nutritional programs in their medical practice.

Welcome to your three indispensable allies—protein, fiber, and fat (which we'll call PFF for short). "I think fiber works best in terms of preventing an immediate rise in blood sugar," says nutritionist Dr. Shari Lieberman.

"The soluble fiber, which dissolves in water, helps slow the absorption of the sugar or starch in a food. That's why an apple, orange, and grapefruit work so well in a low-glycemic meal, because they're loaded with pectin, which is a soluble fiber, and they slow the absorption of the naturally occurring sugars in the fruit and lower the glycemic index," she explains.

You've already learned how fiber slows the breakdown of carbs in your body, but lean proteins and fats can be helpful companions, too, as your meal becomes your fuel. If you're a dessert or white-bread aficionado, reflect a moment on how you eat. On days when you go hog wild over sweets and/or fast-acting carbs, do you skimp or skip shrimp, eggs, chicken, tofu, legumes, fresh fruits and vegetables, olive oil, nuts, seeds, and whole grains?

Chances are, if you're like many Americans who repeatedly stuff their faces with fast-acting foods, you've been neglecting to eat sufficient amounts of protein, fiber, or fat. Together or separately, this dynamic trio can help soften the blood sugar whammy you'd get from carbs alone. Of course, regulation of food intake is a complex process, and many factors are involved, but here's a quick overview of how PFF can partially offset your blood sugar yo-yo predicament.

The Protein Buffer

Protein, first of all, curbs your hunger so you don't overeat and snack too much between meals. Because it takes longer to break down in your body, protein fills you up much more effectively than carbs or fats, and it helps you to stay satisfied longer. In fact, researchers in France, Sweden, and Great Britain have found that high-carb snackers got hungry as quickly as subjects who had no snacks at all, but those who snacked on chicken (protein) stayed full almost 40 minutes longer.

In addition to being satisfying and keeping you full, however, protein also improves your insulin and glucose levels over the long haul. In fact, metabolic researchers have found that protein-rich diets can improve long-term insulin sensitivity whereas low-fat, high-carb diets can influence the progression of insulin resistance, according to Loren Cordain, Ph.D., a professor in the department of health and exercise at Colorado State University and author of *The Paleo Diet*.

Dr. Cordain—who has conducted research over the past two decades linking our modern, carb-laden diet to various diseases—points out that protein isn't stored as fat the way carbs are. In fact, it's difficult and inefficient for the body's metabolic machinery to store excess protein as fat. Extra fats or carbs, not protein, are the foods that most frequently make you fat, he notes.

In fact, dieters and Sugar Kickers find that a "protein chaser" can help out in a pinch, meaning that if you add protein to a higher-carbohydrate food—for example, eating a hard-boiled egg with a couple of crackers—you'll lower the rate at which the carbs convert to sugar in your bloodstream.

"Whenever you add protein with a carb that's high on the glycemic index, it also decreases the immediate blood sugar response," explains Dr. Lieberman. "If you eat a chicken leg with a piece of chocolate cake, I wouldn't count on that decreasing the glycemic index enough, but if you were in a Chinese restaurant having chicken and vegetables, eating those foods would lower the immediate rise in blood sugar that you get with brown rice."

Which brings us to another issue. Yes, as the most careful carb watchers among us have discovered, you can even eat too many high-quality carbs like brown rice, steel-cut oats, or papadam (lentil crackers). Indeed, as I once discovered, even if you overload on complex carbs in any one sitting, you can still get too high a blood sugar response.

"Carbs are carbs whether or not they contain fiber that slows down the absorption of glucose into your bloodstream," nutritionist Vollmuth explains. "That's why I always urge clients to add some protein or a little fat at the same time that you eat the carbs."

Naturally, you just have to use common sense to gauge how much protein, fat, and fiber to use at a meal, Dr. Lieberman explains. "I wouldn't eat a bucket of brown rice with my chicken and broccoli, but eating half a cup of brown rice with steamed vegetables and chicken is going to raise blood sugar more slowly than if you ate the brown rice all by itself. Now, if your Chinese food has a high-sugar sauce on it, remember that the sugar will be part of what raises your blood sugar in addition to the brown rice," she continues.

The Fat Effect

But what about fat's impact on carbs? "When you eat fat with a carbohydrate, it will cause the sugar to be almost time-released into the bloodstream, which is better than a quick spike," nutritionist Vollmuth explains.

"So say you had a little olive oil on a baked potato or some guacamole on tortilla chips. The amount of sugar going into your system is going to be leaked in over time. So instead of a quick spike in blood sugar, which would happen if you ate the chips by themselves, by combining fat with your snack, the sugar is let out in small amounts over time, because fat takes longer to digest than sugar. "That's why we eat foods in combination—because it causes a better biochemical reaction, which is ideal for optimal health," Vollmuth adds.

In the end, however, even adding protein, fat, or fiber isn't going to offset the effects of eating a *junk* carb meal. Sorry to tell you, but it's simply not a good idea to regularly have your cake and eat it, too.

"The bottom line is that if a particular food has an extremely high glycemic index like white bread, sugar cookies, or mashed potatoes, you want to avoid it altogether," suggests Dr. Lieberman, "or eat it very sparingly and only on occasion."

Your Insulin Spikes in Response to Sweets and Quickie Carbs

You now know that after you eat quickie carbs, your blood sugar leaps in reaction. But what happens next? In response to this rise in glucose, your pancreas begins to produce the all-important hormone insulin—alternately called the "master hormone" or "fat-storage hormone." Insulin's role is pivotal because without it your cells cannot use the glucose in your bloodstream for energy. "Insulin helps the cells take in glucose and convert it to energy," according to the National Diabetes Information Clearinghouse (NDIC), a service of the National Institute of Diabetes and Digestive and Kidney Diseases (NIDDK).

Essentially, insulin helps regulate your body's blood sugar level by moving the excess glucose out of your bloodstream and into your cells, thereby lowering your blood sugar and making the glucose available to fuel your body's functions and the activities of daily life.

So after you mindlessly guzzle that soft drink and scarf those cookies, your blood sugar shoots up. And then, as Dr. Willett explains in *Eat, Drink, and Be Healthy*, "[S]wift, high spikes in blood sugar are followed by similar surges in insulin."

In effect, your pancreas responds to this burst of sugar by secreting a proportionate amount of insulin into your bloodstream, explains noted endocrinologist Diana Schwarzbein, M.D.

As she describes it in her book, *The Schwarzbein Principle II: The Transition*, both the insulin and glucose then travel directly into your liver, where "insulin tells the liver cells to open up their doors, or receptors, and let the sugar in." Then, once inside your liver's cells, glucose can be processed through four different pathways.

"Some sugar is used for immediate energy," Dr. Schwarzbein explains.

"Some sugar is stored in the form of glycogen" in the liver and muscles to be used later. And excess sugar is turned into two types of fat—triglycerides and cholesterol.

"This small piece of information—that excess sugars are converted into these two types of fats—tells you that sugars are more damaging to the human body than fats are," she maintains. "High fats in your bloodstream are damaging, too, but [high] levels of sugar in your bloodstream will damage you first."

"These high levels of blood sugar and insulin surges are now implicated as part of the perilous pathway to heart disease and diabetes," Dr. Willett agrees. "The harmful effects of these rapidly digested carbohydrates are especially serious for people who are overweight."

What Goes Up Must Come Down: The Dangers of Fluctuating Blood Sugar

The insulin rush that comes from eating sweets or fast-acting carbs brings about another dilemma. "As all this insulin forces glucose into your muscle and fat cells, blood sugar levels plummet, triggering the unmistakable signals of hunger," notes Dr. Willett.

Ultimately, when you repeatedly gobble and guzzle fast-acting candies, cookies, sodas, or much-like-sugar carbs, you're setting in motion a vicious, health-damaging SUGAR SHOCK! cycle. Let's see how it could play out.

Soon after you pop sugar cookies and soda in your mouth, your body breaks them down and releases glucose into your bloodstream. The spike in your blood sugar triggers your pancreas to crank out a large dose of insulin, which means that the sugar is quickly whisked from your blood, leaving many people with lower-than-normal blood sugar—the condition known as hypoglycemia or low blood sugar.

I'll cover this condition in depth in chapter 13, but for now you should know that your plummeting blood sugar level could not only make you hungry, but also could bring on the blahs, blues, or blubbering, as well as leave you feeling negative, bad tempered, anxious, afraid, depressed, and much more. Meanwhile, this chronic low-blood-sugar condition could set in motion a predictable, health-damaging scenario that causes you to become almost frantic for carbs time and time again.

CELEBRITY FIGHTS SUGAR SHOCK!

"We all know the feeling: It starts with a tiny rumble in your tummy. Soon you have trouble concentrating. You get grouchy and snap at your coworkers or family. Before long you're a heat-seeking missile looking for the fastest source of energy you can get your hands on, often something sugary like a vending-machine candy bar, cookies, or ice cream. You end up consuming a lot of empty calories for no good reason: You still don't have the energy to exercise, and it isn't long before you find yourself reaching for more, as the insulin rush sparks your appetite."

—fitness expert Denise Austin in her book *Fit and Fabulous After 40*

"Within two hours after eating simple carbohydrates like a sweet roll or a bagel, your blood sugar drops too low again, and you experience the mid-morning or midafternoon slump," explains nutritionist Sally Rockwell, Ph.D., author of *Blood Sugar Blues*. "That's when you reach for cookies or candies, which raise your blood sugar again for a couple of hours. You spend the day eating sweets or simple carbs every few hours, because you're just trying to keep going," explains Dr. Rockwell, who counsels sugar or carb addicts, hypoglycemics, diabetics, and depressed people.

Glucagon, the Hormone That Fights Fat and Helps Keep Blood Sugar Stable

Insulin isn't the only hormone that's overstimulated by eating too many quickie, culprit carbs. When you take in too many low-caliber carbs, your hardworking pancreas also secretes glucagon, another important hormone.

Glucagon begins its work when your blood sugar drops below normal. Reproductive endocrinologist Deborah Metzger, M.D., Ph.D., explains: "Glucagon stimulates the breakdown of glycogen, the storage form of glucose, and then you get needed glucose for your body to use. This keeps you from becoming hypoglycemic."

Actually, insulin and glucagon engage in an intricate, artful, back-and-forth dance. "You want to have a normal balance between insulin and glucagon," explains nutritionist Vollmuth. "Insulin puts your sugar into storage (as fat), and glucagon takes it out. In other words, glucagon signals your cells to let stored energy (sugar and fat) out so it can be burned as fuel. But if you secrete too much insulin from eating too many fast-acting carbs, glucagon won't be released, and you won't get its fat-burning effects."

Although glucagon helps regulate blood sugar and mobilize stored fat, it takes a high-protein meal to put it to full use. So when you eat a high-carb meal, you *suppress* glucagon—meaning you probably won't lose weight, note the authors of *SUGAR BUSTERS!* But, after a high-protein meal, you get "a significant increase in the glucagon level," they write. "Glucagon promotes the mobilization of previously stored fat."

Summarizing Your Body's Reaction to Quickie Carbs

To review: The more refined carbs and sweets you eat, the more glucose you dump into your system all at once. This sudden blood sugar spike prompts your pancreas to release a large dose of the "fat storage" hormone insulin, which then helps move your blood sugar (glucose) out of your bloodstream and into your liver. At that point, your blood sugar is either used as energy or stored as glycogen in the liver or muscles or stored as triglycerides (fats) in your blood, cell membranes, or fat (adipose) tissues.

Then, within a short time (roughly two to four hours) after you've eaten those quickie carbs, your blood sugar plunges, leading to a number of unpleasant hypoglycemic ailments—from ferocious hunger to nagging headaches to mood swings.

All the while, the hormone glucagon, which mobilizes stored fat, is unavailable because of your sugar-laden meal. Bear in mind that insulin and glucagon working in tandem are designed to keep your body functioning properly. However, when you're constantly eating fast-acting carbs, you're causing your pancreas, which produces both hormones, to work overtime. Eventually your pancreas poops out, and your insulin-secretion mechanism system goes askew.

"If you continue to consume too many carbohydrates, including refined sugars," Dr. Schwarzbein warns, "the higher insulin levels will eventually cause health problems."

The Gentle Lift That Quality Carbs Bring

While sweets and much-like-sugar carbs cause your blood sugar to shoot up too quickly, tasty, superior, nutrient- and vitamin-rich vegetables, low-sugar fruits, nuts, legumes, and whole grains take longer to process. These carbs convert to sugar *gradually*, feeding glucose to your bloodstream a little at a time—in gentle trickles. In other words, your needed fuel comes at a steady, slow rate.

Let's say you eat some wheat berries. "Your body then has to break through the endosperm layers and the cellular structure of the food," says integrative, nutritionally trained physician Fred Pescatore, M.D., C.C.N., author of *The Hamptons Diet*.

"When you eat refined carbs, that cellular structure is gone. It's the same process with complex carbs like wheat berries, but it's *slower* so you don't get glucose spikes, which cause insulin spikes, which cause insulin drops," continues Dr. Pescatore, former medical director for the Atkins Center for Complementary Medicine in New York City.

"Wheat berries are just better carbs," he concludes. "They're not wasted calories. They provide vitamins, minerals, and nutrients. They tend to be more filling and satisfying. They're more slowly metabolized so you don't have rapid blood sugar swings. And they have fiber, which could help prevent cancer and other diseases."

Cutting or Curtailing Carbs Could Take Off Your Weight

In recent years, researchers have been discovering that the excessive intake of these fast-acting carbs could be a primary cause of the rise in numbers on your bathroom scale.

Nutritionist Dr. Lieberman explains why. "When you eat simple carbs, your blood sugar shoots up fast and then your insulin quickly goes up. When those two things happen simultaneously, you throw a metabolic switch to store body fat that's independent of calories. This has to do with the fact that you consumed foods that became sugar fast."

Ultimately, Americans need to learn that "not all carbohydrates are created equal," points out Kathy Smith, one of the fitness industry's leading wellness experts, with more than 16 million videos sold worldwide.

Indeed, as Smith observes, some intriguing studies show that refined carbs are tied to weight gain. For instance, groundbreaking research from Yunsheng Ma, M.D., Ph.D., assistant professor of medicine at the University of Massachusetts Medical School in Worcester, showed that fast-acting carbs put on weight and have an adverse effect on blood lipids.

In fact, the study created quite a stir upon its publication in the *American Journal of Epidemiology* in early 2005. Dr. Ma and his colleagues found—after weighing, measuring, and analyzing the physical activity of 572 healthy adults—that those who ate more refined grains, starchy vegetables, and similar carbs were significantly heavier than people who ate superior, nutrient-dense carbs such as nonstarchy vegetables, whole grains, nuts, and seeds.

"The *total* amount of carbohydrates is not related to body weight," Dr. Ma explains. "The *type* of carbs is what's important," he adds, noting that another study also found that "diabetics who replaced 'bad carbs' with 'good carbs' significantly improved blood sugar control."

"All carbohydrates are not the enemy," Dr. Ma contends. "But you have to watch for specific kinds of enemies." In other words, as you've been learning, quality carbs—especially from Mother Nature—are your friends, but much-like-sugar carbs are your foes.

We're Not Designed to Eat Quickie Carbs

Numerous experts insist that our bodies are simply not designed to process these fast-acting carbs. Rather, they insist, we're "genetically programmed" to follow a low-carb Paleolithic diet followed by our hunter-gatherer ancestors.

"Both refined sugars and grains weren't even available for the past 2.5 million years. It wasn't until the last 200 years or so that people even began eating them," says Loren Cordain, Ph.D., who has conducted numerous scientific studies demonstrating the many health benefits of eating more like humans did thousands of years ago.

And one of the biggest health benefits to returning to our roots, so to speak, is that we can stay lean.

Excess Quickie Carbs Can Lead to Several Blood Sugar Disorders

As people have been carb gorging and gaining weight in the United States and around the world, we've been witnessing an unparalleled explosion of glucose-metabolism disorders, including hypoglycemia, prediabetes (impaired glucose tolerance or glucose intolerance and impaired fasting glucose), hyperinsulinemia, insulin resistance, metabolic syndrome (originally known as Syndrome X and now increasingly called insulin resistance syndrome), and type 2 diabetes.

Easily more than 65 million Americans—and, according to some experts, possibly as many as 147 million (or one-half the U.S. population)—are afflicted with various blood sugar conditions.

A diet full of sweets and other fast-acting carbs could trigger or exacerbate virtually all these disorders, which are related to the body's inability to effectively assimilate or process the sugars, starches, or quickie carbs that you're consuming.

"It begins with an overproduction of insulin to maintain normal blood sugar," explains reproductive endocrinologist Dr. Metzger. "Over time, the insulin levels can escalate, either leading to hypoglycemia or diabetes, because the pancreas just can't keep up with the demands for insulin."

Dr. Antonio Convit of the Center for Brain Health at New York University School of Medicine amplifies: "You need more insulin to do the same work, as your tissues basically become resistant to your own insulin. That's what happens first. That can start very, very inconspicuously. But after you've been doing this for a while and don't exercise more or lose weight, and you have the genetic predisposition, you can get more insulin resistance or impaired glucose tolerance (which is the same thing as prediabetes)."

Dr. Jonny Bowden, a nutritionist, puts it this way: "It's sort of like the noise level in New York City. When you're constantly exposed to it, you have to shout louder and louder to be heard. When sugar and insulin are so consistently elevated, you have to literally knock louder and louder on the doors of the cells, so to speak, to get them to open up. This reluctance of the cells to open up is called insulin resistance," he continues. "If your cells are resistant to insulin, then the carbs are shuttled into the fat cells, leading to an ongoing cycle of weight gain."

Normally after you eat any kind of carbs (refined or whole), your blood sugar returns to a fairly standard range, points out Dr. Pescatore. "But when you overeat or eat too much sugar and simple carbs, your blood ranges get all screwed up. Insulin is forced to do its work too well and so you end up with a blood sugar disorder."

Interestingly, experts repeatedly emphasize that these glucose-metabolism disorders are relatively new in humanity's history, and they tend to coincide with the introduction of high-speed, machine-enabled food processing and the resultant widespread availability of processed foods in the early 1900s.

"We are metabolically and physiologically the same as we were thousands of years ago, but now you're seeing dramatic numbers of people with insulin resistance, prediabetes, and diabetes," observes nutrition specialist David L. Katz, M.D., M.P.H., an associate professor at Yale University School of Medicine and author of *The Way to Eat* and *The Flavor Point Diet*.

"But," Dr. Metzger maintains, "if you go on a diet and eliminate refined carbs, very often insulin sensitivity returns, and hypoglycemia, prediabetes, or diabetes could go away." (Remember, you *don't want* insulin resistance; you *want* insulin sensitivity.)

The Sequence of Blood Sugar Disorders

"Ideally, we use insulin to soak up available food energy like a sponge. Insulin helps us use food for fuel now and store it as fuel for later. Individuals who effectively release insulin are more fuel efficient," Dr. Katz explains.

He continues, "If you release insulin readily and then are floating in a sea of calories, your release of insulin becomes excessive, which contributes to the dysfunction of insulin receptors in susceptible individuals. You need more and more insulin, and you get into a degenerative spiral, with more and more insulin release leading to more insulin resistance, leading to more release. . . . Eventually, the pancreas cannot keep up with such high demand, and diabetes or other blood sugar disorders develop."

Dr. Katz believes that "the sequence is generally as follows: 1) metabolic efficiency/brisk insulin release (you're healthy), 2) caloric overload (including excessive intake of simple sugars and refined starches), 3) weight gain, and 4) abdominal obesity. Next comes either 5) insulin resistance or 6) impaired glucose tolerance, or they can occur simultaneously. And finally you're hit by 7) diabetes."

Bear in mind that such blood sugar woes don't develop within days, weeks, or even months. "It takes years of day-in, day-out eating refined carbs, and it's usually associated with weight gain," says nutritionist Dr. Lieberman.

A PRIMER ON BLOOD SUGAR DISORDERS

NOTE: Experts single out overconsumption of refined sweeteners and processed carbs as being instrumental in the development of all of the following blood sugar disorders, with the exception of type 1 diabetes.

Healthy: You can eat carbs of any kind and your blood sugar rises and returns to within a normal range. Meanwhile, your insulin levels rise or drop in response to your glucose levels, thereby keeping everything in balance. If you're healthy, your blood glucose levels will range from 70 to 99 milligrams per one-tenth of a liter (milligrams per deciliter) of blood after fasting overnight. In addition, levels of 70 to 140 mg/dL after meals are considered normal or target glucose ranges.

Reactive Hypoglycemia (Low Blood Sugar or Postprandial [After-Meal] Hypoglycemia): Your blood sugar drops abnormally low about two to five hours after eating. You could have one or more of approximately 100 symptoms, including depression, fatigue, heart palpitations, anxiety, carb cravings, headaches, and more. According to experts, you're hypoglycemic if you have a blood glucose level of less than 70 or 50 mg/dL of blood.

Prediabetes (People with this condition have Impaired Glucose Tolerance and/or Impaired Fasting Glucose): Your blood sugar is elevated (higher than normal) but not high enough for you to be diagnosed diabetic. If you're prediabetic, you have fasting levels of blood glucose—between 100 to 125 mg /dL—or your blood glucose is 140 to 199 mg /dL after taking a two-hour Oral Glucose Tolerance Test.

Hyperinsulinemia: You have a high blood level of insulin, which is caused by excessive insulin production by your pancreas. Hyperinsulinemia may be caused by insulin resistance or by a pancreatic tumor. Some experts believe that hyperinsulinemia is the same as insulin resistance and that the terms are interchangeable because you can't have one without the other.

Insulin Resistance: This is a silent condition that occurs when your muscle, fat, and liver cells become insensitive to insulin and no longer use it properly. Your pancreas tries to keep up with your demand for insulin by producing more, but it just can't keep up with your body's need for insulin, so excess glucose builds up in your bloodstream. Genes are partly responsible for insulin resistance, but obesity and physical inactivity can contribute to or aggravate the condition. Insulin resistance and prediabetes usually have no obvious symptoms except central weight gain, and it may take several years before you notice anything wrong.

Type 1 Diabetes: Formerly called insulin-dependent diabetes mellitus or juvenile-onset diabetes, type 1 diabetes is an autoimmune disease that occurs when your pancreas stops producing insulin entirely. If you have type 1 diabetes, you're dependent on insulin injections. Usually, people have an abrupt onset of symptoms, typically before age 30, although it can occur at any age. Type 1 diabetes is estimated to account for 5 to 10 percent of all diagnosed cases of diabetes. (*SUGAR SHOCK!* does not discuss this type of diabetes.)

Type 2 Diabetes: Previously known as non-insulin-dependent or adult-onset diabetes mellitus. Type 2 diabetes, which used to strike people aged 30 and over, is a complex metabolic disorder that is increasingly becoming a disease of overweight kids (even as young as age 6). If you have type 2 diabetes, your insulin production slows down as a result of having to work overtime to stabilize your blood sugar levels. This disease was once known as sugar diabetes, which implies the role that consumption of sweets can have on its development.

Metabolic Syndrome (Syndrome X or Insulin Resistance Syndrome): A constellation of controllable but insidious symptoms that increase your likelihood of developing coronary heart disease, stroke, and diabetes. The phrase "Syndrome X" was first coined and described by Stanford University endocrinologist Gerald Reaven, M.D., in 1988. (I'll discuss this syndrome in more detail in chapter 14.)

The Much-Maligned, Much-Misunderstood Low-Carb Trend

As you no doubt know, in the mid-1990s, low-carb dieting became a huge, nationwide craze, as sales of *Dr. Atkins New Diet Revolution* soared. By late 2004 to early 2005, reports from members of the media and food analysts were concluding that low-carb dieting was dying out or already passé.

But amidst the reports about low carb's demise, most observers were missing the big picture. First of all, despite the naysayers, low-carb dieting in some form or another is here to stay, according to Opinion Dynamics, a market research firm that has tracked the movement since 2003.

"We expect it to stabilize at between 7 to 15 percent of the population [or about 15 million to 33 million people]," says Larry Shiman, vice president of the Cambridge, Massachusetts–based, full-service market research company, which specializes in the food industry. "The legacy of the trend is that for many dieters, low carb still plays a substantial role."

Whether or not carb-restricted diets work (and upwards of 23 studies indicate they do, at least over the short term), the trend has had far-reaching implications. Before he died in 2003, Robert C. Atkins, M.D., was one of the more outspoken physicians to alert the public to the dangers of inferior, fiber-stripped carbohydrates and sugars.

Although the late diet doctor is, of course, best known for launching his much-criticized or much-lauded (depending upon with whom you're talking) low-carb diet, Dr. Atkins clearly deserves much of the credit for educating millions of Americans about the health and weight-loss benefits of eschewing sweets and quickie carbs.

All his books, including *Dr. Atkins' Diet Revolution*, which first hit the bestseller lists in the 1970s, have repeated his self-described "favorite dictum: avoid sugar."

Although many people view the Atkins diet as one that pushes pork rinds, fatty red meat, and butter, they're completely missing the point.

To this day, the Atkins camp contends that the meal plan helps people "learn respect for carbohydrates," points out Colette Heimowitz, M.S., vice president of education and research at Atkins Nutritionals.

"People who go on the Atkins diet or maintenance plan," she insists, "develop *a healthy lifestyle* that incorporates nutrient-dense carbohydrates such as fruits, vegetables, seeds, nuts, and whole grains.

"By always staying beneath their carb tolerance, they maintain their weight-loss goals. You can live with this healthy way of eating for the rest of your life," adds Heimowitz, who has followed "an Atkins carb-watching approach" for 20 years, hoping to avert the fate of her obese, diabetic parents, who both died at an early age.

In addition to drawing attention to perils of quickie carbs, Dr. Atkins pointed out the pivotal role that hormones play in weight loss, and his work paved the way for other diets that stress carb cutting.

"Although all low-carb diets differ in certain respects, all are based on the fact that food has a profound effect on hormones, including the fat-storage and fat-release hormones," explains *Living the Low Carb Life* author Dr. Jonny Bowden.

"The foundation of the low-carbohydrate movement has been the theory that controlling hormones by what foods you eat is at least as important for weight loss as calories are," adds Dr. Bowden, noting that regulating insulin and controlling blood sugar levels are central to the theory of all carb-watching diets.

But Dr. Atkins's seemingly "heretic" low-carb plan did more than just alert Americans to the dangers of processed, "wrong" carbs. It also shook up the traditional medical establishment—a phenomenon brilliantly reported by science journalist Gary Taubes in a controversial, much-talked-about 2002 *New York Times Magazine* article titled, "What If It's All Been a Big Fat Lie?"

Essentially, Dr. Atkins bucked the then-prevailing low-fat, high-carb "dietary dogma" that had been backed since the early 1970s with, as Taubes put it, "an almost religious certainty by everyone from the surgeon general on down."

But, as Taubes and other experts now speculate, by removing or curtailing fats and adding in a bunch of inferior carbs, people gained fat instead of lost it. (More in chapter 14, "The Chronic Big Killers," about how a landmark study recently debunked the efficacy of a low-fat diet.)

The Emphasis on Quality Carbs Endures

More recently, other experts/authors, including Dr. Michael Eades and Dr. Mary Dan Eades in their book *Protein Power*; the four authors of *SUGAR BUSTERS! Cut Sugar to Trim Fat*; Diana Schwarzbein, M.D., in her *Schwarzbein Principle* books; and Fred Pescatore, M.D., in *The Hamptons Diet*, have also sought to educate the public about the health and weight-loss benefits of cutting out inferior, quickie carbs.

In addition, Miami cardiologist Arthur Agatston, M.D., author of the best-selling *The South Beach Diet*, helped raise awareness of the important differences between "good" carbs and "bad" carbs. Although many view the South Beach Diet as low carb, Dr. Agatston disavows that label. "We are not low carb. We are good carb," he insists.

"Low Carb" Is a Misleading Term

At the end of the day, advocates of low-carb dieting and maintaining insist that the term "low carb" is inappropriate and misleading.

"Low carb doesn't mean you're mainlining lard and eating pork rinds all day. It means making healthier choices in carbs and picking better-quality foods," says Lora Ruffner, R.N., who founded the popular www.lowcarb luxury.com website in 1999 and *Low Carb Luxury Magazine* in 2000.

"Low carb means eating more vegetables than you ever did before, more low-sugar fruits such as berries, melons, peaches, and pears, more whole grains, and more fiber. It means *not* eating junk food, especially foods with high-fructose corn syrup and trans fats," insists Ruffner, who says that trimming unhealthy carbs shaved off 100 pounds and "saved" her life after her doctor gave her six months to live.

Carb Consciousness Takes Root

Ultimately, with some guidance and encouragement, Americans are becoming more and more aware of the drawbacks of second-rate quickie carbs and the value of superior, slow-release, quality carbs. And this trend is gaining much more momentum than the low-carb movement ever did. For example, the major food companies now are responding to consumers' desire for whole grains (even though, much to our dismay, they often pack in the sugars, too).

"Consumers are getting smarter," insists Dr. Bowden. "They're learning that a healthy, intelligent, controlled-carb diet low in sugar and junk food is the way to go for both health and weight loss."

And the carb-trimming trend has helped to put this food group into perspective. "If nothing else, low-carb studies made everyone understand that you need moderation in all areas—and carbs is one area where we went overboard," says nutrition expert Bonnie Brehm, Ph.D., associate professor in the University of Cincinnati's College of Nursing, who spearheaded a study showing that a low-carb diet was more effective than a low-fat one for short-term weight loss and it led to improvement in cardiovascular risk factors.

"Maybe now we'll see doctors help people realize that carbs aren't free food. Probably, they will be educating their patients more about why we need to moderate *both* our fat and carb intake," predicts Dr. Brehm.

Sugar Watching Grips the Nation: Is Low Sugar the New Low Carb?

While attention on the low-carb movement was waning, another powerful movement has been gripping the nation. "Low-sugar has become the new low carb," professes Melanie Warner in the May 2005 *New York Times* article, "Low Carbs? Who Cares? Sugar Is Latest Supermarket Demon."

"Carbs were a trend, but the concern about sugar is here to stay," Cathleen Toomey, vice president of communications at Stonyfield Farms, told the *Times*.

In fact, Gus Valen, CEO of the Valen Group, a strategy consulting firm specializing in the food and beverage industry, predicts that "for many years to come consumers will continue to watch their intake of refined sugar and flour."

And, according to the NPD Group's *20th Annual Eating Patterns in America (EPA) Report*, released in 2005, about 21 percent of Americans completely agree with the statement, "A person should be very cautious in serving foods with sugar."

In its survey of grocery shoppers, the Grocery Manufacturers Association, a food industry trade group, found that almost 50 percent of people were looking for products with reduced sugar.

Another study arrived at similar conclusions, finding that 49 percent of Americans report paying attention to sugar content when deciding which foods to eat. The Food for Life study from Yankelovich, Inc., also discovered that, on a typical day, 45 percent of Americans feel they eat too much sugar or junk food.

Although Dr. Sinatra and I applaud the sugar-watching movement, we cringe at the fact that more people are eating—and even overeating—foods filled with potentially dangerous artificial sweeteners such as aspartame, Splenda, and saccharin. (More about this later.)

As Processed Low-Carb Products Disappear, Fresh Carbs Grab the Limelight

One of the biggest lessons of the low-carb movement has to do with the demise of many of the more than 3,000 low-carb products that glutted the market at the height of the low-carb frenzy. These prepared foods were not only chemically *processed*, but often they were neither nutritious nor palatable. Sometimes, they were even high in calories, and every so often, they made you sick. (To be blunt, in our circles, people sneer at these products as "low-carb crap.")

"I got the runs for two days and a stomachache for three after trying a new low-carb breakfast bar at a low-carb conference," reports reproductive endocrinologist Gil Wilshire, M.D., president and chief scientific officer of the Carbohydrate Awareness Council, which supports the scientific basis of carb-controlled diet and nutrition.

Vanessa Sands, former editor in chief of *LowCarb Energy*, contends that these dubious foods "have fallen by the wayside because we don't need them. You could live on a farm and still eat fresh, low-carb foods."

Even so, a smattering of products are still on sale. "I even see them in 'health food' stores," says Dr. Metzger. "Reading the labels makes my coronaries constrict." In fact, Dr. Pescatore believes that "people are never going to get healthy if they over-rely on processed foods of any kind, even if they're low carb. America has to get back to eating *real*, good, wholesome foods and carbs—the way our ancestors did."

5

Take the SUGAR SHOCK!

Challenge

You've now heard Dr. Sinatra's and my stories. You've learned about the differences between inferior and quality carbs. You'll read warnings from hundreds of experts. Of course, what you read here may shock you. You may find it outright preposterous that eating enticing-looking, delectable desserts and quickie carbs could dramatically harm your moods, energy levels, relationships, libido, thought processes, and health.

So I invite you: Don't take my word for it! Question my premise that quickie carbs can endanger you. Take the SUGAR SHOCK! Challenge!

That's right. For three weeks, eat only high-quality protein, veggies, fruits, legumes, nuts, seeds, fats, and whole grains. After those 21 days, provided your doctor gives you permission and you don't have a medical condition such as hypoglycemia or diabetes, allow yourself one single day of indulgence.

Wait! I'm not telling you to pig out. I'm merely saying that you may wish to partake of polite portions of pizza, pasta, candies, pastry, soda, wine, or other "taboo" foods on that designated day.

Next, watch yourself as if you were conducting a lab experiment. Try to learn from it. Write down how you feel later that day, the next day, and two days after eating those "treats." How did your sugar diet affect you? What does your body tell you?

Actually, some forward-thinking schools do just that—they allow their kids a junk-food day. Sure enough, they've found this to be a powerful way to prove the value of staying sugar free.

So test my theory. Take my SUGAR SHOCK! Challenge. Then share your experiences with me on my website or blog at www.SugarShock.com or www.SugarShockBlog.com.

PART 3

WHERE WE ARE: ON A FAST TRACK TO DANGER, DISEASE, AND LITIGATION

6

NOT-SO-SWEET ANGLES ON OBESITY

AND DIABETES

As you'll soon learn, obesity is only a small part of the sugar story. But at this point, it's time to face the unavoidable discussion of our terrifying, runaway obesity epidemic, the onslaught of diabetes, and the role that sugary and refined foods play in their development.

It's unsettling to even contemplate the swelling statistics. More than 65 percent of U.S. adults are overweight or obese, with more than 32 percent (over 66 million) of Americans classified as obese. Furthermore, almost 5 percent of adults were classified as extremely obese, according to CDC's National Center for Health Statistics.

But even adults at the higher end of the "normal" BMI range, with BMIs of 22 to 24, could stand to lose some weight, according to Dr. Walter C. Willett of Harvard. In all, "up to 80 percent of American adults should weigh less than they do," he says.

Perhaps most alarming to health experts is the fact that our nation's kids are steadily gaining weight, with 17.1 percent of children and adolescents 2 to 19 years of age (over 12.5 million youngsters) overweight.

And all that extra flab ultimately is sending people to their graves—from diabetes, heart disease, strokes, and several types of cancer. Indeed, as Dr. Willett puts it so eloquently in his book, *Eat, Drink, and Be Healthy*, "Weight sits like a spider at the center of an intricate, tangled web of health and disease."

In fact, excess weight, obesity, poor diet, and lack of exercise killed 365,000 Americans in 2000, according to epidemiologist Ali Mokdad,

WHAT ARE THE DEFINITIONS OF OVERWEIGHT, OBESE, AND MORBIDLY OBESE?

Wondering where you fit in? The body mass index or BMI is the measure of a person's body fat based on height and weight. For adults, you're "normal" if your BMI is between 18.5 and 24.9; "overweight" if you have a body mass index or BMI of 25 to 29.9; "obese" if your BMI is 30 or more, and "morbidly obese" if your BMI is greater than 40 or you're at least 100 pounds overweight. To learn your BMI, visit the CDC's website at www.cdc.gov/nccdphp/dnpa/bmi/calc-bmi.htm.

Ph.D., chief of the behavioral surveillance branch at the Centers for Disease Control and Prevention (CDC) in Atlanta, Georgia. (By contrast, 435,000 people died from tobacco-related diseases.)

In short, as a group of 10 respected scientists warned in the prestigious *New England Journal of Medicine* in March 2005, "Obesity has been shown to have a substantial effect on longevity." In fact, obese adults are expected to have their life expectancy shortened by two to five years unless aggressive efforts are made to slow the obesity epidemic. As for severely obese people, they'll have their lives shortened by 5 to 20 years.

Overweight and obese children will suffer similarly. "The youth of today may, on average, live less healthy and possibly even shorter lives than their parents," warned the experts, led by University of Illinois demographer S. Jay Olshansky. "Looking out the window, we see a threatening storm—obesity—that will, if unchecked, have a negative effect on life expectancy."

Obesity on the Rise as Junk Food Sales Soar

America and other countries haven't always struggled with growing girth. Indeed, for millions of years, we humans evolved with no hugely significant weight problems. In fact, only in the past 50 years has flab increased.

Until about 1980, obesity rates in this country hovered fairly consistently between 12 to 14 percent. But by 1980, the numbers dramatically rose, with 47 percent of U.S. adults aged 20 to 74 overweight and 15 percent of them obese. By 2002, those obesity statistics climbed even higher, with 65 percent of adult Americans now overweight or obese, as mentioned previously.

About three decades ago, profound cultural changes kicked into motion and set almost two-thirds of this country on the fast track for obesity, according to nutritional epidemiologist Aviva Must, Ph.D., professor of public health and family medicine at Tufts University School of Medicine and a scientist for the Nutritional Epidemiology Program at the Jean Mayer USDA Human Nutrition Research Center on Aging.

"So many things happened at that time," Dr. Must says, noting that in the 1970s, Americans consumed food in smaller portion sizes and totaling several hundred fewer calories a day than today. But then, the shift began: People started eating fewer meals at home, average portion sizes grew substantially, and fast-food restaurants popped up in strip malls, in the heart of the city, and in the suburbs—in short, just about everywhere. What's more, sugary and fat-laden convenience snacks and meals were pretty much ubiquitous, too.

And all of that coincided with a U.S. government recommendation to eat less fat and a lot of carbohydrates. This meant that health-conscious Americans were striving to follow the U.S. Food Guide Pyramid's recommendations to eat 6 to 11 servings a day of bread, cereal, rice, or pasta. But, rather than eat whole grains, folks usually reached for refined, fiber-stripped, processed carbs or sweets.

"Americans were basically told that all fat was bad," Dr. Willett recalls. "By default, you had to eat something, so, even though there was no scientific evidence to support it, people were told to eat massive amounts of carbohydrates without regard to quality."

For example, he says, "we were told to load up on Wonder Bread, corn-flakes, and other breads. As if that wasn't bad enough, they put potatoes in the vegetable group so that, altogether, they were recommending 13 servings [of quick-acting carbs] a day.

"It wasn't just the federal government saying this. This was the conventional wisdom in the medical community," Dr. Willett marvels, noting that the American Heart Association encouraged nonfat foods, even giving the dubious dietary recommendation to switch from nutrient-poor devil's food cake to equally bad-for-you angel food cake.

Of course, nutrition, obesity, and public health experts—sometimes termed "obesity warriors" by the media or, more disparagingly, "nutrition nannies," "diet dictators," or "food police"—cite other obvious reasons for our runaway amounts of adipose tissue: Americans are eating more calories and exercising less. But it is our view that a large percentage of the blame for America's obesity crisis is due to the fact that millions of Americans are overconsuming high-calorie, high-sugar sweets and quickie-carb snack foods on a regular basis.

As Obesity Rises, So Does Diabetes

Increasingly, we're hearing that as more of us Americans become obese, we're experiencing a parallel rise in the incidence of type 2 diabetes, the nation's sixth biggest killer, according to the CDC. Such a close causal connection exists between obesity and diabetes that pediatric endocrinologist Francine Kaufman, M.D.—a former president of the American Diabetes Association, who was instrumental in getting soda sales banned in Los Angeles schools—wrote an important 2005 book, *Diabesity: The Obesity-Diabetes Epidemic That Threatens America—And What We Must Do to Stop It.*

What's more, the nonprofit organization Shape Up America!, founded in 1994 by former U.S. Surgeon General C. Everett Koop to help Americans manage their weight, launched a "Diabesity" initiative to combat the pervasive disease.

Moreover, experts repeatedly point to this link between gaining a lot of weight and developing diabetes. C. Ronald Kahn, M.D., president and director of the Joslin Diabetes Center, points out that American adults have gained a whopping 2 *billion* pounds over the past decade, which averages out to about one pound a year per person. "For every one pound increase in weight, there is a 3 to 4 percent increase in the prevalence of type 2 diabetes, or about 800,000 new cases a year," Dr. Kahn warns.

Diabetes is spiraling so completely out of control that the number of cases tripled just from the mid-1960s to the mid-1990s. In fact, in the past decade alone, the number of cases has nearly doubled, and it's expected to rise a whopping 165 percent by the year 2050. Just check out these alarming statistics:

- The prevalence of type 2 diabetes is three to seven times higher in obese people than in normal-weight adults, according to a joint statement by the American Diabetes Association, the North American Association for the Study of Obesity, and the American Society for Clinical Nutrition in *Diabetes Care*.

■ More than 90 to 95 percent of people with diabetes have type 2 diabetes, which, in many cases, can be prevented by working out and losing weight by eating the right foods.

Internationally, the figures are even more frightening:

■ More than 1 billion people around the world are overweight or obese, according to the London-based International Association for the Study of Obesity.

■ By the year 2025, the number of people with diabetes worldwide is expected to double from 194 million to 333 million, according to the International Diabetes Federation.

The Scary State of Our Nation's Young

Most alarming to parents, experts, and educators alike is how the bodies of America's young are widening more than they're lengthening. At this writing, the United States had more than 12.5 million overweight children aged 2 to 19 years old.

Back in the mid-1980s, a mere 5 percent of children in the nation were overweight or obese. Now, about 30 percent of children and adolescents are at risk for being overweight or obese, or already are, and according to pediatrician Carden Johnston, M.D., former president of the American Academy of Pediatrics, the figure is even higher, perhaps as high as 40 percent.

Still more tragic is that children are increasingly gaining weight at younger and younger ages:

■ More than 10 percent of American *toddlers* aged 2 to 5 are overweight, according to the American Heart Association.

■ Some 19 percent of children aged 6 to 11 are overweight, and 17 percent of adolescents aged 12 to 19 are overweight, according to the CDC's National Center for Health Statistics (NHANES Data).

Given the number of children who are overweight or obese, many are also developing type 2 diabetes and metabolic syndrome. Until recently, type

2 diabetes was known as "adult-onset diabetes" because it generally struck people in middle age. Unfortunately, type 2 diabetes now is becoming a disease of children, even hitting wee ones as young as six.

- In most cases, kids diagnosed with type 2 diabetes are overweight. Inevitably, experts worry, these children's lives will be drastically cut short.

- More horrifying, 2 million adolescents between 12 and 19—or one in six overweight kids—have prediabetes, according to the *Journal of Pediatrics*.

- One in three children born in 2000 is likely to develop type 2 diabetes *unless* he or she starts eating less and more healthily and exercising more. The odds are worse for black and Hispanic children, with nearly one half expected to develop the disease.

- Increasingly, overweight and obese children are developing metabolic syndrome—especially if they continue to gain weight. Yale University School of Medicine researchers reported in the *New England Journal of Medicine* that half of the 439 obese youngsters studied developed various Syndrome X risk factors, including insulin resistance, unhealthy cholesterol, and other metabolic abnormalities.

Now, let's take a look at some not-so-sweet developments and trends that researchers, nutritionists, and junk food critics believe have contributed to our country's obesity epidemic and concurrent health crisis.

Ballooning Portion Sizes Have Become the Norm

In the past two to four decades, corporations have been jacking up portion sizes of everything from cookies to French fries to popcorn to soda. While customers might think they're getting greater value, obesity experts find the phenomenon alarming. They claim that this "portion distortion" is likely contributing substantially to people's extra poundage.

"When you have calories that are incredibly cheap, in a culture where 'bigger is better,' that's a dangerous combination," says Dr. Willett. For example,

- The original Hershey candy bar was 0.6 ounces when introduced in 1908, but current bars range from 1.6 to 8 ounces.

- Twenty years ago, a standard bagel was 3 inches in diameter and around 140 calories. Today's bagels are usually 6 inches in diameter and contain 350 calories, or the equivalent of four slices of bread.

- If you drive an older car, you know that today's soda bottles are simply too large to fit in the cup holders! In the 1950s, Coca-Cola was sold in 6.5-ounce bottles and had 85 calories. In the 1970s the 12-ounce Coke can became the norm. In the year 2000, the 20-ounce bottle, which has 250 calories, became the typical serving size. This means that a typical "serving" of Coke is now a whopping *300 percent larger* than it was in the 1950s. And that doesn't even include the popular, supersized 42-ounce soft drinks promoted at some fast-food restaurants and convenience stores. If you order one of these, watch out: This gargantuan drink gives you 525 calories, more than a regular cheeseburger at McDonald's.

According to a study published in the *Journal of the American Dietetic Association* in 2003, other foods also have swelled in size since the early 1980s and now exceed federal standards:

- Muffins have been supersized from 2 or 3 ounces to between 4 and 7 ounces.

- Cookies have expanded enormously, sometimes eightfold.

- Pasta portions have ballooned to almost six times larger.

- Fast-food chains offer hamburgers, sodas, and French fries that are now two to five times their original size.

Interestingly, the "supersized culture espoused by fast-food chains also has had an impact on how much we eat at home—more!" concludes a study of king-sized offerings that was published in the *Journal of the American Medical Association* and coauthored by nutrition professor Dr. Barry Popkin.

(While we're talking about huge portion sizes, I urge you to rent or buy the Academy Award–nominated documentary, *Super Size Me*. Its producer and star, Morgan Spurlock, ate nothing but McDonald's foods for a

WHEN IN AMERICA, DO AS THE FRENCH DO TO STAY SLIM!

Over the years, you may have wondered how the French get away with eating rich Camembert and Brie cheese, croissants, French bread, foie gras, and butter-drenched escargots and still have lower rates of obesity and heart disease than Americans. American and British scientists like to call this phenomenon the "French Paradox," and some have attributed it to their regular consumption of moderate amounts of red wine with their meals.

University of Pennsylvania psychologist Paul Rozin, Ph.D., and his colleagues, however, took a closer look and found that the American ingrained sense of "bigger is better" may be largely responsible for our more portly proportions. When scientists compared packaged products in Paris and Philadelphia, they found that *nearly all items, especially those containing sugar*, were larger in the United States.

Philadelphia also was home to larger portion sizes at restaurants and at "all-you-can-eat" dining places. For example, a scoop of Häagen-Dazs ice cream was 25 percent bigger in Philly than Paris, a candy bar was 41 percent larger, and a Coca-Cola was 52 percent larger. Likewise, recipe serving sizes over here in the United States are bigger.

But, in the study's only amusing finding, French toilet paper squares are larger!

month, supersized only when asked, and quickly gained 25 pounds. The Oscar-nominated film offers an intriguing exposé of the health and obesity risks of fast-food diets.)

Convenience Calls and Dining Out

Another development that insiders believe has led to increased consumption of sugar is our fast-paced, "grab it, get it, and go" culture. Frenzied, stressed-out, in-a-rush Americans frequently rely on inexpensive, readily available, sugary, fatty, packaged snack foods. In fact, prepared, processed foods, frozen foods, and baked goods accounted for more than 40 percent of supermarket sales in 2000. (Produce generated a mere 9 percent of sales.)

Moreover, many people gravitate specifically toward ostensibly "healthy" quick snacks such as protein bars, which are often laden with high-fructose corn syrup and/or other sweeteners. Or maybe they'll buy some low-fat "goodies" that are likely filled with sugar and not even necessarily low calorie. Or they'll grab quickie-carb crunchies that, 9 times out of 10, have used some kind of sweetener. Obviously, all those extra snacks can lead to episodes of SUGAR SHOCK!

Coupled with our desire for convenience is a parallel trend. Indeed, about 64 percent of all meals are eaten outside the home. And much of that budget goes to fat-filled, processed fast foods, inevitably containing fast-acting carbs as a major component of the meal (think hamburger buns, fries, and onion rings).

"Americans spend more money on fast food than on higher education, personal computers, computer software, or new cars. They spend more on fast food than on movies, books, magazines, newspapers, videos, and recorded music—combined," Eric Schlosser reveals in *Fast Food Nation*.

What's more, in almost all cases, as noted earlier, all this dining out means people also are unknowingly putting into their bodies processed foods often pumped with hidden sugars. "People are consuming products that they wouldn't even dream have sugar in them," says food scientist Russ Bianchi.

"The perfect example is roaster chickens, which are injected with water, salt, sugar, fructose, starch, and preservatives. You're thinking, 'I'm tired and I'll surprise my family by bringing one home.' How could that be wrong? Who would even think there's sugar in them?"

SUGAR SHOCKER! SUPERSIZING PACKS A BIG-CALORIE WALLOP

Most Americans find it hard to pass up the chance for *more*. And whenever we buy food at a movie theater, convenience store, or fast-food joint, we're nudged to do just that. Notice how often you're asked, "Would you like to make that a jumbo size, sir, for just a few pennies more?" or "Care for a supersized portion, madam?"

Call it a "value meal," supersizing, or just getting more bang for your buck, but when you add it all up, you're faced with one undeniable fact—a humongous increase in calories, sugar, and/or fat. Thanks to the enlightening report, *From Wallet to Waistline: The Hidden Costs of Super Sizing*, issued by a coalition of health organizations, here's an idea of how saying yes to supersizing piles on the calories:

For example, if you opt for a Classic Cinnabon instead of a Minibon, you pay "only" 48 cents more but get 370 extra calories or 123 percent more. Or, if you move from a regular portion to 7-Eleven DoubleGulp Coke, you pay a mere 37 cents more, but get an extra 450 extra calories, more than you'd get in a McDonald's Quarter Pounder.

And if you can't resist a medium movie theater popcorn instead of a small, you'll pay only 71 cents more but get 500 calories—a whopping 125 percent more calories and two days' worth of saturated fat for the buttered popcorn. (And this isn't the jumbo size.)

"Americans are constantly induced to spend a little more money to get a lot more food," says Margo Wootan, director of nutrition policy for the Center for Science in the Public Interest.

But when it comes to eating food, *bigger isn't better.* In fact it often means overeating.

Sure, this so-called value marketing helps food companies turn a profit, but all it does for the consumer is widen his or her waistline.

Americans Go Low Fat and Fat Free but Consume More Carbs

Another movement that has no doubt contributed to obesity is our pursuit of foods that are low in fat, but that end up being high in refined grains and/or sugar. Indeed, as mentioned earlier, beginning in the late 1970s, many Americans, assuming they were making the correct dietary choices, began to follow the U.S.-government-sanctioned recommendation that we eat *less* fat and *more* carbs.

- This meant that health-conscious Americans were possibly eating or trying to eat 6 to 11 servings a day of bread, cereal, rice, and pasta.
- But, rather than eat whole grains, folks usually reached for refined, fiber-stripped, processed carbs or sweets.

> ## EXPERT VIEWPOINT
>
> *"One of the most unfortunate unintended consequences of the fat-free crusade was the idea that if it wasn't fat, it wouldn't make you fat. I even had colleagues who were telling the public that you can't get fat eating carbohydrates. Actually, farmers have known for thousands of years that you can make animals fat by feeding them grains, as long as you don't let them run around too much, and it turns out that applies to humans [too]. We can very easily get fat from eating too many carbohydrates."*
>
> —renowned Harvard researcher Walter C. Willett, M.D.

Urged to curtail fat, many Americans mistakenly assumed that any foods labeled "low fat" were inherently healthier and lower in calories than their full-fat versions. The result? Consumers began buying and eating excess amounts of low-fat cookies, crackers, yogurt, and more.

The problem? When fat is taken out, in most cases, more sugar is added to provide flavor, bulk, and texture to these reduced-fat foods. Not only are many such foods *not* lower in calories, but, on top of that, with the fat removed, it's harder to feel full—so you want to eat *more*.

"Food manufacturers are good at labeling processed foods as '99 percent fat free,'" says Victor Zammit, Ph.D., a professor of experimental diabetes at the Warwick Medical School in Great Britain.

"What they don't say is that they have 15 percent more sugar. Many people may deliberately select low-fat processed foods, thinking that they are making a really healthy choice."

The upshot? Eating a lot of low-fat products often means that you're eating processed foods and more sugar, and that, in turn, can lead to weight gain.

The Trend to Drink Sweet Soda and Fruit Drinks

Now let's discuss another well-entrenched American habit—that of guzzling soda as if it were water. Unlike H_2O, however, soft drinks are so sweet that Michael F. Jacobson, Ph.D., executive director of the nutrition advocacy group the Center for Science in the Public Interest (CSPI), calls soda "liquid candy."

Just check out these numbers:

- In the last 50 years, soft drink consumption among people of all ages has increased a colossal 500 percent, according to the USDA.

- In 1947, companies produced an average of about one hundred 12-ounce cans for every man, woman, and child in this country. By 1997, that number had soared to 575 cans per person, according to the National Soft Drink Association, which has since changed its name to the more innocuous-sounding, non-soda-oriented American Beverage Association (ABA).

- In 2004, Americans drank slightly more than 52 gallons of carbonated soft drinks per person, the ABA reports.

Regular (nondiet) soda is now sweetened primarily with high-fructose corn syrup (HFCS), and a typical 20-ounce bottle of soda contains about 16.87 teaspoons of the popular sweetener. (Some researchers now finger HFCS as a leading cause of the fattening of America. More about this shortly.)

But nutrition gurus aren't fingering soda alone for our burgeoning obesity. Sweet drinks of any kind, including fruit drinks and juices (usually laced with high-fructose corn syrup), also can pave the way for disease, health advocates argue.

In fact, a study of 73,345 people aged two and up, published in *The American Journal of Preventive Medicine*, demonstrated a stupendous boost in sweetened beverages such as soda, fruit mixes, fruit juices, and sports drinks from 1977 to 2001. The average person was downing 135 percent more calories from sweetened beverages, 38 percent fewer from milk, and taking in an extra 278 calories per day.

"Extensive research shows that consuming these soft drinks and fruit drinks increases weight gain in children and adults," says coauthor Dr. Barry Popkin of the University of North Carolina at Chapel Hill.

Actually, people could be drinking *more* than the study found, because people might have underreported their consumption. Reducing the intake of soft drinks and fruit drinks "would seem to be one of the simpler ways to reduce obesity in the United States," Dr. Popkin advises.

Kids, in particular, are guzzling soda like it's water. For instance, soft drink intake increased a behemoth 187 percent for boys and 123 percent for girls from 1964 to 1996. At the same time, fruit drinks with less than 10 percent juice increased 112 percent for boys and 65 percent for girls, according to the *Journal of Nutrition*.

So what is driving this quest for sugary drinks?

Three factors contribute to this alarming upswing in soft drink consumption, Dr. Popkin believes. "Portion sizes have increased, a higher proportion of people are drinking soda, and the number of times a day people are drinking soda has grown," he says. "The changes have gone on across all age groups in the United States."

Artificially Sweetened "Diet" Soft Drinks Take Off, Too

While sugary soft drinks are being snapped up, so are artificially sweetened "diet" sodas, a trend that worries Dr. Sinatra and me.

- In 2004, approximately 180 million Americans over 18 downed low-calorie, artificially sweetened, sugar-free beverages and foods, up from 68 million in 1984, according to the Calorie Control Council.

- About 58 percent of people picked diet soda, and 53 percent chose sugar-free or light noncarbonated soft drinks.

Whether coincidental or not, this trend toward drinking artificially sweetened sodas coincides with the fattening of America. And this phenomenon leads some experts to suggest that "diet drinks" might hinder rather than promote weight loss and control. More about this in chapter 22, which is devoted to frequently asked questions (FAQs).

As High-Fructose Corn Syrup Takes Off, Obesity Soars

In the 1970s and 1980s, most major American food manufacturers began replacing sugar (sucrose, made from sugarcane or beets) with such corn-based sweeteners such as high-fructose corn syrup (HFCS).

High-fructose corn syrup now is found in an astonishing array of processed goods, including soft drinks and fruit juices, as well as condiments, breads, cookies, breakfast cereals, pasta sauces, frozen foods, jams, and jellies.

Food manufacturers made the switch from cane- and beet-based sugar to corn-based HFCS because it's far cheaper to produce than sucrose. Not only that, but high-fructose corn syrup is sweeter, is easier to handle during processing, has a longer shelf life, and keeps baked goods soft while giving them a warm, toasty color.

Interestingly, as the use of high-fructose corn syrup has soared, America's obesity problem has also spiraled out of control. In fact, journalist Greg Critser, author of the intriguing *Fat Land: How Americans Became the Fattest People in the World*, observes that the lower-priced high-fructose corn syrup has allowed food producers to increase portion sizes without sacrificing profits. Ultimately, he notes, overconsumption of HFCS is "skewing the national metabolism toward fat storage."

Now, a growing body of research and articles support that statement. Indeed, one examination of our sweetener consumption patterns, which was published in the *American Journal of Clinical Nutrition*, found that in a mere 20 years (from 1970 to 1990), consumption of high-fructose corn syrup leaped by more than 1,000 percent, "far exceeding the changes in intake of any other food or food group."

This review of medical literature on the subject, headed up by the internationally renowned obesity and diabetes authority George Bray, M.D., Boyd professor at the Pennington Biomedical Research Center of the Louisiana State University System and professor of medicine at LSU Medical Center, concluded that the "increased use of HFCS in the United States mirrors the rapid increase in obesity."

The commentary explains that beverages with HFCS don't raise our blood glucose levels as well as sucrose. But a rise in blood glucose is what stimulates insulin production, which is necessary to turn glucose into energy and to signal satiety. What's more, beverages sweetened with high-fructose corn syrup also "may enhance caloric overconsumption," the paper concludes. And that scenario leads to obesity.

Normally when we're getting calories from one food, we consume fewer calories from all other foods. But it doesn't work that way with any beverage and certainly does not seem to work that way with high-fructose-sweetened beverages, according to Dr. Bray and his coauthors, Dr. Barry Popkin and

Samra Joy Nielsen. These HFCS-containing beverages don't trigger the body's signals of satiety and so they interfere with the body's natural ability to balance its calorie intake. "Sucrose in beverages will do the same, but it is probably not as 'sweet' and thus doesn't drive intake as much," says Dr. Bray.

Another study published in the *Journal of Clinical Endocrinology & Metabolism* also suggests that there is a hormonal mechanism by which consuming a diet high in chemically produced fructose could lead people to increase their caloric intake and gain weight. A team of researchers from the University of California at Davis (UC Davis), the Monell Chemical Senses Center, the University of Pennsylvania, the University of British Columbia, the USDA, and the University of Cincinnati concluded that fructose fails to trigger the usual hormonal responses that turn down appetite and increase metabolic rate and that this could lead people to take in more calories and gain weight.

The researchers—who were led by principal investigator Peter J. Havel, D.V.M., Ph.D., a nutrition and endocrinology researcher at UC Davis—compared how consuming beverages sweetened with either 100% fructose or 100% glucose, along with normal meals, affected hormonal responses over the next 24 hours.

As Dr. Havel explains, "We found that consuming fructose-sweetened beverages with meals resulted in *decreased* secretion of insulin and *reduced* production of leptin. Both of these hormones help regulate food intake and body weight." (Insulin, as you learned earlier, is needed to regulate blood sugar levels by moving glucose out of the blood and into the cells. It also stimulates the production of leptin by the body's fat cells. Over the long term, leptin helps to suppress appetite, regulate food intake, and burn fat.)

In addition, as this study and others indicate, "when fructose is ingested, it goes directly to the liver, where it is more prone than glucose to being metabolized and converted into fat and, therefore, raises triglyceride levels for many hours after consumption," Dr. Havel says.

Still other studies have shown that long-term fructose consumption can raise LDL (bad cholesterol) levels. "All of these results," Dr. Havel contends, "suggest that long-term consumption of diets high in fructose could lead to an increased risk of developing cardiovascular disease."

Meanwhile, additional researchers from the University of Florida speculated that a high-fructose diet could trick the body's metabolism, thereby causing rapid weight gain. The study also suggests that "fructose may have a major role in the epidemic of metabolic syndrome and obesity due to its ability to raise uric acid." High levels of uric acid causes lower levels of nitric oxide, which leads to poor glucose metabolism, which, in turn, increases one's risk of metabolic syndrome.

The study debunks the concept that people become overweight just because they eat too many calories and don't exercise enough. "Our data suggest [that] certain foods and, in particular, fructose may actually speed the process for a person to become obese," said Dr. Richard J. Johnson, lead author of the study, which appeared in *Nature Clinical Practice Nephrology* and the *American Journal of Physiology-Renal Physiology*.

More researchers at the University of Cincinnati, writing in *Obesity Research*, also found that fructose could promote weight gain. In fact, for this study, mice drinking fructose-sweetened water and soft drinks ultimately had 90 percent more body fat than mice consuming just water.

"We were surprised to see that mice actually ate less when exposed to fructose-sweetened beverages, and therefore didn't consume more overall calories. Nevertheless, they gained significantly more body fat within a few weeks," said study author Dr. Matthias Tschop.

Still additional researchers writing in *Pediatrics* reported that they found dramatic evidence that the empty calories in soda and noncarbonated soft drinks promote weight gain in overweight teenagers.

Researchers Speculate That Too Much HFCS Leads to Diabetes

For years, fructose has been considered safe for diabetics because it doesn't trigger a rapid rise in blood sugar. Now, however, research reveals that overconsuming fructose and high-fructose corn syrup could actually be *more harmful* than sucrose for the very reason that it was originally considered safe.

In fact, one review report from scientists from Harvard Medical School, Harvard School of Public Health, CDC, University Hospitals of Cleveland, Brigham and Women's Hospital, and Inter-Medic Medical Group in North Port, Florida, published in the *American Journal of Clinical Nutrition* suggested that corn syrup and refined carbohydrates may actually be at least partly to blame for the huge increase in type 2 diabetes in the United States over the past few decades.

The researchers found that although Americans have been eating approximately the *same amount* of carbohydrates (500 grams per day) from 1909 to 1997, we're now eating *different* types of carbs—fewer fiber-filled whole grains and more refined, processed, fiber-stripped grains and sugars, mostly in the form of high-fructose corn syrup.

"The basic gist of the study is that declining carbohydrate quality as measured by the declining fiber content and the increase in high-fructose corn syrup paralleled the upward trend in type 2 diabetes," explains study leader Lee Gross, M.D., of the Inter-Medic Medical Group in North Port, Florida.

Interestingly, the American Diabetes Association, in a statement in *Diabetes Care* in 2002, reversed its position on fructose. Although the ADA still allows sucrose, it recommended that diabetics avoid fructose except in the small amounts that naturally occur in fruits or vegetables. The ADA's reason? Because of "concern that fructose may adversely affect plasma lipids."

Both Dr. Sinatra and I applaud the ADA's reversal and we believe that the organization was justified in its recommendation, because compelling research illustrates the harms of chemically derived fructose.

The Great Fructose Debate: Doctors Versus Insiders Dish Different Views

As high-fructose corn syrup has been demonized in recent years, some doctors and, of course, the corn industry, have been claiming that the sweetener isn't much different from sucrose and that it's unfair to single it out as a primary cause for obesity and other diseases.

Rather, they argue, both sweeteners are potentially devastating to our health. "There's no evidence to suggest that high-fructose corn syrup is any worse than sucrose," says Dr. Willett. "The real issue is too much sugar."

David Ludwig, M.D., Ph.D., director of the Optimal Weight for Life (OWL) obesity program at Children's Hospital Boston, also argues that high-fructose corn syrup, (most of which is 55 percent fructose and 45 percent glucose) and sucrose (which is 50 percent fructose and 50 percent glucose) are "biologically the same. Sucrose is just as bad as high fructose corn syrup," maintains Dr. Ludwig, an associate professor of pediatrics at Harvard Medical School.

Dr. Michael Jacobson of the Center for Science in the Public Interest believes that the HFCS discussion is confusing people. "It's unfortunate that some consumers have been distracted by false concerns about HFCS and lost sight of the fact that we're consuming far too much sugar in the form of both HFCS and table sugar (sucrose). We should be consuming a lot less of both."

But those familiar with the corn refining process heatedly disagree and claim that arguments such as those cited above are based on inaccurate information. "To argue that corn-derived fructose is metabolized the same as sucrose is medically and scientifically flawed," maintains Russ Bianchi, CEO of Adept Solutions, a global food formulation firm.

"Even the medical, peer-reviewed *Circulation Magazine* did a landmark study back in 1998, which concluded that fructose derived from corn does metabolize differently in the body and immediately triggers the build-up of triglycerides (the primary building block for LDL or 'bad' cholesterol)," notes Bianchi, who has been to many sweetener refinery plants and witnessed the manufacturing process for both sugar (from cane and beet) and high fructose corn syrup (from corn).

One industry insider, who prefers to remain anonymous, angrily contends that the corn industry is capitalizing on the confusion generated by the misleading term "fructose," which causes most consumers to assume wrongly that corn-derived fructose is from fruit.

"Refined man-made fructose is not the same as fructose found in fruit or sucrose," the expert says, rattling off a number of differences between fructose and sucrose. "The body of evidence is irrefutable. One of the biggest differences is in sweetness. HFCS is 1.41 times the sweetness of sugar on an equal weight, meaning that it's 40 percent sweeter than sugar. High-fructose corn syrup is not from fruit, it's a starch; it does not exist in nature (it's chemically refined to an artificial hydrocarbon); and it's therefore not recognized by the body."

In addition, people need to know, the source says, that "sucrose is recognized by the body and converted to blood glucose. Fructose and glucose are not from the same source; they don't have the same molecules; they don't use the same refining process; they don't have the same metabolic effect; they don't have the same physical characteristics under heat or cold; they don't have the same flavor, aroma, PH, or stability; and they don't have the same prices. (Sugar costs about 30 cents a pound, HFCS is about 10 cents a pound.)

"You can find further proof that sucrose and high fructose corn syrup are different in the corn lobby's claim that HFCS doesn't raise blood glucose and has low or no glycemic response on a glycemic index scale, at a rating of 20, yet sugar has a ranking of 100 on the GI. That's an 80-point difference.

"How can the corn industry claim that fructose doesn't raise blood sugar, but sugar from cane or beet does? It's the equivalent of calling an apple an orange. What the corn lobby is doing is trying to confuse rather than convince you because they know that they've been outed," the source continues. "Such spin tactics are typical; the corn industry has borrowed from the disinformation playbook of the tobacco industry, who claimed for over 70 years their products were not harmful."

Insiders believe what all this ultimately boils down to is money. "Nestle, Coke, Pepsi, Cadbury Schweppes, Hershey, Kraft, ConAgra, ADM, Cargill, M&M/Mars, Tyson, Campbell's, etc.—there isn't a mainstream food company that isn't using high-fructose corn syrup," one source points out. "They're making a profit at the health expense of the consumer."

Marketing of Sweets and Quickie-Carb Snacks Influences Our Buying Patterns

Clearly, companies making soda, cookies, crackers, cereals, candies, donuts, and other sugary and quickie-carb foods are caught in an awkward predicament. Naturally, they have a mandate to increase sales, but that goal runs completely counter to the health of our nation's citizens.

"Food companies grow by selling more food, not less," observes renowned nutritionist Marion Nestle, Ph.D., M.P.H., who formerly headed the Department of Nutrition and Food Studies at New York University.

"They aren't sitting around trying to figure out, 'How can we make Americans fatter?' They're trying to do well in a competitive economy," adds Dr. Nestle, author of *What to Eat: An Aisle-by-Aisle Guide to Savvy Food Choices and Good Eating*; *Food Politics*; and *Safe Food*. "If people eat less, it's bad for business," succinctly notes Dr. Nestle, no relation to the food company.

Food and beverage companies find beefing up marketing efforts an effective way to snag new customers, who, they hope, are loyal for life, ensuring continued sales. For example, former Coca-Cola Chairman Douglas Ivester told shareholders, in a now-famous statement in Coca-Cola's 1997 annual report, about his company's goals to make their sugary beverage "the preferred drink for any occasion, whether it's a simple family supper or a formal state dinner."

Furthermore, Ivester outlined plans to "build pervasiveness" for its products, which included putting Cola Classic and its other brands "within reach, wherever you look: at the supermarket, the video store, the soccer field, the gas station—everywhere."

Such ubiquitous, omnipresent marketing tactics helped prompt Yale eating-disorders and obesity expert Dr. Kelly Brownell and consumer advocate Michael F. Jacobson, Ph.D., to put forth a controversial proposal that state governments enact small taxes on nutritionally lacking junk food.

Meanwhile, as author Greg Critser observes in his book, *Fat Land: How Americans Became the Fattest People in the World*, "such promotional campaigns can be highly effective" because of the fact that "the soft drink industry spends upward of $600 million annually to promote its trash (compared with the National Cancer Institute's paltry $1 million budget for promoting fruit and vegetable consumption)."

The Celebrity Connection

Another absolutely appalling, thoroughly disappointing development in recent years is that a plethora of well-known singers, models, sports figures, and actors—who are, of course, idolized by impressionable kids and revered by many awestruck adults—have sold out by signing lucrative deals with major companies just to urge us to consume nutrient-deficient junk foods and beverages that can send us into SUGAR SHOCK!

- Singers Britney Spears and Beyoncé Knowles have plugged Pepsi-Cola. So have baseball players Alex Rodriguez and Vladimir Guerrero.

- Model Cindy Crawford has pushed both Pepsi and Pizza Hut.

- Baseball player Sammy Sosa and singer Christina Aguilera put their backing behind Coca-Cola.

- Basketball star Michael Jordan lent his clout to selling Gatorade.

- Venus and Serena Williams smilingly favored Wrigley's Doublemint chewing gum.

- Actress Christina Applegate allegedly revealed to a reporter, "I did a commercial once where I ate 50 bowls of Frosted Flakes." (Are we supposed to be sympathetic that she was forced to take a sugar overdose?)

Even entire sports teams have backed sugary foods.

- A Snickers-brand candy-bar TV commercial takes place in the Chicago Bears' locker room.

- Coca-Cola is a sponsor of the San Francisco Giants.

- And Frosted Flakes is "the official cereal of the National Hockey League."

With all that star power plugging sugary, fatty foods, how can we expect our children to willingly gravitate toward nutritious fruits, vegetables, nuts, seeds, organic meats, and whole grains?

Dr. Sinatra and I can't help but wonder: Would the nonprofit Produce for Better Health Foundation, which promotes the worthwhile 5-A-Day the Color Way program, be able to fork over enough bucks to nab a big name (such as those above) to back these quality-carb foods?

If anything, why don't some celebrities willingly donate their time to make healthy foods "cool" and "hip" as they do when putting their weight behind valuable diabetes organizations?

We hereby challenge any and all big-name personalities to do just that.

Fighting for the Hearts and Tummies of the Next Generation

What most angers and horrifies us, along with nutrition experts, pediatricians, children's advocacy groups, and parents, is that many corporations go after our nation's young to inculcate brand loyalties for life.

"Kids are major consumers of sugary and fatty junk food so the industry is positioning the goods toward them," observes Dr. Adam Drewnowski, director of the University of Washington's Center for Public Health Nutrition.

Marketing to kids "comes with its very own research enterprise, rationale, budget, and code of ethics," Dr. Marion Nestle explains in *What to Eat.*

As can be expected, Dr. Nestle notes, "marketing enormously influences kids' choices of brands and food categories, particularly of the heavily advertised breakfast cereals, soft drinks, candy, snacks, and fast foods."

In fact, research on how to reach kids with their food messages is "simply breathtaking in its comprehensiveness, level of detail, and undisguised cynicism," she continues.

Psychologist Susan Linn, Ed.D., author of *Consuming Kids*, says that "marketing to kids has escalated exponentially since the 1980s. Corporations are spending about 150 times what they were nearly 25 years ago.

"We regulate marketing to kids less than any industrialized democracy," adds Linn, a Harvard Medical School psychiatry instructor, who, in 2000, cofounded the coalition Campaign for a Commercial-Free Childhood (CCFC), whose long-term goal is to put an end to targeting kids with potentially harmful advertising messages.

"The food industry is clearly under a lot of pressure," she says. "They're acting a lot like the tobacco industry did in the 1990s. There's a possibility that [down the line], we'll have regulation of junk food marketing to kids." (We'll cover the Big Tobacco comparisons soon, in the next chapter.)

"Self-regulation by corporations has clearly failed. Corporations should not be the guardians of public health," adds Linn, associate director of the Media Center at Judge Baker Children's Center in Boston, Massachusetts.

Let's look now at some shocking marketing statistics:

- The food industry spends at least $15 billion a year targeting children, according to the Campaign for a Commercial-Free Childhood (CCFC). The Institute of Medicine, part of the National Academies of Sciences, put that marketing figure at $10 billion a year in 2004. This is up from $7 billion a decade ago, according to CSPI.

- Children are seduced by a nonstop parade of television ads—some 17,000 to 40,000 per year, according to varying estimates. And these figures don't even include pervasive "product placements" of junk food in films and TV shows.

- About 70 percent of TV commercials advertise sugary, fatty, salty foods. Rarely can you find ads enticing our young to eat fruits and vegetables.

- Kids are also targeted on the Internet, on school buses, in classrooms and cafeterias, at the movies, on DVDs, and even via cell phones.

The insistency, consistency, and almost urgency of all this marketing seems unstoppable, as the CCFC points out.

- Just about every major media program for kids has a line of licensed merchandise that sells breakfast cereals, snacks, candy, and fast food.

- Many toys are really junk food ads in disguise. Take, for example, Coca-Cola Barbie and McDonald's Play-Doh.

- To establish what CCFC calls "cradle-to-grave brand loyalty," marketers zero in on tots and toddlers by licensing toys, accessories, and even baby bibs with popular characters.

Sadly, our nation's young are sitting targets for marketers' exploitative means. In fact, a child doesn't even understand the concept of advertising until about age eight, and young kids just can't differentiate between commercials and program content, according to the CCFC. Even older kids sometimes don't know that product placement is at work.

Much to our chagrin, sophisticated marketers "often use older children's desire to fit in with their peers and tendency to rebel against authority figures as selling points for their products," the CCFC observes. "A recent Pepsi ad celebrated teens who had been arrested for downloading music illegally."

Previously, health advocates also were horrified by a dubious marketing tactic by soda companies to reach parents of nutrient-needy babies: they licensed their logos to a large manufacturer of baby bottles. "Infants and toddlers are four times likelier to be fed soda pop out of those bottles than out of regular baby bottles," fumed Dr. Michael Jacobson, CSPI's executive director. (As Linn and Jacobson now note, this much-criticized marketing approach was eventually phased out, we suspect because of pressure from groups such as the CCFC and the CSPI.)

Other Countries Set Higher Priorities on the Well-Being of Their Kids

Despite our alleged civilized democracy, what's happening in the United States seems backward. By contrast, a number of countries around the world protect their children with stringent TV advertising rules and regulations.

- Sweden and Norway ban advertising to kids under 12.

- Ireland prohibits TV commercials for fast food and candy.

- Italy forbids advertising during cartoons, and characters can't show up in ads before and after programs in which they appear.

- Austria, Belgium, Luxembourg, and Norway bar advertising before, during and after children's TV programs.

- Finland and Germany won't allow companies to try to persuade a child to buy a product with a direct offer. It's also a no-no in Finland to run TV ads where sales pitches are delivered by familiar cartoon characters or children.

- In Denmark, figures and puppets appearing in children's programs can't push products in ads.

- In the United Kingdom, children's TV personalities and characters cannot pop up in TV ads before 9 p.m., and merchandise based on kids' programs can't be advertised two hours before or after the program.

- Marketing to children in schools is illegal in Belgium, France, Portugal, Luxembourg, and Vietnam.

But back here in America, that continual ad exposure influences people's food preferences and choices. And marketing to our nation's young is big business.

Marketing to Kids Is Highly Lucrative for Food and Beverage Companies

Despite claims to the contrary, marketing to children pays off handsomely.

- Children aged 4 to 12 themselves made $30 billion in purchases in 2002. That's a phenomenal increase over 1989's spending figure of $6.1 billion.

- Youngsters 12 to 19 spent $170 billion in 2002—or about $101 each week per teen.

- In all, children under 12 influence $500 billion in purchases per year.

So how do these teens spend that discretionary money? Sure enough, sweet foods reigned in popularity. "Half chose candy, more than one-third chose soft drinks and ice cream, and about one-fourth bought fast food," explains nutritionist Dr. Nestle in her book *Food Politics*.

Specifically, reports Nestle, "soft drink companies unapologetically name 8- to 12-year-olds as marketing targets. Advertisers encourage marketing directed to 9-year-olds as a logical consequence of the fact that children—and girls in particular—are maturing earlier."

In fact, corporations have devised ways to win over young people by hooking up with organizations that cater to them. Coca-Cola, for instance, is paying $60 million over 10 years to the Boys & Girls Clubs of America for exclusive marketing rights in more than 2,000 clubs, and the National PTA embraced Coca-Cola as one of its "proud sponsors." Both moves raised the ire of two consumer interest groups, Commercial Alert and the Center for Science in the Public Interest.

All of these marketing tactics enrage children's advocacy groups. In fact, Linn's group, Campaign for a Commercial-Free Childhood (formerly Stop Commercial Exploitation of Children), represents a national coalition of health-care professionals, educators, advocacy groups, and concerned parents. Another big player is Commercial Alert, which seeks to keep commercialism from "exploiting children and subverting the higher values of family, community, environmental integrity, and democracy."

The Battle to Ban Soda and Other Junk Food from Our Schools

The situation that most infuriates health and family groups across the political spectrum is that corporations sell their processed, often sugary snacks or sugary beverages on school grounds.

Consumer advocate and social critic Ralph Nader describes this ploy as "relentless marketing to the youth that bypasses parents."

"Parents used to be the main guardians against excessive sugar intake by their children," Nader said in a phone interview. "Parents would say, 'No, you've had enough candy.' 'No, you're not going to have ice cream.' Now, with direct marketing to children at a very young age, that parental function has been seriously eroded. So these little kids are essentially defenseless," insists Nader, cofounder of Commercial Alert.

"It is wrong to use the public schools to deliver private propaganda to impressionable schoolchildren," adds Gary Ruskin, Commercial Alert's other cofounder and executive director.

"The purpose of school is to teach kids to read, write, add, and think— not buy junk food like soda pop, candies, gum, and fast foods," Ruskin protests, calling both obesity and diabetes "marketing-related diseases."

Dr. Walter Willett of Harvard also aptly argues, "Soda, like smoking, simply has no place in schools."

What it comes down to, bemoans Harvard endocrinologist and researcher David Ludwig, M.D., Ph.D., is that "we as a society have really abdicated responsibility for teaching kids how to eat right and how to have an active lifestyle."

But, since about the year 2000, in large part because of the rapidly growing obesity and diabetes epidemics, a rebellion has been brewing against soft drinks and junk food in schools, so much so that the beverage industry finally buckled under pressure and took some action, albeit suspicious.

In fact, scores of health experts, activists, and groups across the political spectrum, including the aforementioned Commercial Alert, CSPI, and CCFC, as well as the American Family Association, Eagle Forum, U.S. Green Party, and Center for Media Education, have been banding together to convince corporations to stop selling soft drinks and junk food in schools.

Even the American Academy of Pediatrics (AAP), whose members include 57,000 primary care pediatricians and pediatric specialists nationwide, took a stand against soft drinks and urged school districts to consider restricting the sale of them "to safeguard against health problems that result from overconsumption."

Specifically, family groups seek to abolish highly lucrative "pouring rights," contracts whereby soft drink companies fork over millions of dollars to school districts by making payments over a 5-to-10-year period in return for the exclusive rights to sell their soft drinks in vending machines on school premises and at school events.

This financial arrangement is particularly loathsome to health advocates. As he recounts in his book, *The Food Revolution: How Your Diet Can Help Save Your Life and Our World*, author John Robbins found, "In one such deal, a school district in Colorado actually requires teachers to push Coca-

Cola consumption in classrooms whenever sales fall below contractual obligations."

The Drive to Give Channel One the Boot

In addition to kicking soda out of the schools, activists are also seeking to get rid of the controversial Channel One News, the daily commercial news program that beams 12 minutes of programming—including some two minutes or more of commercials—into schools nationwide. At last count, about 40 percent, or some 12,000 middle, junior, and high school classrooms, about 8 million students nationwide, watch Channel One during classroom time.

Incensed health advocates and children's advocacy groups complain that the service, launched in 1989 and now part of the Channel One Network, a PRIMEDIA Inc. company, blatantly serves up captive student audiences to companies plugging soda and sugary foods, as well as movies, video games, and other products.

For instance, 27 percent of commercials in 100 shows aired on Channel One during the five-year period from 1997 to 2002 were for junk food or sweet drinks such as Mountain Dew, Pepsi, Mug Root Beer, Snickers, Twix, Juicy Fruit Gum, Hostess Cupcakes, and Gatorade, tallied up Jim Metrock, president of Obligation, Inc., a Birmingham, Alabama–based children's advocacy media watchdog group.

. . . But the Tide Has Turned as Soft Drinks Are Banned from U.S. Schools

Although a battle still lies ahead of them, junk-food-in-the-school opponents are encouraged by the tremendous swell of support and some recent successes. In fact, one by one, school districts around the country have been banishing soft drinks, if not sugary foods, from their premises, although some, we've been dismayed to discover, still allow sales of sugary sports drinks and fruit drinks, as well as potentially dangerous, artificially sweetened beverages.

But let's look at some of the outstanding wins. California, Maine,

Texas, Arizona, Arkansas, Louisiana, New Jersey, Connecticut, New York, and Tennessee all now have some kind of soda and/or candy restrictions in place in the schools, reports Gary Ruskin of Commercial Alert. Furthermore, he notes, a number of cities across America have taken strong stands, including Seattle, Oakland, Philadelphia, Nashville, Chicago, and Los Angeles.

As various cities and states have been booting out sugary drinks or foods (or at least limiting sales), the beverage industry has been beleaguered, to say the least.

Finally, in August 2005, after much angry, cautionary rhetoric and mounting pressure from health advocates and obesity warriors, the American Beverage Association—the group that used to be much more appropriately called the National Soft Drink Association—announced plans to ban sugary soda from elementary and middle schools and to restrict sales in high schools.

While this new policy was a step in the right direction, it unfortunately had a number of major flaws. Furthermore, some health advocates brand it as "a shameless publicity stunt" on the part of the soda industry.

Then, in May 2006, the nation's three top soft drink companies, faced with threats of a lawsuit from the Center for Science in the Public Interest advocacy group, announced that they would voluntarily stop selling caloric soda and iced teas in school vending machines and cafeterias at public schools nationwide by the 2009–2010 school year.

The much-ballyhooed deal was brokered by the Alliance for a Healthier Generation, a collaboration between former President Clinton's William J. Clinton Foundation and the American Heart Association.

All the major soda companies signed on—Coca-Cola, PepsiCo Inc., and Cadbury Schweppes (which sells Dr Pepper and Snapple), as well as the trade group, the American Beverage Association, which represents, as its website explains, "producers, marketers and distributors of virtually every nonalcoholic refreshment beverage you can name."

Under the deal, some 35 million kids nationwide will be given healthier drink choices. Only water, nonsweetened juice (which still is laden with natural sugar), and low-fat milk will be available to elementary and middle school children during school hours and after-school activities.

Insiders say the agreement came about after six months of behind-the-scenes negotiating and meetings between nutrition advocates and attorneys, including CSPI litigation director Stephen Gardner and tobacco lawsuit veteran Richard A. Daynard, who was representing the Public Health Advocacy Institute.

Michael Jacobson, Ph.D., executive director of the Center for Science in the Public Interest applauded the move and announced intentions to drop its planned soda lawsuit.

Unfortunately, though, the deal was far from perfect. Sugary sports drinks such as Gatorade and Powerade, erroneously called or considered "healthy drinks" by some nutritionally uneducated members of the press, will still be allowed. And potentially dangerous diet drinks also will be for sale. At press time, it was unclear whether or not sugary, calorie-filled fruit drinks would be offered.

Nonetheless, as Daynard declared, "This is the first major victory for the obesity litigation strategy. This would have not happened but for the threat of litigation."

But while noting that the agreement illustrates the power of the growing kick-soda-out-of-the-schools movement, other children's advocates were less enthusiastic.

"It's really a desperate attempt by soda companies to stay in the schools," says Commercial Alert's Ruskin, who found fault with the fact that the deal doesn't address advertising in schools—on Channel One, and on scoreboards and vending machines.

Furthermore, both Ruskin and Michele Simon, founder of the Center for Informed Food Choices, worry that the plan has no enforcement mechanism, no oversight, and no accountability. "Is Bill Clinton going to run around to every school to make sure the policy gets implemented? Industry isn't interested in having government pass laws telling them what to do, so now they're saying that they're taking care of things voluntarily," contends Simon, a public health attorney. "They want to make it seem like we don't need these laws."

When all is said and done, however, the tide has turned against sweets-purveying advertisers. In fact, the marketing services consultancy firm Yankelovich, Inc., found that 61 percent of Americans surveyed in 2004 feel that marketing and advertising are "out of control" and 65 percent back "more limits and regulations on marketing and advertising."

SUGAR SHOCKER! BIG APPLE SNAPS UP SNAPPLE IN DUBIOUS DEAL

New York City banished soda, candy, and other sugary snacks from public schools in September 2003. Instead, the Big Apple signed a $166 million deal with Snapple, a division of Cadbury Schweppes, to be the exclusive beverage vendor for the city's 1,200 public schools, with rights to sell all-new 100% juice blends and bottled water in vending machines. The five-year deal brings $8 million to city school coffers.

Consumer advocates and well-known *New York Times* journalist Marian Burros greeted the move with skepticism, if not outrage, because the new high-fructose-corn-syrup-containing Snapple drinks aren't much different than HFCS-filled, noncaffeinated sodas.

"Problem is, the new drinks have even more calories and sugar, and are marginally better than soda only because Snapple has added vitamins and trace amounts of other nutrients," Burros wrote. Besides, she argued, nutritionists "have long cautioned that children should not drink more than 4 to 12 ounces of juice a day, depending on their age, because it has a lot of sugar and calories without the fiber found in whole fruit and, with the exception of orange and grapefruit juice, not much else."

Indeed, "the bottom line is that the Snapple drinks are basically sugar water. That doesn't make them good for you. That makes them *marginally better than soda*," adds Dr. Jonny Bowden, author of *The 150 Healthiest Foods on Earth*. In short, critics charge, the Snapple deal wasn't so sweet after all.

Americans Are Flat Out "Nutritionally Illiterate"

Other alarming developments are occurring while celebrities are pushing sugary, fatty foods: portion sizes are careening out of control; consumption of high-fructose-laden products is skyrocketing; soft drinks are being removed from schools only to be replaced by unnutritious diet drinks and sugary sports drinks, folks are grabbing meals or snacks on the run; and runaway unethical marketing continues unabated.

Most Americans are flat-out nutritionally naïve. Indeed, "nutritional illiteracy has reached epic proportions," according to the "Food for Life Study," released in spring 2006 by the marketing consultancy Yankelovich, Inc.

Even more appalling, the average American gives herself or himself a failing grade of D (68 out of 100) on a scale of A to F on how he or she eats when at home. The typical U.S. resident is more damning when revealing eating habits while away from home. Most Americans brand themselves with an awful F—48.5 on a scale of 100, found the Food for Life Study, reportedly "the first in-depth analysis of consumers' attitudes and behaviors toward diet, nutrition, and preventive health care."

What's more, another survey from StrategyOne, released around the same time, found that most Americans (63 percent) are simply confused about what constitutes proper nutrition because of all the conflicting information out there.

America's Dietary Habits and Pervasive Enticements Create a Serious Dilemma

Talk about a colliding of interests. As public health advocates, physicians, and nutrition experts warn us, if people don't start scaling back on portion sizes, quit downing sweet soda and sports drinks, and begin changing their sedentary, quickie-carb-eating patterns, our nation's already escalating obesity epidemic and diet-related health problems could intensify.

As we well know, it can be a challenge to make positive dietary changes, especially given that we're continually tempted by a barrage of persuasive ads, aggressive marketing, and even free samples of sugary or much-like-sugar foods.

We concede that sellers of sweet, refined foods are fighting to survive, if not thrive, but let's bear in mind that the rest of us are fighting to stay healthy and trim at the same time. Not an easy problem to resolve.

Dr. David Ludwig of Harvard succinctly sums up our collective dilemma: "What we're up against is this: the forces of private profit are being put above the interests of public health."

7

Is "Big Sugar" the Next "Big Tobacco"?

What a difference a few years can make. Back in August 2000, the satirical publication and website *The Onion* elicited chuckles, chortles—and even some confusion—with its seemingly far-fetched spoof class-action lawsuit against "Big Chocolate." Today, with such eerily similar cases already filed or considered against fast-food giants and companies, that satire has lost its sting, and the piece now seems prophetic.

But in the year 2000, many readers, we suspect, were amused by *The Onion's* fictitious news story about the Hershey Foods Corporation being ordered to pay a monstrous $135 billion in restitution fees to 900,000 obese Americans in five states for "knowingly and willfully marketing rich, fatty candy bars containing chocolate and other ingredients of negligible nutritional value." It was entertaining to many when a fictional Pennsylvania Attorney General pronounced: "Let this verdict send a clear message to Big Chocolate. If you knowingly sell products that cause obesity, you will pay."

Reality and Fiction Collide

Fast-forward seven years and that *Onion* spoof could be a bona fide news story. Indeed, what may have been laughable in 2000 is plausible today. On the one hand, food companies now argue that it's just plain absurd, if not unreasonable, to hold them accountable for consumers who knowingly overeat their foods and then get obese or ill. On the other hand, an increasing number of outraged and offended obesity experts, consumer watchdogs, and public health advocates charge that food manufacturers, with their pervasive, often tactless marketing tactics and advertising ploys, are essentially persuading, if not "making," people buy and possibly eat too much of their sugary, fatty, or nutrition-lacking foods.

Indeed, in this new climate, an increasing number of experts are contending that large food producers may be liable for health problems that their products could be causing in certain members of the public. Although many people may find these arguments to be on shaky legal grounds, they raise strong ethical questions about the role of corporate responsibility. In fact, if the trend continues, both attorneys and lawmakers may decide to take a closer look (if they haven't already) at the part corporations may play in harming the health of our citizens with their nutrient-deprived food products.

Some industry observers insist that when food corporations bombard would-be, unsuspecting customers with sensual, pleasurable images or messages about cereals, fast foods, cookies, candies, chips, ice cream, and other junk foods, they may be to blame because, in a way, they're thwarting people's sense of personal responsibility and choice.

In fact, scientists affiliated with the University of Cambridge in the United Kingdom released a study in the *Journal of Neuroscience* in May 2006, which supports this point of view. They found that photos and TV commercials of tempting foods could, in fact, help explain why some people become overweight or obese and develop eating disorders.

Using the latest magnetic resonance imaging (MRI) technology, researchers from the Medical Research Council Cognition and Brain Sciences Unit in Cambridge showed people pictures of appetizing foods (e.g., chocolate cakes), bland foods (e.g., broccoli), and disgusting foods (e.g., rotten meat), while measuring brain activity in regions of the brain that respond to food cues (such as the amygdala, orbito-frontal, ventral striatal, and midbrain regions). Curiously, the researchers found that some folks are more responsive to tempting food images.

The study's lead author, John D. Beaver, Ph.D., formerly a member of Dr. Andrew Calder's Emotion Group at the Medical Research Council Cognition and Brain Sciences Unit, notes that "previous studies in this area assumed that brain activation patterns are similar in all healthy individuals. But our new findings demonstrate that even in healthy individuals, some peoples' brain reward centers are more sensitive to appetizing food cues.

"The variation in people's brain response to appetizing food cues was closely related to the individual's personality trait that has been previously linked by psychologists to eating disorders and obesity," he continues.

Dr. Beaver and Andy Calder, Ph.D., a senior scientist at the Brain Sciences Unit, pointed out that differences in brain activation to appetizing food cues "help explain why some individuals experience more frequent and intense food cravings and are more likely to be overweight or obese and are more vulnerable to developing certain disorders like binge-eating. This is particularly pertinent to understand the rapidly increasing prevalence of obesity, as people are constantly bombarded with beautiful images of appetizing food items through television advertising, print ads, vending machines, or product packaging in order to promote food intake."

"Clearly, some people are more susceptible to a company's advertising messages," says Dr. Calder, speaking by phone. "What we don't know is how easy or hard it is to control these urges.

"The advertising industry is capitalizing on the fact that this basic human urge is more strongly expressed in some individuals just as the cigarette industry capitalizes on it," he continues.

"Seeing a chocolate cake engages the same reward mechanisms that are involved in other addictions. These brain regions are also activated by cocaine addicts viewing a visual image associated with cocaine, cigarette addicts viewing cigarettes, and so on. Some people are just more susceptible to these cues than others."

But he adds, "Reward sensitivity isn't the full story. It is one of many factors that can dictate or explain obesity."

Physician Ian Campbell, an expert in obesity from Nottingham, England, and medical director of the UK's leading obesity charity, Weight Concern, told the BBC that this research shows that "an involuntary exaggerated neurophysiological response to pictures of desirable food presented through clever advertising makes it incredibly difficult for some affected individuals to resist.

"The message is clear. While individuals must retain a responsibility to do their best to control their intake of [junk] foods, this responsibility must be shared by the food manufacturers and advertisers."

"In practice, what this means," Dr. Campbell explained to me, "is that the food industry must become much more responsible in the way they market high-fat, high-sugar foods. Otherwise much of what clinicians and patients can achieve in the consulting room is rapidly undermined by irresponsible advertising."

Legal Assaults Against "Big Food" Make Headlines

In a society plagued by runaway obesity and associated medical problems, tobacco litigation veterans and public advocates have been gearing up for the past few years to launch legal assaults against major food companies for their role in exacerbating and encouraging America's health nightmare.

Already, several prominent cases against the food industry have been successful. For instance, BanTransFats.com, headed by attorney Stephen Joseph, filed a lawsuit against Kraft to stop the marketing and sales of trans fat–laden Oreo cookies to children. "After the corporate giant agreed to remove the artery-clogging substance, I dismissed the lawsuit," he explains. Next, Joseph targeted McDonald's (in two lawsuits) for defrauding the public about the level of trans fat in its cooking oil. "The cases eventually settled, with McDonald's agreeing to pay $1.5 million to notify its customers that it hadn't switched to a trans fat–reduced oil, as previously promised, and another $7 million to the American Heart Association to fund a trans fat education program," Joseph adds.

Taking legal action against the food industry isn't new. For example, in 1983 the Committee on Children's Television, Inc., various consumer groups, and individuals brought a lawsuit in California against General Foods for deceptively advertising breakfast cereals such as Cocoa Pebbles, Sugar Crisp, Alpha Bits, Fruity Pebbles, and Honeycomb to children. Plaintiffs argued that calling them "cereals" was misleading. Rather, they contended, they're "more accurately described as sugar products, or candies" since they contain 38 to 50 percent sugar. Although the case was later settled, the California Supreme Court ruled that ads implicitly claiming that cereals are healthful or nutritious made potential targets for litigation.

Now, lawyers on both sides are gearing up for many more such cases. "I think collectively food and obesity are going to be the next Big Tobacco," asserts John Banzhaf III, who pioneered lawsuits against the tobacco industry and led the fight to remove cigarette advertising from TV. "But it's going to happen more quickly, with a time compression," adds

Banzhaf, a professor of legal activism at George Washington University Law School.

Tobacco litigation pioneer Richard Daynard also is optimistic that such Big Food lawsuits could succeed. "Back in 1985, it seemed like a fantasy to sue the tobacco companies," recalls Daynard, a Northeastern University law professor. "But look what happened," he adds, referring to the 1998 decision that forced the four largest tobacco companies to pay more than $240 billion to all 50 states over a period of 25 years.

With obesity fast approaching cigarette smoking as the single largest cause of preventable death, high-profile legal strategists believe they have valid grounds for litigation. They're pursuing several angles, including over-aggressive marketing, advertising aimed at children, unfair or deceptive marketing practices, soda companies' exclusive pouring rights contracts, and misleading and inaccurate labeling (such as advertising a product as "low fat" without stating that it's high in sugar and calories).

Then, there's the addiction argument, fueled by the fact that compelling new evidence has been pouring in (as I'll discuss in chapter 9) suggesting that, like Big Tobacco, manufacturers of processed, sweet desserts and fast foods may be making their foods just too darn "palatable"—a word that to most people means "I just can't get enough of it." In fact, new research indicates that some formulations from food companies may interfere with our satiety signals so that, as a result, we eat more than we want or need.

Whether or not the allegations are true, processed-food antagonists charge that some corporations have been adding more sugar and other chemicals to their products in order to tempt consumers to buy and eat more. In fact, insiders say, food companies have been conducting studies of the role played by appetite, hunger, opioids (the brain's own feel-good chemicals), and other factors on the choices we make.

But why go to court over sugary or fast foods?

"Lawsuits create media, which changes public perception, which changes consumer demand," Daynard told me. "For example, heavy marketing of high-sugar sodas to kids in schools is legally questionable. This looks a little like Joe Camel. But unlike the tobacco industry, the food industry can play fair *and* still make money."

John Coale, another tobacco litigation veteran, also believes that lawsuits targeting marketing to children and adolescents are "fertile ground.

SUGAR SHOCKER! SWEET TO SMOKE

If you smoke, do you ever wonder why your cigarettes taste so sweet? Well, sugars are "used extensively by the tobacco industry to ameliorate the effects of inhaling smoke," reveals biochemist, whistleblower, and former tobacco executive Jeffrey Wigand, Ph.D. "Sugars are particularly helpful to reduce harshness or irritation or acridity of smoke," adds the former vice president for research and development for Brown & Williamson Tobacco Corporation, whose *60 Minutes* interview exposing tobacco industry malpractices was the inspiration for the 1999 movie, *The Insider* starring Russell Crowe and Al Pacino.

Indeed, sugar is the largest single additive to cigarettes, coming to about 3 percent of the total weight, according to TARNIVAL (Tobacco Education Through Art & Science) and ASH (Action on Smoking and Health). Sweetened or flavored cigarettes allow smokers to inhale more and more, and more easily absorb the desired nicotine dose. "When burned, sugar produces acetaldehyde, a chemical that interacts with the brain's neurotransmitters," the TARNIVAL website points out. "Once the ability of acetaldehyde to increase nicotine addiction was discovered, the sugar levels in cigarettes rose dramatically as tobacco companies took advantage of the new knowledge to hook younger smokers with good-tasting and highly-addictive cigarettes."

"That acetaldehyde, plus nicotine, make the tobacco even more addictive," says Dr. Wigand, who now heads a nonprofit foundation, Smoke-Free Kids, to reduce teen tobacco use. "It's easy to get children to smoke cigarettes because the taste approaches sweetness. Sugar is one of many components used to make cigarettes more candylike. Unfortunately, the sweet taste helps hook some 3,000 to 5,000 kids a day. Ninety percent of smokers begin before age 20," he claims. "The average onset of cigarette smoking in the United States is 12 to 13 years old, and even younger overseas."

Kids are bombarded with ads for junk foods. There's no restraint from the food companies.

"If you can link misleading advertising to childhood disease, you've got yourself not only a lawsuit, but a movement," continues the founder of

Coale Cooley, a Washington, D.C.–based mass tort law firm. "We're not bringing down the food industry next Tuesday, but there are legitimate legal issues here."

Companies Unveil Antiobesity Programs As Threats of Legal Action Loom Large

Despite the fact that food sellers publicly proclaim such lawsuits "frivolous," they appear to be taking the risk of litigation very seriously. For starters, beginning in 2003, they've been arming themselves with tactics to thwart them. For example, representatives from some of the largest food manufacturers, including Coca-Cola, Frito-Lay, KFC-Yum! Brands, and Krispy Kreme, even attended at least one conference on how to prevent and defend obesity lawsuits.

Even more noticeable is the fact that a number of major food companies and fast-food chains have been unveiling a flurry of antiobesity measures and unrolling more healthful food options. Indeed, lawyers and junk food foes such as Coale, Daynard, Nader, and Dr. Nestle find it particularly intriguing that just as the threats of litigation are occurring, these corporations are taking action. In fact, they wonder if these moves are a way of defending themselves against Big Tobacco–like lawsuits.

Often accompanied by much-heralded announcements, companies publicly shared plans to alter product components, revise marketing practices, sell smaller portions, establish fitness initiatives, and introduce new menu items. For instance:

- Kraft Foods announced that it would abolish in-school marketing to children, change some recipes, and introduce smaller portion sizes.

- McDonald's stopped offering supersized fries and soft drinks, unfurled a multiyear Balanced Lifestyles platform featuring national commercials that encourage consumers to be more active, and introduced McDonald's Go Active! Happy Meal, which includes a salad, a fountain drink or water, a Step with It! Stepometer (pedometer), and an informative booklet by fitness expert/exercise physiologist Bob Greene, who is Oprah Winfrey's personal trainer.

- The Boys & Girls Clubs of America (BGCA), the Coca-Cola Company, and Kraft Foods announced TRIPLE PLAY, a new after-school health and wellness activity offered at the clubs. The $12 million, five-year program is purported to be "the largest health and wellness endeavor ever undertaken by the BGCA clubs and the first youth-focused program of its kind developed in collaboration with the U.S. Department of Health and Human Services."

- Pepsi-Cola announced that its "school-selling policies were examined in light of the obesity issue," bottlers are directed "not to sell carbonated soft drinks to students in elementary schools," and it does not make "up-front payment for school contracts."

Leonard Marquart, Ph.D., R.D., assistant professor of nutrition at the University of Minnesota and a consultant and former senior scientist at General Mills, Inc., offers an insider's view of the dilemma food sellers now face: "The pressure right now is greater than ever to develop products that will sell but be healthier. That's not an easy thing to do," he says. "Companies need strong nutrition departments to lead them through this."

Lawsuits Don't Need to Win to "Succeed"

Anti-junk-food advocates say that the potential for lawsuits and the embarrassment they could generate might be enough to bring about massive changes. In light of these developments, the outcome of litigation might even be superfluous, say some observers such as consumer advocate Ralph Nader.

"These lawsuits highlight the issue, educate the people, spill more information out into the public domain, encourage whistleblowers, produce depositions, and provide a good alert function, *regardless* of whether or not they succeed," Nader proclaimed in a phone interview with me.

Nutritionist Dr. Nestle agrees. "It doesn't matter if lawsuits win, lose, or draw," she says. "They've already had a huge effect in making food companies examine their food products. All big companies are carefully looking at their product mixes and their marketing practices to children."

Moreover, Banzhaf argues, plaintiffs wouldn't even have to prove all of their arguments conclusively in order to win. "If you have enough reputable evidence in major scientific, peer-reviewed journals, that could be enough," he speculates, noting that damaging the reputation of a company—or threatening to harm it—could prompt changes from the food industry.

"If there's one lesson to be learned from the Miles 'light' cigarette lawsuit brought against Philip Morris, it is that the stock markets can severely punish the perception of deceptive marketing practices or misrepresentation," says London-based JP Morgan senior food analyst Arnaud Langlois.

"Even if nothing illegal emerges during the process of trials (assuming they get to that stage), we believe food companies may find it embarrassing to see courts shedding light on some of their marketing practices," Langlois continues.

"Were children the main targets? Were obese people targeted? As far as the equity market is concerned, the risk is that, once litigation starts being taken seriously, the equity 'story' starts to be driven by news flow associated with litigation rather than fundamentals."

Big Tobacco Is Often Behind Big Sugar

Although we're talking about lawsuits against food manufacturers, obesity and eating disorders expert Kelly D. Brownell, Ph.D., points out that the tobacco industry actually controls important parts of the foods industry.

"Nabisco, a massive company once connected with R.J. Reynolds, is now owned by Kraft, as are Planters, Oscar Meyer, and many other companies," Dr. Brownell writes in his book, *Food Fight: The Inside Story of the Food Industry, America's Obesity Crisis, and What We Can Do About It.* "Kraft in turn is the largest food company in the [country], but is itself [almost completely] owned by . . . [Altria Group, Inc., formerly known as tobacco giant] Philip Morris."

Insiders are now struck by the similarities between what once faced Big Tobacco and what now faces Big Sugar. "Saying that all these heavily sweetened drinks or foods cannot harm you is the moral equivalent of the tobacco industry claiming for decades that their products had no causal relationship to heart disease or cancer," laments one knowledgeable source, who desired anonymity for fear of reprisal in the workplace.

It's Not Nice to Fool Consumers:
The Legal Volleys Begin

Not surprisingly, while I was writing this book, experts told me about a dozen legal volleys (i.e. class action lawsuits) already proposed against companies making sugary foods and drinks or fast food.

For instance, some attorneys filed consumer class-action lawsuits against the J.M. Smucker Co. in various states, including Illinois, Arizona, California, Florida, and Wisconsin. The lawsuits alleged that the company's line of "Simply 100% Fruit" products was deceptive, because the products don't contain 100 percent fruit as billed and the main product component is fruit syrup from a variety of fruit sources. The cases—which eventually reached a nationwide class settlement—came soon after or around the time the watchdog consumer group the Center for Science in the Public Interest (CSPI) publicly criticized the Orrville, Ohio–based company for misleading consumers.

"Calling these spreads '100 percent fruit' is 100 percent fraudulent," CSPI's legal affairs director Bruce Silverglade charged in a May 13, 2003 press release. Silverglade contended, for instance, that Smucker's Simply 100% Fruit Strawberry Spreadable Fruit was only 30 percent actual strawberries and that the majority—70 percent—came from fruit syrup derived from apples, pineapples, lemon juice concentrate, pectin, red grape juice concentrate, and other unspecified "natural ingredients."

The J.M. Smucker Co. counters. Calling "a product '100% Fruit' when all the ingredients of the product are, in fact, from fruit, is in no way fraudulent," a company spokesperson wrote in an e-mail to me, noting that the following description was added to labels: "Sweetened with fruit syrup from apple, pear, or pineapple juice concentrate." (The spokesperson also "vigorously" denied claims that the company "violated any law" and asserted that its product "meets all federal labeling requirements. Our ingredient statements have always communicated that a combination of fruit ingredients make up Simply 100% Fruit.") Incidentally, when I visited the company's website right before press time, all 15 flavors of the product had been renamed "Simply Fruit," with the "100%" claim completely removed.

In spring 2005, soon after reading an Associated Press article revealing that new versions of popular kids' breakfast cereals aren't any lower in sugar than the old versions, Jennifer Hardee, a San Diego mother of two, sued Kraft Foods Co., General Mills Cereals, LLC, and Kellogg USA Inc. Hardee's suit—which has since been settled—sought class action status on behalf of all duped California consumers who bought the new cereals. It alleges that the cereal companies' new "low-sugar" claims on cereals were deceptive and deliberately misleading and that they falsely advertise the cereals as nutritionally superior.

And in early 2006, the Center for Science in the Public Interest, the Campaign for a Commercial-Free Childhood, and two Massachusetts parents, Sherri Carlson of Wakefield and Andrew Leong of Brookline, publicly announced plans to file a lawsuit in a Massachusetts court against Viacom, which owns the children's TV giant Nickelodeon, and the Kellogg Company to stop them from marketing sugary, fatty, salty, nutrient-lacking foods to young children.

"Nickelodeon and Kellogg engage in business practices that literally sicken our children," said CSPI executive director Michael F. Jacobson in announcing the proposed lawsuit, which seeks to ban ads aimed at children for Kellogg junk foods on Nickelodeon, and prevent such beloved Nickelodeon characters as Dora the Explorer or SpongeBob from appearing on packaged junk foods.

The threatened lawsuit seeks to address several marketing offenses. For example, of 168 TV food commercials reviewed that appeared on Nickelodeon, 88 percent were for foods of poor nutritional quality; of 27.5 hours of Saturday morning programming, 98 percent of Kellogg's ads touted nutritionally lacking foods, and of 80 Kellogg foods found in the supermarket with kid-friendly on-package marketing, 84 percent were for low-quality foods. Interestingly, the announcement of this planned lawsuit, which was in settlement discussions as this book was going to press, came six weeks after the Institute of Medicine's landmark report, which found that food advertising aimed at kids gets them to prefer—and request—foods high in calories and low in nutrients.

In publicizing the lawsuit, CSPI's press release quoted Sherri Carlson, a mother of three, who lamented Nickelodeon's "enticing junk food ads. Adding insult to injury, we enter the grocery store and see our beloved Nick characters plastered on all those junky snacks and cereals. This irresponsible marketing to young children undermines my efforts as a parent and must be stopped."

Although the CSPI gave "formal notice of intent to sue" Viacom and Kellogg, at press time for this book, the organization still had not filed a lawsuit, because discussions were under way with Kellogg, according to CSPI litigation director Stephen Gardner.

More Legal Action on the Horizon

Observers and legal experts believe legal action is just beginning. "Regardless of the merits, it's likely that lawsuits against the food and beverage industry will continue," says attorney Harold K. Gordon, partner at Jones Day, who wrote an overview article, "Class Action Food Fights," in the *New York Law Journal.*

All in all, are beleaguered food corporations worried about potential lawsuits? "You'd never get them to admit it. Certainly not to our audience," says London-based analyst Jason Streets, formerly with UBS Warburg. "But some corporations have set up internal committees to look at the issue of obesity, or they've been talking with the World Health Organization to learn what they can do about it."

Interestingly, some insiders also believe that legal actions or threats of them could eventually harm sales of sugary products. "Ultimately, companies who sell primarily sugary or fatty products face the biggest challenges and long-term risks," contends Streets. "In my view, it's almost inevitable that sales of high-sugar, high-fat products will decline. It starts now, and it'll be gradual, but over the next 10 years, we'll see a significant reduction."

8

STRANGE BEDFELLOWS:
SUGAR, SEX, AND POLITICS

According to some irate insiders, at least one reason why we've landed in this dismal quagmire of skyrocketing obesity and sugar-related health woes is because companies processing sweeteners and food manufacturers using them have successfully wielded their influence over members of both the U.S. government, which makes nationwide dietary recommendations, and the World Health Organization (WHO), which is empowered to recommend ways to combat obesity and promote good health. Certainly, this is a complicated topic, but here are five different examples (taken over a period of several years), which reveal how the sugar and processed-food industries and the U.S. government (specifically because of lobbying and financial contributions) are influencing decisions that affect the sugar, corn, or processed-food industries—and ultimately could harm our health.

The Sugar Industry's Extraordinary Access to Government

In her provocative book, *Food Politics: How the Food Industry Influences Nutrition and Health*, Dr. Marion Nestle cites the "most stunning example" of access to upper echelons of the U.S. government, which is revealed in "of all unexpected places, the *Starr Report*." This official document, which, of course, recounts former President Clinton's dalliance with White House intern Monica Lewinsky, proves that on the afternoon of President's Day holiday, Monday,

February 19, 1996, President Clinton "told [Ms. Lewinsky] that he no longer felt right about their intimate relationship, and he had to put a stop to it."

The *Starr Report* reveals that as he was ending their liaison, "the President had a [private] call from a sugar grower in Florida whose name, according to Ms. Lewinsky, was something like 'Fanuli.' In Ms. Lewinsky's recollection, the President may have taken or returned the call just as she was leaving." The *Starr Report* then confirms that "the President talked with [prominent sugar grower] Alfonso Fanjul of Palm Beach, Florida, from 12:42 to 1:04 P.M. Reportedly, Mr. Fanjul had called the President on a federal holiday because Vice President Gore had just announced a plan to tax Florida sugar growers," Dr. Nestle writes in *Food Politics*. "The proposed tax would help pay for federal efforts to restore parts of the Everglades that had been polluted by sugarcane runoff. Furthermore, the House was debating whether to phase out sugar subsidies. The *Time* [magazine] reporters [covering the story] noted that the tax was never passed. Their account concluded, 'That's access.' "

"I thought it was astonishing that someone who donates a lot of money to political parties was able to get through to the president personally, on a federal holiday, when he's quite otherwise occupied," Dr. Nestle revealed to me in a phone interview.

"You and I could not do that. Lobbying . . . is done secretly, behind closed doors," she added, noting that financial contributions not only provide access, but also result in policies favorable to donors.

Dr. Nestle also investigated the connection between contributions from political action committees (PACs) and congressional votes on sugar subsidies. Not surprisingly, she found that the largest contributions from sugar PACs went to congressional members who voted for the subsidies. She also uncovered that the larger the PAC contribution, the more likely our elected officials were to support sugar industry positions. In addition, Dr. Nestle reports, "Month-by-month analyses of the history of legislation on sugar and peanut subsidies demonstrate an increase in contributions to both parties just prior to votes."

The Sugar Industry Fights WHO's Report

Our second example has to do with the World Health Organization (WHO) and the Food and Agriculture Organization (FAO) of the United Nations, which, in spring 2003, jointly issued a draft of the "Report of the Joint WHO/FAO Expert Consultation on Diet, Nutrition and the Prevention of Chronic Diseases." The draft suggested dietary changes, including limiting the consumption of "free" sugars to less than 10 percent of caloric intake. ("Free" signifies sugars that are added to foods you don't think of as sweet, such as mayonnaise, some mustards, ketchup, processed meats, peanut butter, and many snack foods.)

The recommendation set off a storm of protest. Rather than applauding the report, the U.S. Department of Health and Human Services issued a scathing 28-page critique concluding that the WHO document was scientifically flawed. Then the Washington, D.C.–based Sugar Association, which represents sugar growers, vowed to use "every avenue available to expose the dubious nature" of the recommendations, even asking members of Congress to challenge the United States' $177 million in contributions given annually to the WHO.

Consumer and nutrition groups were outraged. The Center for Science in the Public Interest blasted the Sugar Association, calling its tactics "thuggish" and describing its threats as blackmail rather than lobbying.

The distinguished Dr. Marion Nestle and Dr. Kelly D. Brownell, director of the Yale Center for Eating and Weight Disorders, wrote a scathing *New York Times* editorial decrying the U.S. government's reaction. They called it "blatant pandering to American food companies that produce much of the world's high-calorie, high-profit sodas and snacks, especially the makers of sugars, the main ingredients in many of these products.

"When food industry executives or government officials complain about the lack of sound science, self-interest is generally at work," Drs. Nestle and Brownell pointed out in their editorial. "Internationally known scientists drafted the WHO report. The report comes to obvious conclusions. Threatened by such conclusions, food companies and their friends in government try to pick apart the science, ridicule the process, and delay action, just as the cigarette industry did for so many years."

Drs. Nestle and Brownell's letter continued: "Senators Larry Craig and John Breaux, co-chairmen of the Senate Sweetener Caucus, asked Health and Human Services Secretary Tommy Thompson to call on the WHO to 'cease further promotion' of the report, while trade associations for the sugar, corn refining, and snack food industries questioned the report's legitimacy and asked for Mr. Thompson's personal intervention. They got it.

"By making its position on the WHO indistinguishable from that of the food industry, the Bush administration undermines the efforts of more forward-thinking food companies and threatens public health," Dr. Nestle and Dr. Brownell wrote. "Its action underscores the need for government to create a wall between itself and the food industry when establishing nutrition and public health policy. Recommendations to cut back on sugars may not please food companies, but it's time to stop trading calories for dollars."

The final WHO plan that was launched on April 23, 2003, and approved on May 22, 2004, was considerably weaker than its earlier draft. Critics contend that heavy lobbying by the sugar and food industries caused some key policy recommendations to be left out: You will *not* find suggestions 1) to limit free sugars to 10 percent or less of your caloric intake, 2) to restrict or ban junk food advertising to children, 3) to reduce consumption of soft drinks, or 4) to support policies that promote production and marketing of fruits, vegetables, and legumes.

Nutrition advocates concede that the WHO's global strategy does present some positive suggestions, including calling for food and beverage ads to "not exploit children's inexperience or credulity," discouraging "messages that encourage unhealthy dietary practices," and limiting "the availability of products high in salt, sugar, and fats in schools." But let's face it, this global strategy would have been much more powerful, effective, and appropriate if it had included the four points outlined above.

The Sugar Industry's Efforts to Influence WHO's Work to Combat Obesity

We can shed more light on sugar politics, thanks to the British publication *The Observer*, which uncovered an internal 2004 document written by the British head of the sugar-industry-funded World Sugar Research Organization. The memo outlines a strategy for getting the sugar group into World Health Organization (WHO) meetings by providing substantial funding to gain nongovernment organization (NGO) status.

The document also shows that the sugar organization "analyzed whether the key WHO officials are hostile to its interests," and it highlights the sugar group's "desire to win over policymakers who will have a big influence on countries that are trying to improve their national diet," *The Observer*'s health editor, Jo Revill, reported.

Not surprisingly, the internal document dismayed both WHO officials and health-minded advocates, who believe, as *The Observer* put it, that the sugar industry "is trying to subvert attempts to introduce policies aimed at reducing sugar levels."

When shown the document, Professor Philip James, chair of the London-based International Obesity Taskforce, reportedly told *The Observer*, "This is a ruthless and vicious strategy to undermine the work being done around the world to enable people to have healthier diets. Does the sugar industry really believe it can bribe the WHO? Has it come to this?"

Politics and Industry Interests Play a Role in New Dietary Guidelines, Critics Charge

Our fourth politically charged example has to do with the latest *Dietary Guidelines for Americans*, jointly released on January 12, 2005, by the U.S. Department of Health and Human Services (HHS) and the U.S. Department of Agriculture (USDA). Published every five years since 1980, the guidelines are intended to "provide authoritative advice for people two years and older about how good dietary habits can promote health and reduce risk for major chronic diseases." But in this instance, good intentions collided with industry interests, according to nutrition insiders, who say that intense lobbying by food industry and advocacy groups—rather than solid science—had much to do with the creation of our nation's new dietary recommendations.

Although health advocates applaud some of the advice, such as eating more fruits, vegetables, and whole grains, and exercising more (up to an hour and a half per day), they find other tips nebulously presented and downright disappointing. For example, the USDA and HHS make vague, unspecific suggestions like "choose foods and beverages with little added sugars or caloric sweeteners" or "limit the intake of saturated and *trans* fats, cholesterol, added sugars, salt, and alcohol."

Rather, critics argue, the USDA and HHS guidelines should be more specific about which foods and beverages we should choose and how much we should limit other foods and drinks. Health advocates also charge that the new government-sanctioned guidelines have some glaring omissions and flaws, especially when it comes to sugary foods, sweet beverages, and refined grains.

"They really did not address soft drinks and fruit drinks in a serious manner, for instance," says nutritionist Dr. Barry Popkin.

"The recommendations kowtow to the sugar industry by not taking a stronger stance on sugar," adds Lee Gross, M.D. "They don't provide a recommended daily cap on sugar consumption," adds the director of diabetes and nutrition education for Fawcett Memorial Hospital in Port Charlotte, Florida.

Critics also claim that the new dietary recommendations don't go far enough when it comes to whole grains.

"The new guidelines still imply that eating half of your grain products in a refined form is okay, when this is not optimal," says Dr. Walter Willett. "The word 'enriched' should really be called 'depleted,' and these refined starches should really be in the use-sparingly category. Thus the cup is half full," Dr. Willett adds, noting that lobbying groups clearly had an influence in "deciding who is on the committee and the spin on the guidelines."

Likewise, nutrition specialist David Katz, M.D., of Yale finds the guidelines "deficient because they don't tell you what you shouldn't eat. They don't say, 'Don't eat sugary breakfast cereals like Froot Loops, Cap'n Crunch, or Cocoa Puffs, or don't eat refined carbs or fatty foods like Pop-Tarts, Doritos, French fries, greasy hamburgers, sausages, bacon, and processed deli meats— foods that deliver sugar, salt, or trans fats.'

"The dietary guidelines are not a work of pure science but a compromise between science and politics," Dr. Katz maintains. "They're partly for consumers and partly for the food industry. Those compromises favor the food industry when it comes to guidance about what *not* to eat."

According to insiders, those who wield behind-the-scenes power to influence the outcome of the U.S. dietary guidelines and other governmental policies include food companies and biased food-industry groups, often with innocuous, unbiased-sounding names such as the Sugar Association, Corn Refiners Association, International Food Information Council, Calorie Control Council, American Cocoa Research Institute, and the benevolently named American Council for Fitness and Nutrition.

The head of this last organization, whose members include the Coca Cola Company, PepsiCo, Kraft Foods, Cadbury Schweppes, the Snack Food Association, the American Beverage Association (formerly the National Soft

Drink Association), and the Sugar Association, reportedly once stated that soda-and-candy-filled vending machines in schools don't play a role in the obesity crisis. "You can take every vending machine out of schools, and I don't believe you'd touch the obesity issue in children," Dr. Susan Finn, chairwoman of the American Council for Fitness and Nutrition, said, according to a Knight-Ridder Newspapers account.

Another influential, outspoken lobbying group is the Center for Consumer Freedom, which Dr. Kelly Brownell describes in *Food Fight*. "Dressed up to appear to defend consumers and basic freedoms, the Center for Consumer Freedom opposes actions that would hurt food or tobacco companies," Dr. Brownell writes, noting that the organization was started with tobacco money and is now a coalition of restaurant and tavern owners that "attacks people who argue for policy changes to improve nutrition."

Ultimately, some observers suspect that consumers will pay scant attention to the government's dietary advice in any case. "I don't think many people read them or understand them, because the government puts very little muscle into marketing them," obesity and eating disorders expert Dr. Brownell told the *New York Times*. "If you ask 10 people on the street do they know about this or previous guidelines, no one will know anything," Dr. Brownell remarks, "but if you ask them what candy melts in your mouth not in your hand, 9 out of 10 will know."

U.S. Farm Policy Helps Trigger Obesity

As I was just completing my final editing for *SUGAR SHOCK!*, one final, politically explosive document emerged, which flat-out blames the U.S. government's preferential farm policies for significantly contributing to the obesity epidemic. The damning, much-needed 14-page report, "Food without Thought: How U.S. Farm Policy Contributes to Obesity," issued by the nonprofit, nonpartisan Minneapolis-based Institute for Agriculture and Trade Policy (IATP), astutely explains that Americans have been gaining weight, in large part, because for the past 50 years, U.S. food policy has been driving down the prices of a few farm commodities, particularly corn and soybeans, so that they're "artificially cheap." At the same time, the IATP pointed out, prices for higher quality fruits and vegetables, grown with little government support, have steadily increased.

As the paper explains, these low prices have prompted a surge in production and sales of food substances that are really cheap to produce. For instance, inexpensively priced high-fructose corn syrup (HFCS) has skyrocketed in popularity in recent years. (As I pointed out in chapter 6, HFCS has skyrocketed in popularity and has been added to more and more food products in recent years, and researchers are now increasingly citing it as a potential contributor to obesity, in part, because it appears to be processed differently in our bodies and can lead to fat storage.)

Meanwhile, lower-priced soybeans have been used to make unhealthy trans fats, which are often found in nutrient-deficient, processed baked goods and other food products. (In theory, trans fats are being used less lately because of both bad press about their dangers and new label regulations that took effect in January 2006.)

The report concludes: "Whether by intention or not, current farm policy has directed food industry investment into producing low-cost, processed foods high in added fats and sugars. These foods are often more available and more affordable than fresher, healthier choices and, not coincidentally, U.S. consumers are now eating many more added sweeteners and oils than is healthy. Our misguided farm policy is making poor eating habits an economically sensible choice in the short term."

Mark Muller, coauthor of the report and director of the Environment and Agriculture Program for IATP, which works "to keep farmers on the land to ensure a safe and healthy food system," said in an interview that the investigation was conducted because people weren't getting the complete story as to why Americans are becoming obese and ill.

"Food marketing is only part of what's happening. Our study connects the dots and take things a step further. We point out that the low price of corn and soy is what's hurting our health," Muller explains.

"What's driving these corporations to advertise junk foods is that they can make the most profits off of them," Muller continues. "The sugars and bad fats are the cheapest foods out there. And farmers are growing corn and soy because that's what the food companies want."

In other words, "The food industry and consumers are following the distorted market signals driven by our farm policy."

The IATP paper makes a number of health-promoting recommendations to make U.S. food policy more equitable, including ensuring fair prices for all crops; encouraging school and government procurement policies that favor healthy foods; developing market incentives for increasing healthy food consumption; offering farmers financial incentives for raising or growing more healthy foods such as organic produce and grass-fed dairy and livestock; and emphasizing the connections between public health, food, and farm policy.

Let's hope that this important document is spread all around Capitol Hill and that it helps generate a change in our U.S. food policies.

Can Food Industry Interests Be Served and Good Health Programs Result?

Sadly, as the above examples illustrate, the bottom line and political power are often at odds with the health and welfare of our nation's citizens. Given the realities of doing business in America—the processed-food industry needs to make money to survive—it's simply unrealistic to expect the interests of we, the people, to come first.

While Big Sugar and Big Food are taking some positive steps to confront the epidemics of obesity, diabetes, and other diet-related illnesses, Dr. Sinatra and I strongly urge and encourage you to educate yourself so that you won't have to take them at their word when they say that their sugary, processed-food products are okay to consume.

PART 4

HOW SUGARY FOODS COULD MESS WITH YOUR MIND AND EMOTIONS

9

PROOF POURS IN: NEW STUDIES SHOW THAT YOU CAN BECOME DEPENDENT ON SWEETS

Who would have dreamed having a sugar habit could be so hilarious? You see, once upon a time, in the make-believe world of animated television, in a brilliant, funny episode of *The Simpsons*, the beloved character Marge decides to shun the sweet substance after her hometown of Springfield earns the dubious distinction of the "World's Fattest Town."

In this smartly sarcastic "Sweets and Sour Marge" episode, the crusading Marge takes on the "Motherloving Sugar Corporation" for "ruining the whole town's health" by making "harmful foods." She then goes door to door to recruit neighbors for her class action lawsuit against "Big Sugar."

For instance, Marge brings on spaced-out Disco Stu, who admits, "I've been hooked on the white stuff since the seventies." Then, in an uproarious, laugh-out-loud TV moment, Stu greedily inhales sucrose through a rolled dollar bill as if it were a line of cocaine.

The spoof continues as "whistle blowers" are trotted out in court. "Well, we knew perfectly well it was addictive," testifies a professor working on a top-secret "Hoiven Maven" project. "Candy was just a sugar delivery system. We thought we were God."

At first, all rejoice when Marge wins her case, but when the judge bans all forms of sugar from Springfield forever, pandemonium sets in.

"Sugar, need sugar," plaintively cry the jittery, frantic townspeople.

Marge's desperate-for-sweets hubby, Homer, even plots with other sugar-clamoring men and becomes a sugar bootlegger, smuggling in the substance "from the island of San Glucose." (Pretty clever, eh?)

When the sweet shipment arrives, Marge warns her spouse, "Homer, you'll be condemning this town to a life of obesity and diabetes." Reluctantly, he then jettisons the sugar into the harbor.

Ultimately, frenzied residents jump in to guzzle the sweet, fish-filled water, and Marge finally sadly realizes, "Everyone looks so happy. Maybe I should stop trying to change the world."

The episode concludes as the judge rescinds his ban, and sugar-craving townspeople, including Homer and his kids, leap into the harbor to slurp the sweet brine.

Sure, this TV scenario may seem like nothing more than a clever cartoon. But, let's face it: Millions of people—like *The Simpsons* characters—get downright desperate for their next sugar "fix" when they're in the grips of sugar cravings.

There, at the neighborhood supermarket, you may witness a child throwing a temper tantrum if he or she doesn't get a candy bar. Or, you may have a teenage boy who impatiently waits for school to get out so he can scurry over to 7-Eleven for a large sugary drink. Our editor on this book even watched her young relative lick sugar off a bowl after polishing off the sprinkled strawberries.

And sure enough, when they do decide to try to break free of sugar's addictive qualities, many folks feel much like Marge Simpson—frustrated, hopeless, and even angry at "Big Sugar" for incessantly beckoning them with formidable temptations, which lurk everywhere.

"We're getting our first Krispy Kreme doughnut shop here soon," Marie T., 43, of Calgary, Alberta, wailed to members of my free, online KickSugar group in early 2003. "I don't know where they're building it, but I just hope it isn't close to me. I just wish people would take sugar addiction seriously," Marie bemoaned. "Too many people laugh it off, but they wouldn't laugh if you told them you were a drug addict or an alcoholic."

Therefore, it's impossible to dismiss *The Simpsons* episode as fanciful fiction. Rather, it cleverly illustrates our world's overpowering, almost universal reliance on sweets. Few of us are immune to their allure.

In fact, a slimmed-down Tom Arnold admitted to Ellen DeGeneres on

TV that cutting sugar out of his life was harder for him than kicking the drug "crack."

"[Quitting crack] was a walk in the park compared to getting off sugar. Because sugar is everywhere," Arnold complained. "[But] crack you gotta go looking for."

Arnold's story may sound like an exaggeration, but it echoes the feelings of sugar junkies everywhere. Just mention sweets and you'll unleash a torrent of tormented tales.

"I totally feel like an addict," laments Lisette L., 27, of Newport Beach, California. "My drug of choice is sugar. After I have sugar, especially chocolate, I get an intense rush and a delicious high. I get happy, relaxed, and euphoric for about an hour.

"But, then suddenly everything comes to a screeching halt, and I crash like a cocaine user coming down. I love sugar—but I hate it at the same time, because it makes me feel weak and out of control."

And Jodi D., 36, of Park Hills, Kentucky, confesses a common sentiment of ex "abusers": "I don't eat sugar, but I am addicted to it. Just like an alcoholic is one drink away from drinking again, I am just one dessert away from my sugar days again."

But not everyone is as aware as Lisette and Jodi of his or her excessive, unhealthy attachment to sweets. All around us, I contend, millions are unknowingly hooked and trapped in a SUGAR SHOCK! cycle that has them spinning like hamsters on an exercise wheel from which escape is an enormous challenge.

How Many of Us Are Unwittingly, Unknowingly Hooked?

It's impossible to know how many people worldwide compulsively grab for refined sweets and quickie carbs, but some medical experts cite extremely high figures.

"I bet you at least 70 percent of Americans are addicted to processed carbs and sugar," speculates Fred Pescatore, M.D., former medical director for the Atkins Center for Complementary Medicine in New York City and author of *The Hamptons Diet*.

Nutrition-minded physician Joseph Mercola, D.O., author of *Sweet Deception* and creator of the number-one natural health website www.mercola.com, suspects that "as many as 80 percent of people are addicted to refined sugar and grains."

And preventive medicine specialist Michael Lam, M.D., M.P.H., A.B.A.A.M., medical education director for the Academy of Anti-Aging Research, guesses that as many as 90 percent of us are addicted. "Not to be hooked on sugar and refined carbohydrates is abnormal nowadays. You really have to try not to do it," says Dr. Lam.

Experts Troubled by Long-Term Ramifications of Sugar Addiction

More and more, medical experts are alarmed by our excessive consumption of sweets and refined carbs, a habit that, they believe, could send many to an early death.

"Sugar addiction and carbohydrate addiction are epidemics of modern-day humans in America and other countries," worries drug addiction and obesity expert Forrest Tennant, M.D., Ph.D., founder of five weight-loss/carbohydrate-dependency clinics in Northern California, who, in 1991, lost weight and restored himself to health by discovering and kicking his own carb and sugar addiction.

"For years, I've tried to convince fellow members of the American Society of Addiction Medicine that sugar and carbohydrates can be addictive. Obesity treatment is failing because practitioners ignore people's carbohydrate-dependence problems."

Neuroscientist Candace B. Pert, Ph.D., former physiology and biophysics professor at Georgetown University Medical Center in Washington, D.C., and author of the groundbreaking book *Molecules of Emotion*, voices a similar concern.

"In my lectures, I often used to show a slide of sugarcane. I ask my students, 'What's the difference between it and cocaine or heroin?' Relying on refined sugar as a pick-me-up can be as addictive and, in terms of long-term health effects, can be quite dangerous," says Dr. Pert, who, as a graduate student in the early 1970s, achieved acclaim for discovering the opiate receptor, a cellular binding site that is tied to addictive behavior.

> ## SUGAR SHOCKER! UNDER LOCK AND KEY
>
> It's hard to believe, but, as William Dufty recounts in *Sugar Blues*, refined white sugar was locked up back in the 16th and 17th centuries in Europe and America. At the time, the substance was so expensive (the equivalent of about $30 a pound or a year's salary for the average working man) that it was considered a delicacy reserved for the very wealthy, and the nobility certainly didn't want their servants stealing such an exorbitantly expensive substance. To this day, Unani healers or hakims in Afghanistan reportedly keep sugar under lock and key, believing it to be a narcotic.

Scientists Have Known This for Years

For more than 50 years, scientists have been exploring the relationships between hunger, satiety, food intake, appetite, and endogenous opioids (the body's own feel-good chemicals), or, in other words, how highly palatable foods can trigger reactions in our brain that cause us to overeat. In 1955, Jaques Le Magnen, a French scientist, published several groundbreaking studies on the subject. In 1979, two British researchers, James McCloy and R. F. McCloy, postulated that food in the gut stimulates the release of feel-good endogenous opioids upon which we become dependent, thereby causing us to overeat. And by the 1990s, researchers were uncovering more and more convincing evidence of a link between food palatability, opioid release, and overeating.

"There's now good evidence that these high-palatability foods trigger biochemical cravings for more," says British scientist Robert Matthews, a visiting reader in science (the U.S. equivalent of an associate professor) at Aston University in Birmingham, England, and former science correspondent for the *Sunday Telegraph*.

"They officially deny it, but food-industry researchers told me they now fear that they've created foods that undermine the body's natural abilities to control food intake, and this helped propel the global obesity epidemic," adds Matthews.

Neal Barnard, M.D., author of *Breaking the Food Seduction*, charges that "food companies selling sugary products are as manipulative as tobacco companies. They're trying to make the foods as seductive as possible. A chocolate manufacturer spends hours and hours and hours and millions of dollars trying to figure out the most seductive combination of fat and sugar that triggers chocolate addiction and makes it impossible to break it. Or a soda manufacturer has pushed up serving sizes and made sure that addictive ingredients such as sugar and caffeine are left in the mix.

"They're in business for one reason only—to make money. These are addictive products. That's all there is to it," argues Dr. Barnard, founder and president of the Physicians Committee for Responsible Medicine, a nonprofit organization that promotes preventive medicine and conducts clinical research.

"So many people imagine that if a food calls out to them much more than someone else that it's because they had a bad childhood or that they have weak willpower or an oral personality. To that I say, 'Nonsense,'" Dr. Barnard insists. "Certain foods simply have physical properties that cause them to be addictive, more so than other foods. The problem is physical, and the answer to it is physical."

For millions, Dr. Barnard's comments ring true. But remember that since we're all biochemically different, sugary foods won't hold the same kind of overwhelming allure for everyone. Of course, it's up to you to figure out just how attached you are to sweets.

Interestingly, many cutting-edge appetite researchers belong to an international organization called the Society for the Study of Ingestive Behavior, which is committed to advancing scientific research on food and fluid intake. Upon visiting the group's website, however, you learn that the organization's sponsors include companies that make sugary and much-like-sugar foods, including Nestlé SA, Proctor & Gamble, Unilever, and MasterFoods. "One can't help but wonder about the links between academics and the sources of funding," worries scientist Matthews.

We Can't Say We Haven't Been Warned

A handful of vocal medical experts have been trying to get the word out for years. Back in 1975, William Dufty, in his compelling bestseller *Sugar Blues*, acknowledged his "kinship" to junkies and convincingly maintained that the

CONFESSIONS OF A HAPPY SUGAR KICKER

"Sugar is a trigger for me. When I have some, I just can't stop. But, when I stay away from sugar and other refined carbs, I don't have those kinds of food binges." —Myra P., 45, Monroe, New York

"difference between sugar addiction and narcotic addiction is largely one of degree.

"After all, heroin is nothing but a chemical," he wrote. "They take the juice of the poppy and they refine it into opium and then they refine it to morphine and finally to heroin. Sugar is [also] nothing but a chemical. They take the juice of the cane or the beet and they refine it to molasses and then they refine it to brown sugar and finally to strange white crystals."

As I noted earlier, for years, the popular but maligned diet guru Robert C. Atkins, M.D., also cautioned against repeatedly overconsuming sweets and refined carbs, because doing so sets you up for an "addictive situation."

"It isn't simply that a jelly donut tastes good to you and you'd like to have it," he explained in *Dr. Atkins' New Diet Revolution*. "No, your body absolutely roars with anxiety and passion for that jelly donut. And then you know. You've activated an addiction, just like an alcoholic with his bottle.

"This isn't shameful, it's physical, it's chemical, it's metabolic, and that's precisely why you must avoid it," he wrote. "Most of you already know that for a significant portion of your life carbohydrates have been stronger than you. Don't trifle with them."

In 1993, Rachael F. Heller, M.A., M.Ph., Ph.D., and Richard F. Heller, M.S., Ph.D., also raised the public's awareness about the addictive qualities of inferior carbs with the release of their book *The Carbohydrate Addict's Diet*, which is dedicated to "the untold numbers of carbohydrate addicts who, deep down, have always known that it was not their fault." And in 1998, with the publication of *Potatoes, Not Prozac*, Kathleen DesMaisons, Ph.D., also garnered a following for her sugar-is-addictive conclusions.

Research Provides Proof That Sugar Dependency Is Real

Although the research is still in its embryonic stages, a group of revered, veteran scientists at universities and institutions throughout the United States, Canada, and Europe are reporting on laboratory-controlled animal behavior that sheds new light on the overpowering attraction exerted by dessert or "highly palatable" sweet foods.

Internationally renowned neuroscientist Bartley G. Hoebel, Ph.D., a Princeton University professor, is at the forefront of this research. He has spent four decades examining how the brain controls appetite and addictive behavior. Since 1996, he has spearheaded a series of studies on the effects of sugar, and his astounding results are capturing attention throughout the world.

Initially, Dr. Hoebel's intention was to study the effects of various appetite-suppressant drugs on sugar intake. For a few hours every day, rats were given a 10 percent sugar-and-water solution. The idea was to let their sugar intake plateau and then observe changes induced by the drugs. But the study took an unexpected turn when, after only a few days, the very *idea* of sugar triggered Pavlovian responses in the rats.

"It got to the point where I'd walk into the room, and they'd get really excited and worked up, because they knew the sugar was coming," recalls a chuckling Carlo Colantuoni, who worked with Dr. Hoebel while a senior at Princeton University and was the first author on two of his studies.

"The rats would run to the front of the cage and try to get the sugar. Sometimes, when I stuck the nozzle of the sugar-water bottle in front of the cage, they got so excited that they'd rip the stopper right off the bottle, and sugar water would go everywhere."

The researchers noticed other strange behavior as well. "When the rats got chow and sugar water at the same time, they would turn away from the food and spend more time slurping on the sugar water. They were drinking as much as the rats that got 24-hour access to the sucrose solution," Colantuoni remembers.

Because of the rats' excessive interest in the sugar water, Dr. Hoebel's research group switched gears and began to look into what, if any, neurochemical changes it triggered in their subjects and whether they experienced symptoms of withdrawal when it was withheld. They then created a feeding schedule that many humans follow, albeit inadvertently. They didn't eat for 12 hours and then missed breakfast. For the next 12 hours, they received food and either a 10 percent or a 25 percent sugar solution. Ultimately the rodents binged on sugar when it became available and ate less food.

"This is very similar to what many women and some men put themselves through," Colantuoni adds. "They starve in the morning, miss many meals in a row, and end up doing crazy bingeing."

The researchers then gave the rats the opiate blocker naloxone. When humans or rats addicted to morphine or heroin receive naloxone, they instantly go into withdrawal.

Curiously, within a half hour of being administered naloxone, the rats' "teeth started chattering," Dr. Hoebel recalls. "They waved their heads back and forth. Their forepaws quivered. They acted anxious in a maze test.

"These are all signs of sugar withdrawal," he explains. "They weren't as pronounced as what we see with morphine, but it was withdrawal.

"This suggests that sugar triggered production of the brain's natural opioids or morphinelike compounds. But they didn't have opiates [drugs]; they just had sugar. The rats were getting addicted to their own opioids like they would to morphine or heroin. Drugs give a bigger effect, but it's essentially the same process."

What Princeton's Sugar-Dependent Rats Teach Us about Overeating and Bulimia

So what can we learn from these sugar-guzzling rats?

"Our results imply that some people can get overly dependent on sweet foods, especially if they periodically stop eating and then binge," Dr. Hoebel explains. "It's probably like alcohol. Most people in the world who drink alcohol aren't addicted. But some do become dependent and then have trouble controlling their intake."

Dr. Hoebel suspects that his team's sugar-dependency studies could help explain bulimia—eating and then purging by vomiting or taking laxatives to prevent weight gain. Recent research has shown that bulimic women often binge on sugary, rich foods like donuts, cookies, candies, pies, chocolates, and soft drinks, but when they choose nondessert foods like salads and vegetables,

CONFESSIONS OF A HAPPY SUGAR KICKER

"At work meetings, someone would bring donuts, and, of course, I'd have one. Then, heaven help me if there were any left over. I became fixated on them until they were gone. If there was one left at the end of the meeting, I'd pick it up on my way out. It was this way with all sweets, every day. The first sweet thing to cross my lips always started an avalanche. No matter how much I hated myself, I couldn't seem to stop."

—Anita F., 44, Ottawa, Canada

they usually don't go overboard. "The research implies that some people with eating disorders might have an addiction," he says.

In addition, the experiment's "big ticket" (as Colantuoni puts it) was that, during withdrawal, the rats experienced neurochemical changes in the part of the brain called the nucleus accumbens. Basically, just like heroin-addicted animals going into withdrawal, acetylcholine (a neurotransmitter associated with aversion) was increased, and the release of the brain chemical dopamine (a neurotransmitter involved with motivation and reward) decreased.

Canadian Rodents Go Gonzo for Sugar and Get Gnarly When It's Removed

After Dr. Hoebel's rats were becoming dependent on sucrose in New Jersey, more rodents were clamoring for sugar in Canada. Interestingly, neither research team was aware of the other's work. Their results, however, bear remarkable similarities.

Like at Princeton, the first of many sucrose experiments at Laurentian University in Sudbury, Ontario, began by happenstance. "We were exploring how pregnancy leads to shifts in taste among female rats—you know, the famous pickles-and-ice-cream phenomenon. But we couldn't proceed with the study because the rats drank so much sucrose," explains Michael Persinger, Ph.D., a neuroscience and psychology professor, who has been studying the relationship between brain activity and behavior for 35 years.

92-YEAR-OLD FITNESS ICON JACK LALANNE WAS ONCE A SUGAR JUNKIE

At 92, Jack LaLanne remains in remarkable shape, but as a child and teen, he was a scrawny, pimply, angry, downcast, suicidal, bulimic, and hard-core sugar addict.

Already at age three, he became hooked when his mother put a cloth dipped in sugar water and cornstarch into his mouth. "I'd suck on it, and by the time I was four, my baby teeth had rotted out, and soon all I wanted was sugar, sugar, sugar," he recalled, in a fun, entertaining phone interview with me.

"At 15, I was a full-blown sugarholic. I had terrible headaches every day. I got failing grades at school. I was 30 pounds underweight. I was constantly tired and had 'pooped-out-itis'. I had an uncontrollable temper. I did and said things that I wish I'd never done. I had no friends. Kids used to beat me up and make fun of me. I was unhappy, worried, and miserable all the time. It was like hell on earth.

"I used to eat a quart of ice cream, put my finger down my throat, heave it up, then have some more. I would eat cakes, pies, ice cream, soda pop, everything with sugar in it," LaLanne remembers.

"My mother gave me regular foods, and I wouldn't eat them. I'd steal junk food from the kitchen and go into the backyard to eat in secret. I was just like an alcoholic."

LaLanne's turning point came after attending an inspirational lecture by health food pioneer Paul Bragg. "He said you should obey nature's laws, and one of the big ones was to eat foods in their natural state. So I immediately cut out all white sugar and white flour," he recalls.

"The minute I cut them out, my whole life changed. My headaches went away. I got good grades in school. Within months I joined the Berkeley YMCA, became an athlete, and gained weight. It was a rebirth.

"In my mind, nothing on this earth is more addictive than refined sugar," LaLanne insists. "So many people worldwide are hooked on sugar, but they just don't realize it. I'm convinced that people are hit with diabetes, cancer, arthritis, rheumatism, and most diseases because they're not eating properly and not getting enough exercise. If I sound like a nut, I'm a damn healthy nut. I'm 92, and I feel like I'm 32."

"Much to my surprise, the rats drained the entire sucrose bottle," he recalls. "At first, we thought the bottles were leaking. So we gave the rats larger bottles, but they still kept drinking. So we supplied them even bigger bottles. They were insatiable.

"When they were awake, the rats sucked on a sucrose bottle once every five minutes—sometimes even more. They didn't quit. They just kept drinking and drinking like the Energizer bunny."

Not only did the critters become reliant on sugar, but they also consumed 33 percent more food. "And when we took away the sugar, all the rats got really irritable and nippy," Dr. Persinger observes. "They became aggressive to the other rats and to the experimenters, and their eyes bulged."

As with humans, some rats became more fiercely attached to the sweet drinks. "Half the rats didn't just nip; they tried to gnaw at our fingers. The worst bites I ever received were from those rats," Dr. Persinger recalls. "This nippiness is typical of addiction. It's called withdrawal-induced aggression."

The rats exhibited other typically addictive behaviors, too. For instance, they drank more sucrose in stressful situations such as when they were moved to different cages, when their sleep cycle was disrupted, or when their feeding schedule changed.

The Laurentian team's research study, which appeared in *Psychological Reports*, clarifies, "The voracious nature of the sucrose consumption was evident daily when the bottles containing the water and the sucrose were removed, refreshed, and returned."

Another curious reaction, Dr. Persinger notes, is that "when the sucrose was brought back after a few minutes away, the rats would grab at, bite at, and claw at the nozzle of the sucrose bottle so it wouldn't be taken away again."

And some 10 percent of the rats spurned plain water, pushing the bottle out of the cage. "They wanted sucrose water or nothing," says study coauthor Michael Galic.

The Dopamine Connection

Theories abound among addiction specialists as to why some of us get hooked on sweets while others don't. Some experts cite allergies as the cause of all addictions. Other camps point to genetic factors, environmental influences such as peer pressure, a family history of sugar abuse or alcoholism, anxiety, depression, poor eating habits, stress, hormones, and the need to "self-medicate." One researcher even claims that economics (i.e., sweets are cheap) is responsible for hooking people on sugary foods.

Here's a closer look at the cutting-edge dopamine/genetics theory. Many experts believe that substance abusers turn to sugar, drugs, or alcohol to compensate for faulty biochemistry, such as lower levels of dopamine, serotonin, or beta-endorphins.

Dopamine is released when you experience pleasure, which may be when you eat sweets or when you make love, and that dopamine rush makes you want to repeat the activity that caused it again and again.

The Cutting-Edge DRD2A1 Gene Theory

Two leading experts on how gene theories relate to addiction are Kenneth Blum, Ph.D., and Ernest Noble, Ph.D. In 1990, they discovered the "reward gene" (the dopamine receptor gene, DRD2A1) that is associated with severe alcoholism. Since then, individually, together, and alongside other researchers worldwide, they have amassed a mounting, convincing body of evidence to implicate DRD2A1 in other addictions as well, including cocaine, nicotine, and now sugar.

"Our brains are normally hot-wired so that they need dopamine to allow us to achieve pleasure states," explains Dr. Blum, an adjunct professor at Wake Forest University School of Medicine in Winston-Salem, North Carolina. "You're compromised when there's a genetic foul-up or dysfunction with the wiring system and the neurotransmitters that allow you to get dopamine released. Then, you're going to look for anything that will give you a dopamine boost. So alcohol, cocaine, heroin, PCP, and sugar all do it—only sugar is a little less potent than alcohol or drugs.

"Many brain chemicals directly impact an individual's romance with sugar. Dopamine is the final common pathway in terms of the brain's reward center." According to Dr. Blum, "one-third of the U.S. population has a gene variant that causes low dopamine," a phenomenon he calls "Reward Deficiency Syndrome" (RDS).

Brains of the Obese Look Like Those of Drug Addicts

Addiction researchers Nora D. Volkow, M.D., and Gene-Jack Wang, M.D., also found a dopamine-addiction-sugar connection. Their findings, which appeared in *The Lancet*, concluded that obese people, like substance abusers, have fewer receptors for DRD2 (dopamine receptor D2) than people of normal weight.

"It's very similar to what you see in drug addiction," says Dr. Volkow, a psychiatrist and former director of Brookhaven's Neuroimaging Center, who is now director of the National Institutes of Health's National Institute on Drug Abuse (NIDA).

"We suspect that obese people feel compelled to eat more high-energy foods like sweets to feel satisfied to compensate for their low dopamine state," explains Dr. Wang, lead scientist on the study. "By eating more, they're trying to stimulate dopamine 'pleasure' circuits in their brains just as addicts do by taking drugs."

Chocolate, the Most Addictive Sweet of All

We crave it, rave about it, and save it for later—if we can. Melt-in-your-mouth chocolate is the most frequently desired food in the United States today. In fact, Americans savor some 3 billion pounds of it every year, or roughly 12 pounds per person.

" 'Gotta have it' is the driving thought of an addict—a drink, a drag, a hit, a line, a pill, another piece of chocolate. This urgent inner demand overrides all others, undermines reason, resolve, and will. It does not stop until it is satisfied. And then, it starts again." Thus wrote Ronald A. Ruden, M.D., Ph.D., in *The Craving Brain*.

Does this describe you and chocolate? Take heart. You're not alone.

"It is becoming apparent that certain food substances, most notably chocolate, may effect similar physiological and psychological reactions in susceptible people," write Kristen Bruinsma, M.S., and Douglas L. Taren, Ph.D., in their article, "Chocolate: Food or Drug?" that appeared in

AND YOU THINK TODAY'S WOMEN ARE HIGH CHOCOLATE MAINTENANCE?

To what extremes chocolate lovers will go! Anne of Austria allegedly married Louis XIII of France in 1615 only if she could bring her own stash of chocolate with her. And in 1774, when Louis XVI ascended to the throne, Marie-Antoinette appointed her own personal chocolatier, who created tasty culinary concoctions, including chocolate with powdered orchid bulbs.

the *Journal of the American Dietetic Association*. Such foods, the article states, end up "blurring the once distinct line between foods and drugs."

"Chocolate isn't a drug. It's the whole drugstore," quips Dr. Barnard, author of *Breaking the Food Seduction*. By "drugstore," Dr. Barnard is referring to the fact that chocolate contains not only sugar and fat, but also psychoactive substances:

- *Theobromine:* A stimulant that literally means "food of the gods."

- *Phenylethylamine (PEA):* An amphetamine-like compound that's also chemically similar to the street drug "ecstasy."

- *Anandamide:* A chemical related to marijuana's active ingredient whose name means "internal bliss."

- *Caffeine:* A 1.4-ounce Nestlé Crunch bar has some 10 milligrams of caffeine or one-tenth the amount in a cup of coffee.

Chocolate's "Power" over Many

World-renowned appetite expert Marion Hetherington, Ph.D., chair of the psychology department at the University of Liverpool in Great Britain and author of *Food Cravings and Addiction*, finds that people use chocolate to serve many functions, despite the fact that it's ultimately ineffective.

For some, eating the substance is a way to self-medicate and battle depression. For others, "their habit disrupts their lives," Dr. Hetherington says in a phone interview from the U.K.

"One woman said she couldn't keep chocolate in the house. When she got strong cravings, she mixed cocoa and butter to create chocolate and would eat that. Another interviewee reported that whenever she got a strong craving, she would go on a bicycle ride to the nearest town four miles away. People will go to extreme lengths to get chocolate. That's very, very similar to what you find in bulimia."

Dr. Hetherington was alluding to the fact that people with the eating disorder of bulimia tend to lose control and get into a destructive cycle of binge eating—often consuming large amounts of high-calorie dessert foods such as chocolate in a short period of time—and then follow up with purging, either through vomiting, laxatives, or exercise.

In another study of "chocoholics," Dr. Hetherington found that subjects demonstrated addiction traits such as "salience, conflict, relief, relapse, tolerance, and withdrawal."

She concludes: "Since chocolate provides pleasure, contains psychoactive ingredients, and may be considered a forbidden fruit, it is possible that some individuals abuse or binge on chocolate, as [people] might abuse other substances such as drugs or alcohol."

The Evidence Mounts

Other researchers worldwide also found intriguing connections between drugs, alcohol, and a sweet taste. "We just keep getting more and more evidence that these are tied together in some way," says Marilyn Carroll, Ph.D., a psychiatry and neuroscience professor at the University of Minnesota in Minneapolis, who found that animals substitute sweets for drugs.

For instance, at the University of Wisconsin-Madison Medical School, neuroscientist and psychiatry professor Ann E. Kelley, Ph.D., has found evidence that the brain chemistry of rats on sweet, fatty foods shows distinctive, long-lasting changes.

"Our data show that if rats eat a sweet, chocolaty, high-fat food for three hours a day for two weeks, the gene expression for enkephalin decreases in the nucleus accumbens. This means that the brain is adapting to the effects of the food," explains Dr. Kelley, chair of the university's neuroscience training program.

"You get the same thing if you give alcohol, heroin, or morphine to a rat every day for several weeks," she explains. "Our studies suggest that, in some people, overindulging in high-sugar foods *may* cause brain alterations similar to those observed in addiction. Perhaps overindulging in these foods primes the system to want more."

Seeking Solace in Sucrose

When substance abusers kick their habit, they appear to boost their intake of sweets. "The sugar solution is a kind of a substitute for the drug," says Robin Kanarek, Ph.D., a psychology and nutrition professor and dean of Tufts University's Graduate School of Arts and Sciences program.

"The relationship between sweets and drugs has been known about for a while in less-than-scientific circles," agrees Blake Gosnell, Ph.D., an expert in taste preferences and drug taking and basic research director at the Neuropsychiatric Institute in Fargo, North Dakota.

SUGARY MOVIE MOMENT

The Man with the Golden Arm, 1955, starring Frank Sinatra and Kim Novak

Sinatra: "The most gorgeous day I ever saw. . . . I got a craving for something sweet. You got anything sweet?"
Novak: "Sugar."
Sinatra: "Gimme." [She pours sugar into his cupped hands.]
Sinatra: [Licks the sugar.] "More."
Novak: "Eeeww. How can you?"
Sinatra: "Ohhh, I never felt this good in my life. I feel like all the things inside me settled into place . . ."

In fact, when lecturing about his research, Dr. Gosnell shows a revealing clip from the Otto Preminger drug-addiction drama, *The Man with the Golden Arm*. In it, dope addict/card dealer Frankie Machine (Frank Sinatra) spends a harrowing night kicking drugs cold turkey. After enduring withdrawal, guess what he *craves*?

Of Sugar, Drugs, and Alcohol

Alexey B. Kampov-Polevoy, M.D., Ph.D., first noticed this gimme-sugar-now tendency among patients with alcohol problems. "I was trying to be nice by offering candies," he recalls. "Most people were taking one or two, but some started taking them until they cleaned the whole plate. Then, I realized that they had a problem," says Dr. Kampov-Polevoy, now a research assistant professor in the psychology department at the University of North Carolina's Bowles Center for Alcohol Studies.

In all, Dr. Kampov-Polevoy has conducted more than a dozen studies showing that a preference for sweets is systematically linked to a craving for alcohol in rats and humans alike. For example, he found that newly abstinent alcoholics preferred sweeter solutions than the control subjects did. And he also made another fascinating discovery: Preferences for sweets, combined with novelty seeking, can predict whether or not a person is an alcoholic.

SUGARY MOVIE MOMENT

Days of Wine and Roses, 1962, starring Jack Lemmon, Lee Remick, and Jack Klugman

In this scene, recovered alcoholic Jim Hungerford (Jack Klugman) talks to Joe Clay (Jack Lemmon) about his alcoholic wife, Kirsten Arneson (Lee Remick).

"Joe, do you remember how you told us about Kirsten's obsession with chocolate candy when you first met? A perceptive psychologist could have told you right then that she was a potential alcoholic."

So what do sugar, drugs, and alcohol have in common? "One popular theory is that sugar, drugs, and alcohol all activate similar reward-related parts of the brain," Dr. Gosnell suggests.

Dr. Carroll agrees. "Sugar and drugs are similar in the way they affect the brain."

And Dr. Kampov-Polevoy believes that "sweets stimulate the brain's opioid system and trigger the release of opioids such as beta-endorphins and dopamine."

Some experts believe that this yen for sweets signals that most alcoholics experience hypoglycemia, a phenomenon noticed by the late Dr. Atkins. In fact, he maintained that "sugar provides the same temporary lift that alcohol once did."

Psychiatrist Abram Hoffer, Ph.D., M.D., for example, told me he has "never seen an alcoholic who wasn't hypoglycemic. I stopped checking after hundreds of patients tested positive. I couldn't find a normal blood sugar tolerance curve." Dr. Hoffer also said he was "a personal friend" of the late AA (Alcoholics Anonymous) cofounder Bill W., who himself personally triumphed over his own sugar cravings and hypoglycemia symptoms by quitting sweets and coffee, eating ample protein, and taking large niacin doses.

Sugar and the Gateway Theory

Although sugar may not be addictive in exactly the same way as hard drugs, some experts speculate that sweets may act as a "gateway" substance.

EXPERT VIEWPOINT

"For some people, sugar can become an object of addiction. When people are miserable, depressed, and in pain, the risks of addiction go up. For people who are happy, interested, motivated, and involved, their chances of becoming addicted are slim, even when exposed to sugar, cocaine, etc."
—Howard J. Shaffer, Ph.D., C.A.S., director of Harvard Medical School's Division on Addictions and a psychologist who has studied and treated addictions for three decades

"I think when children get hooked at a young age on soft drinks, candy, junk food, and caffeine, it can set up a pattern of craving," Dr. Carroll believes.

"They learn early to develop this addictive behavior from carbohydrate craving and excessive eating. Coding patterns and memories form in their brain, and that can transfer to addiction to other substances, but not in everyone, of course."

Hope Is in Store!

Happily, a growing number of nutrition-oriented treatment programs, often run by naturopaths, chiropractors, osteopathic physicians, nutritionists, eating disorder specialists, or holistic M.D.s, are having astounding success by taking innovative approaches to help people lick their carb addictions, as well as eating disorders such as bulimia and binge eating. These programs are unique in the sense that most seek to rebalance the individual's biochemistry through diet.

"When people normalize brain and body chemistry, they're much less vulnerable to relapse," says Julia Ross, executive director of the Northern California–based Recovery Systems, which uses nutrition therapy, counseling, and education to help people conquer sugar, weight, alcohol, and drug problems.

Meanwhile, at Dr. Tennant's five carbohydrate-dependency/weight-control clinics in California, the first thing staff members do when a new client arrives is to determine if he or she has carbohydrate dependency and/or hypoglycemia.

"We use the word 'dependency' rather than addiction to soften the blow. We're trying to break through people's denial and establish rapport. When you call someone an 'addict,' you get an automatic turnoff. By using the term 'dependency,' we get through denial amazingly fast. We tell them, 'You're dependent upon carbohydrates for a great deal of controlling your emotions and your behavior.' They say, 'By gosh, I sure am,'" adds Dr. Tennant, whose clinics use "standard addiction medicine techniques" to help their patients lose weight and gain control of their lives.

If you're feeling addicted to sweets, you may feel vindicated and validated at last. With this new information, you can take charge. But having been where you are now, I need to be brutally honest: It's easy to fall prey to sugar's seductive charms. You need to be vigilant. You need to stand strong. Most of all, you need to know that you can succeed.

When tempted, perhaps you could follow Lisette's tactic: "I have to constantly tell myself, 'You've come too far to take orders from a cookie!' "

10

SUGARY SNACKS CAN MINIMIZE
YOUR MEMORY

From 2000 to 2003, Kate H. of Vero Beach, Florida, felt tormented and trapped in a brain that wouldn't think straight. She felt overcome by confusion, spaciness, and chaotic thoughts.

"Both my daughters knew when 'the brain fog' was hitting me, because I would get a dazed, glazed, 'out-there' look. It got to the point where I was losing my balance and I would have to go through my house holding on to furniture," she recalls.

Desperate for answers, Kate, then 53, went to her family physician. "I was afraid I was getting early-onset Alzheimer's, because both my parents suffered from this disease. My doctor sent me to a psychologist." Since she was also dealing with the tragic loss of her husband to a drunk driver, the therapist wrote off her fuzzy thinking as yet another symptom of depression. But, says Kate, "I knew it was something deeper."

It wasn't until she "walked into a wall, right there in the doctor's office," that her mystified family physician began to take her seriously. Thinking she had multiple sclerosis, he sent her for a CAT scan and an MRI. Both tests, however, indicated that she had a "healthy brain."

Despite the fact that her dazed-and-confused symptoms are indicative of poor blood sugar control, not once did her doctor ask her what kind of foods she was eating. In the end, relief came not from her puzzled doctor but because she finally took a friend's long-standing advice to quit sugar.

"I simply hadn't been ready to do it, because in my family, everything revolved around food, especially sweets. We were big bakers. We'd make pumpkin pie, pecan pie, cherry cheesecake, chocolate peanut-butter fudge, lemon meringue pie, rice pudding, Mexican wedding balls, scones, butter cookies, oatmeal cake, and homemade breads."

As it turned out, Kate had been putting herself into constant SUGAR SHOCK! by consuming not only large quantities of sweets but also too many processed, much-like-sugar carbs and getting only scant amounts of protein. For example, she'd eat a meal of "French bread or homemade rolls [not whole grain], smothered with butter, along with lots of pasta, and topped with three little shrimp."

On June 17, 2003, Kate quit refined sugars and carbs. The result? Her brain fog lifted after just one week. Without even trying, she eventually also peeled off 33 pounds. Today, she thinks "more clearly than ever before," and has ample energy for her profession as a miniaturist who builds doll-houses for collectors.

According to experts, Kate's predicament is shared by millions. Indeed, new research theorizes that anyone with poor or impaired blood sugar control is at risk for memory woes and that blood sugar issues such as diabetes, prediabetes or impaired glucose tolerance, insulin resistance, and hypoglycemia could be caused or exacerbated by eating too many sweets and refined-flour products, as well as by not exercising.

Brain Basics

Weighing in at a mere three pounds, our brain is the seat of our intelligence. It helps us remember things, controls our behavior and movement, and helps us interpret information provided by our five senses. While our brain comprises only about 2 percent of our total body weight, it uses up some 30 percent of the calories we take in. Remember, as you learned in chapter 4, our brains need glucose (sugar) to survive, but fast-acting, inferior, processed carbs and sweets can mess up your brain, not help it.

In fact, one recent study conducted by researchers at the University of Wales shows that people who eat superior, complex carbohydrates for breakfast (such as slow-cooking oatmeal and high-fiber breakfast cereal)

CONFESSIONS OF A FORMERLY FUZZY-BRAINED SUGAR KICKER

"If I eat sweets, I can't concentrate or think clearly. Now that I'm not eating sugar, my mind is sharper and my short-term memory recall is better."

—Lisa J., 44, New York City

have better memories than those who begin their days with low-caliber carbs (such as donuts and pastries).

"Unlike other tissues in the body that have multiple fuel sources, the brain depends on sugar (i.e., glucose) for 99 percent of its energy," explains Dr. Antonio Convit of the New York University School of Medicine and the Nathan Kline Institute.

"Carbohydrates converted to blood sugar supply the brain with the fuel it needs. The brain can't use anything else. It can't use fatty acids or amino acids like other parts of the body."

But while our brains need glucose for fuel, it's the type of fuel or food supplied that matters, observes Dharma Singh Khalsa, M.D., president and medical director of the Alzheimer's Prevention Foundation International, a nonprofit organization that takes an integrative medical approach to preventing and reversing Alzheimer's disease.

"Sugar is good for the brain *only* if it comes from complex carbohydrates that are released slowly," explains Dr. Khalsa, author of the best seller *Brain Longevity*, as well as *The Better Memory Kit, Food as Medicine*, and *Meditation as Medicine*.

"Refined carbohydrates and sugars cause your blood glucose levels to swing wildly. For maximum efficiency, your brain needs a *steady* supply of glucose, and this is best achieved with a diet rich in complex carbohydrates and at least 30 grams of fiber each day," continues Dr. Khalsa, who calls white sugar, white bread, white flour, and other white foods "alarm foods," because they're false stimulants with no nutritional value, and they prompt "a stress reaction" in your body.

Studies Confirm a Link between Blood Sugar and Brain Function

Some ongoing and recent scientific studies are now paving the way for new insights into how sugar can affect our brains. In one groundbreaking study published in the *Proceedings of the National Academy of Science*, Dr. Convit and his research team looked at 30 healthy, nondiabetic, nondemented people, with an average age of 67 and a normal mental aptitude. Researchers administered to them an intravenous Glucose Tolerance Test and drew their blood often over a four-hour period. In addition, the subjects got an MRI to learn the size of their hippocampus, the part of the brain responsible for learning and memory. Then they measured how quickly the participants metabolized sugar and how well they did on memory tests.

When the results were tabulated, "our study demonstrated that people who did not process their blood sugar normally [prediabetics whose blood sugar stayed high longer after a meal than it should] performed *worse* on

ARE *YOU* AT RISK FOR A SUGAR-RELATED MEMORY PROBLEM?

Wondering why the name of that corner video store slips your mind, despite the fact that you've been going there for five years? You could be one of millions with high or low blood sugar levels and not even know it. That's why it's so important to:

- Get annual physical checkups, including fasting glucose tests, especially if you spend most nights in front of the tube while noshing on potato chips and chocolate.
- Quit overeating processed carbs and sweets. Instead choose superior carbs, lean protein, and healthy fats.
- Exercise regularly and lose weight, if necessary.

Just by making these important lifestyle changes, many are able to reverse or reduce memory or concentration problems.

memory tasks than those who had normal blood sugar control. In addition, people with poor blood sugar control had a smaller hippocampus," explains Dr. Convit, who is conducting follow-up research "to determine if the shrunken hippocampus is causally related to poor glucose regulation."

Essentially, he explains, "if the way we regulate sugar in the body is not optimal, it's likely that the brain is not getting all the fuel it needs when it needs it. The longer the sugar stays in the bloodstream after a meal, the more the person has impaired glucose tolerance, and it's that impairment that has been associated with poor memory.

"When the brain is working properly, it uses sugar very quickly for its fuel and the glucose levels in the brain dip. Every time your brain is activated or you're thinking about something, the sugar levels in the part of the brain that's working are dropping.

"It's perhaps that ability to bring more glucose quickly to the brain when you need it that may be impaired with people who have diabetes or prediabetes," Dr. Convit explains. "And that's why they have more problems with cognitive function, because when they need to bring in extra glucose to compensate for the dips, they can't do it."

Already, some 25 medical studies show that diabetics have more memory and learning problems than the general population, Dr. Convit says. But what's particularly intriguing about his research is that he studied *nondiabetics* and found that those people whose elevated blood sugar levels were not high enough to be considered diabetic also experienced memory problems.

What's especially scary is that these days, children with type 2 diabetes are also experiencing cognitive difficulties, points out Dr. Convit, who is now studying children between ages 14 and 18 with type 2 diabetes to determine how well their brains work.

"Up until 10 years ago, the predominant type of diabetes cases in children was type 1 diabetes. About 40 percent of the new cases have type 2 diabetes, and they're predominantly obesity related. We've found preliminary evidence that these children have significantly more cognitive problems—15 to 20 percent more—than kids the same age [who are] also obese but don't have diabetes. This is going to impair their ability to do well in school, which could affect how well they do in life. It's not just obesity that's causing the problems, but metabolic problems due to the diabetes that's causing the cognitive problems," he adds.

Dr. Convit's research results raise the possibility that losing weight by eating fewer sweets and fast-acting carbs and other nonnutritive foods, along with exercising (which also helps control blood sugar levels), may help *reverse* some memory loss that accompanies aging.

"Up to now, most people have associated poor blood sugar control only with diabetes, heart disease, and stroke. But now we know that when glucose isn't processed normally, it has ramifications on brain function as well," he explains.

"You can lose some of your brain function if you don't exercise sufficiently and eat properly," Dr. Convit concludes. "What our grandmothers and our mothers have been telling us for a long time is true—exercise, eat well, and don't get heavy. Couch potatoes may now have a new incentive to exercise and get their weight down."

A team of Canadian researchers from the University of Ottawa led by psychology professor Claude Messier, Ph.D., has made similar findings concerning the link between blood sugar and brain function. One study, which was published in the *Neurobiology of Aging*, looked at 57 healthy, nondiabetic people aged 55 to 84 who took a Glucose Tolerance Test. Dr. Messier and his colleagues measured the length of time the glucose stayed in the subjects' bloodstream and then examined two groups—one with good blood sugar control and the other whose control was impaired. Participants of both groups were then asked to recall a list of names provided by the researchers. "We found that those who didn't metabolize their sugar normally performed worse on the memory tests," says Dr. Messier. "Those with normal blood glucose levels performed very well on them."

Studies Show a Link between Poor Blood Sugar Control and Alzheimer's Disease

If fuzzy-headed forgetfulness isn't enough to motivate you to jettison your secret stash of candies and cookies, more groundbreaking research linking insulin resistance to Alzheimer's disease might. For some time, scientists didn't know why people with diabetes were at greater risk of developing Alzheimer's disease and other types of dementia than the rest of the general population. (Dementia is any mental disorder characterized by impairment of memory, judgment, and abstract thinking, as well as personality changes.)

Recent research by scientists at the Joslin Diabetes Center in Boston suggests that the reason could be related to insulin resistance in their brain cells, which affects the way those cells function. As mentioned previously, insulin resistance, a main cause of type 2 diabetes, is a disorder that occurs when your body's cells lose their sensitivity to insulin and no longer use it normally to control blood glucose levels, requiring your pancreas to produce more and more in order to compensate.

In their study, the Joslin researchers compared the metabolic processes of normal mice with those of a second group that had been genetically altered to reduce the number of insulin receptors in their brains. The altered mice experienced reduced insulin activity signaling the proteins in their brains. As a result, they developed an increase in the amount of chemical modification (phosphorylation) of tau proteins that is a hallmark of brain lesions in Alzheimer's disease. (Tau proteins are essential to healthy brain-cell function; in cells affected by Alzheimer's, however, the tau proteins show an increase in phosphorylation and this alters their function, eventually leading to other changes in how the brain cells can signal.)

The researchers aren't prepared to say that diabetes alone actually *causes* Alzheimer's disease. "Diabetes may cause some of the early biochemical changes found in Alzheimer's disease," explains C. Ronald Kahn, M.D., president and director of the Joslin Diabetes Center, "but those early changes probably aren't enough by themselves to cause Alzheimer's."

Scientists do, however, believe that further research is needed to clarify how the effect of insulin resistance on the brain cells interacts with other genetic and biochemical problems to trigger various dementias. "We hope to begin to uncover common mechanisms that could play a role in the onset of the disease," Dr. Kahn says.

The Link between Free Radicals and Alzheimer's Disease

Meanwhile, other studies conducted at the State University of New York at Buffalo demonstrate that eating sugary foods and quickie carbs may not only boost production of harmful free-radicals but lower levels of vitamin E, known to be a helpful free-radical scavenger, thus causing inflammation of the arteries that could increase one's risk for stroke and Alzheimer's.

Free radicals are harmful by-products of normal cell activity that can cause inflammation of the blood vessels and ultimately block blood flow to the brain, thus contributing to serious health problems, including stroke, heart disease, and cancer.

"Your brain needs a blood supply just like your heart and any other major organ in your body," says Paresh Dandona, M.D., Ph.D., distinguished professor of medicine and director of the Division of Endocrinology, Diabetes, and Metabolism at SUNY-Buffalo.

"If your brain cannot get the blood supply it needs, aging may become accelerated. Free radicals accelerate hardening of the arteries everywhere in the body, including the brain," explains Dr. Dandona, who spearheaded a study that was published in the *Journal of Clinical Endocrinology and Metabolism*.

"We've known for some time that eating certain foods, particularly those containing the antioxidant vitamins A, C, and E can help protect against damage from free radicals," Dr. Dandona says. "But our studies established for the first time that if you take sugar, you will get an increase in free radical generation. The free radicals are highly reactive, interacting with other cells and damaging them."

Curiously, Dr. Dandona's interest in the subject began while studying overweight subjects whose harmful free radical levels went down after they restricted dietary intake and lost weight within a short period of time. This observation led him to wonder if certain types of food could produce harmful free radicals.

In another study, Dr. Dandona found that "glucose increases inflammation and free radical generation within an hour of taking 75 grams of a glucose drink. [The] discoveries were important because many obese people have type 2 diabetes, and diabetics are known to have higher levels of dangerous free radicals. Long-term diabetes leads to fallen cognitive abilities probably due to the free radical generation and inflammation," he speculates.

"Those free radicals could damage all tissues in the body, and if you have an excess of sugar in your body, you're doing this continuously," continues Dr. Dandona, who was startled by another discovery—that DNA in the white blood cells of diabetics is damaged by free radicals. "This may have implications for vascular disease and cancer.

"Even now, people don't really appreciate the fact that food is the major contributor to free-radical generation in the body," adds Dr. Dandona, whose McDonald's study in the *American Journal of Clinical Nutrition* attracted considerable attention when it showed that a 900-calorie fast-food meal resulted in free radical generation and inflammation for more than three hours. By contrast, a meal of fruit, fiber meal, protein, and healthy fats didn't produce any inflammation or oxidative stress.

Dr. Dandona has also conducted research suggesting that sugar may be linked to Alzheimer's disease because it causes harmful inflammation. After giving subjects a sweet glucose drink, he found that the solution "caused an increase in inflammation that lasted three hours. What this means is that the inflammation damages the lining of the blood vessels, which can inhibit a healthy flow of blood to the brain. Diminishing blood flow, which robs the brain of necessary oxygen, could put you at a higher risk for Alzheimer's disease, as well as heart disease and stroke."

Mark Hyman, M.D., author of *UltraMetabolism: The Simple Plan for Automatic Weight Loss* and editor-in-chief of *Alternative Therapies in Health and Medicine*, actually contends that "sugar is probably the biggest cause of inflammation in our society. Inflammation is the biggest cause of cancer, heart disease, and Alzheimer's disease."

Experts are now interested in learning more about how the long-term effects of glucose may affect the risk of Alzheimer's disease and other forms of dementia, which lead to loss of cognition, memory, reason, judgment, and language.

If the theory that excessive sugar consumption plays an important role in the development of these conditions is true, the implications for our aging population could be profound. That's because some 4 million Americans aged 65 and up are now plagued by this most common cause of dementia. In fact, 14 million older Americans are expected to get it by 2050, according to the National Institute on Aging's Alzheimer's Disease Education and Referral Center.

Befriending Your Brain

So there you have it. Our brains rely on sugar or glucose to function, but it's the *type* of foods or carbohydrates we eat that can help us remember, or lead us to forget—those vital bits of information. So, if you want to think clearly and get "brain power," you must eat high-quality foods. In fact, Dr. Khalsa of the Alzheimer's Prevention Foundation International has the right idea when he recommends eating colorful vegetables and fruits (which are rich in the antioxidants that protect cells against free-radical damage); foods high in omega-3 fatty acids such as fish, flax oil, and spinach; whole grains like brown rice and whole wheat bread; and "clean protein" from fish, soy, legumes, and free-range, organic meats. Interestingly, Dr. Khalsa was also one of the first in the United States to recommend that people learn valuable stress management techniques such as meditation, exercise, and yoga to prevent and help treat memory loss.

As scientists continue to investigate ways in which improper sugar metabolism may be related to memory loss and loss of cognitive skills, the advice ought to be clear: We should cut back on sugars and refined carbs and exercise regularly, for the sake of our brains.

11

SWEETS CAN SOUR YOUR MOODS

Social worker Kelly S., 28, used to binge daily on cakes, cookies, and ice cream. But soon after taking that first bite of a "sweet treat," she would swing from a thrilling, euphoric "sugar high" into a dismal, pessimistic misery. To make things worse, she ballooned to 100 pounds over her ideal weight. "For me, sugar causes depression, anxiety, and irritability," admits the self-described sugar addict, who is the daughter of an alcoholic and the granddaughter of a diabetic.

After reading a book by food addiction author Kay Sheppard, Kelly began to suspect that the quickie carbs she'd been overeating were triggering her mood swings. To test the theory, she eliminated sugar, refined carbs, and alcohol, and within three months, her depression lifted, emotional calm returned, and she eventually shed 100 pounds.

This jolting sugar-mood reaction is also familiar to Devorah R. "If I have just a piece of cake or a brownie, my joy quotient takes a dramatic dip," confesses the script consultant and former movie-studio executive.

"After eating sugar, I get cranky, short fused, and agitated," she says. "Don't let me negotiate that deal or return that phone call, because my little sugar binge will erase my natural grace.

"And it doesn't matter what kind of sugar I consume, whether it's sucrose, fructose, or more 'natural sweeteners' like maple syrup or honey. All of them take me down a dark—albeit seductive—alley, where it's hard to ward off negative thinking. I might reach for sweets because I'm feeling down, but after the quick rush, I descend into a darker mood. When I'm on sugar, I'm downbeat; when I'm off sugar, I'm upbeat. It's that simple."

Sound familiar? Your feelings may not be as pronounced as Kelly's or Devo's, but perhaps you, too, are caught in a harmful cycle, where you unsuccessfully bury your blues beneath a mound of chocolate ice cream. Although you may feel better briefly, inevitably you'll need another sugar boost hours later.

Do Sweets Smash Our Spirits?

At one time or another, many of us turn to sugary snacks or much-like-sugar carbs for solace and comfort. We unthinkingly use such sweets to fend off our melancholy, ease our edginess, and lessen our angst. But what most of us don't realize is that those very same fast-acting carbs that *temporarily* make us feel so good can quickly take us from that deceptively elated high to a crushing low.

Compelling recent research shows that cramming down sweets and processed carbs has a devastating downside for many people, especially those sensitive to sweets. In fact, junk-food junkies report recurring feelings of despair, desolation, and hopelessness, and the more they consume fast-acting carbs, the more depressed they become. Then, the worse they feel, the more they turn to sweets to give them that deceptive, short-lived high. And so the vicious cycle continues, with the quickie-carb habit simply fanning the flames of depression.

Indeed, some experts believe that America's escalating consumption of cakes, cookies, chips, candies, and other quickie carbs—in short, SUGAR SHOCK!—plays a potentially pivotal role in our plummeting moods and mounting unhappiness.

To some nutrition authorities, it's no coincidence that as more people gravitate to processed carbs, more and more of us are plagued by depression and anxiety disorders.

Julia Ross, author of *The Mood Cure* and *The Diet Cure*, calls mood-destroying dessert foods and white-flour starches "the gruesome twosome. They're really more like drugs.

"Many of our clients have been freed from the moodiness they've endured for years, simply by dropping these two items from their menus. No supplements, no other changes, dietary or otherwise, required," continues Ross, who runs the San Francisco–area Recovery Systems Clinic.

A Look at Depression's Depressing Figures

At this point, it might be useful to look at some statistics, which reveal that as our consumption of processed foods has increased, so have our rates of depression: More than 57 million people 18 and older—or about one in four adults—have a diagnosable mental disorder in any given year, according to the National Institute of Mental Health (NIMH). This is roughly 26 percent of the U.S. adult population.

Now see other alarming figures:

■ Each year, anxiety disorders afflict 40 million American adults (or about 13 percent of U.S. adults aged 18 to 54).

And those are just the stats for the anxious among us, not the depressed.

■ Then, about 9 percent of the U.S. population aged 18 and older have a depressive disorder in any given year. Some 12 million depression sufferers are women—roughly twice the rate of men.

(Note, however, that many who suffer from depression also suffer from anxiety and vice versa.)

Now, let's look at the younger population. Check out these sobering figures, which have been growing steadily:

■ Studies suggest that one in five children and adolescents may have a diagnosable mental, emotional, or behavioral disorder, according to the Department of Health and Human Services (DHHS).

■ At any point in time, 10 to 15 percent of children and adolescents suffer some symptoms of depression, according to the National Mental Health Information Center of the U.S. Department of Health and Human Services.

Sugar's Depression Reaction around the World

The potential link between our sugar intake and plummeting mood is so beguiling that one group of researchers has tracked both depression and sugar consumption rates in six countries around the world: New Zealand, Canada, Germany, France, the United States, and Korea. Interestingly, the study found that those countries with the highest rates of depression also had the highest rates of refined sugar consumption.

Reporting in *Depression and Anxiety*, the researchers concluded that there was a "highly significant correlation between sugar consumption . . . and the annual rate of depression." For instance, New Zealand, where people consumed nearly 500 calories per capita per day of sugar, had the highest depression rate, with almost 6 percent of the population affected. And in Canada, with a depression rate of a little more than 5 percent, people consumed nearly 400 calories per capita per day from sweets.

"Although speculative, there are some . . . reasons to consider that sugar consumption may directly impact the prevalence of depression," conclude the study's authors, Arthur Westover, M.D., at the time a resident physician in psychiatry at Southwestern Medical Center in Dallas, and Lauren B. Marangell, M.D., associate professor of psychiatry, director of clinical psychopharmacology, and director of Mood Disorders Research in the psychiatry department at Baylor College of Medicine in Houston, Texas.

Dr. Marangell and Dr. Westover admit they can't conclude that high sugar consumption *causes* depression, but they aren't ruling it out either. "It's just far too early to tell. Maybe that's the case, maybe not," Dr. Westover told me.

"The study also raises some interesting questions about the relationship between diabetes and depression," adds Dr. Westover, who would like to further investigate the carb–bad-mood hypothesis.

The link between diabetes and depression is nothing new.

"More than normal rates of depression can already be detected" in patients with diabetes, say researchers from Finland and Germany, who revealed even further proof. Their study, which was published in the *British Medical Journal*, suggests that even before they develop type 2 diabetes, people with insulin resistance and impaired glucose tolerance are getting depressed.

U.K. Researchers Recognize the Obvious Food-Mood Connection

While scientists in the United States have explored some intriguing connections between what we eat and how we behave, experts in Great Britain and Scotland have increasingly taken a leading role in recognizing this link.

"Food is very important to mental and emotional health, but not many people are aware of the food-mood connection," laments the formerly depressed nutritional therapist Amanda Geary, 42, speaking from Great Britain, where she founded the Food and Mood Project. Her project was funded by a Millennium Award from Mind, the country's leading mental health charity.

Geary, author of *The Food and Mood Handbook*, told me that she now shuns the sugary breakfast cereals, biscuits, cakes, and wheat-based foods that she believes once brought on her low moods, leading her to spend much of her time in bed.

Meanwhile, over in Scotland, medical experts, school personnel, and parents are similarly aware of the role nutrition can have on children's moods and concentration. For instance, the Inverness-based Food and Behaviour Research (FAB Research), a Scottish group cofounded by researcher Dr. Alex Richardson, cosponsored a one-day conference, "Diet, Behaviour and the Junk Food Generation," which examined the relationships between diet, behavior, and learning in school-aged children.

And still two more charities in Great Britain have been working hard to draw attention to what they believe is a mental health crisis caused by what people eat. The Mental Health Foundation, a London-based research and policy-influencing think tank, and Sustain: the alliance for better food and farming, jointly released a landmark 2006 report, "Changing Diets, Changing Minds: How Food Affects Mental Health and Behaviour."

Courtney Van de Weyer, a researcher for Sustain's Food and Mental Health Project, said to me via phone from Great Britain that she and colleagues had reviewed around 500 research studies published in peer-reviewed scientific journals to illustrate how changes in the food system—people eating few whole grains, mostly refined carbs, few vegetables and fruits, more sugar and salt, and so on—"may be partly responsible for the rise in mental health and behavioural problems at the same time."

The report acknowledges, of course, that poor diets aren't the causal factor for all mental health problems, behavior disorders, or mood fluctuations, but it singles nutrition out as "a highly plausible and important contributory factor in both the cause and treatment of these conditions."

Is SUGAR SHOCK! Driving Us to Depression and Anxiety?

Experts often point to our nation's dramatic shift in consumption patterns from more natural to processed foods as evidence that helps explain our upswing in depression and other mental health disorders. Because people aren't eating as healthily, they're suffering from nutritional deprivation, and hence depression is skyrocketing, Julia Ross, M.A., explains in her book, *The Mood Cure*.

"We're in a bad mood epidemic [and we're] a hundred times more likely to have significant mood problems than people born a hundred years ago. And those problems are on the rise," Ross observes.

"Adult rates of depression and anxiety have tripled since 1990, and over 80 percent of those who consult medical doctors today complain of excessive stress. Even our children are in trouble, with at least 1 in 10 suffering from significant mood disorders. Our mood problems are increasing so fast that, by 2020, they will outrank AIDS, accidents, and violence as the primary causes of early death and disability."

When you look at the escalating figures for our consumption of sucrose

---

CONFESSIONS OF A SUGAR KICKER

"Sugar makes you into someone you're not, if you're sensitive to it. I went for years from being the life of the party after eating sweets to suffering the inevitable crash and turning into this other person who was grumpy, tired, anxious, unsociable, and lacking self-esteem. For years, I read up on illnesses to find out what was the matter with me. The real, sugar-free person turned out to be surprisingly normal: cheerful, energetic, sensible, and steady. Life without sugar is great: It's the real thing."

—Ruth M., 53, England

and corn sweeteners and put them next to our swelling stats for depression and mood disorders, the evidence suggests that a connection exists. Isn't it curious that we've become a nation of antidepressant-popping folks just as our consumption of added sweeteners has soared to the point that refined foods and sweets now comprise about one-third of our daily calories?

Sugar and the Chemistry of Your Brain

Experts aren't entirely clear about why people get the blues. Many, however, believe that depression is largely caused by a malfunction in the brain's chemistry, dysfunctional cognition (negative thinking), social pressures, and a genetic susceptibility, although there's still a lot to be learned about how it is linked to neurotransmitters, stress, genes, hormones, diet, and nutrients.

In simple terms, your brain cells communicate using special message-carrying chemicals called neurotransmitters that travel across tiny gaps between cells to "receptors" on neighboring cells. Each type of neurotransmitter has a special shape that allows it to fit into a nearby receptor, like a key in a lock. When the neurotransmitter "key" fits into the matching receptor "lock," the cell fires and sends the message on its way.

Scientists point to serotonin, beta-endorphins, and dopamine as among the most important mood-related neurotransmitters responsible for telling your brain: "Relax!" "Calm down!" "Be happy!" When you have the right amount of these chemicals, you feel cheerful, calm, focused, and optimistic. But when the level of these vital chemicals drops, messages can't get across the gaps, and brain communication slows down.

Although they disagree on whether dopamine, beta-endorphins, or serotonin is the catalyst, scientists speculate that when you eat those deceptively tasty dessert snacks or heavily processed much-like-sugar carbs, within a couple of hours your brain releases feel-good neurotransmitters.

Yearning for the White Stuff When We're Feeling Down in the Dumps

One of the most compelling questions scientists have is whether or not people try to "self-medicate" when they feel depressed. To learn if that was the case,

Larry Christensen, Ph.D., chair of the psychology department at the University of South Alabama in Mobile, studied 113 male and 138 female college students. Sixty-seven percent reported that they craved sugar-rich foods when feeling anxious, depressed, tired, or moody. As soon as they ate something sugary, most (79 percent) felt better right away—happy, relaxed, or energetic.

"We looked at their reported feelings before and after they ate carbohydrates," explains Dr. Christensen, author of *Diet-Behavior Relationships: Focus on Depression*. "They reported more distress before and less afterward. We found that as their cravings increased, so did their emotional distress. And, the higher the cravings, the more emotionally distressed they were. After they ate the sugary foods, their moods improved, but not for long," he continues. "Ultimately, they got a quick lift in their moods, but it rapidly dropped again, because the food was only a temporary fix. There's that circular pattern taking place. That's why they need something like therapy, eliminating sugar from their diet, or psychopharmacology to break that circularity and create a permanent improvement in mood."

Curiously, those students who longed for something sweet reported far more intense cravings than their friends who desired protein. And the ones who clamored for the very sweetest of carb snacks reported the strongest urges to eat them.

When people—and even animals—are depressed, they tend to crave sweet "rewards" more, agrees Welsh psychology professor Paul Willner, Ph.D. In one study he conducted, depressed volunteers reported an intense desire to eat chocolate, and their depression increased the intensity of their cravings. "There is considerable evidence that food cravings in general, and chocolate-craving in particular, are associated with mood disturbance," Dr. Willner observes, noting that this occurs among nondepressed individuals as well.

If You're Sugar Sensitive, Your Moods Fluctuate More

If you know people who seem immune to sugar's calling, it could be because they have higher tolerance levels, explains nutrition expert Elizabeth Somer, M.A., R.D., author of *Food & Mood* and *The Food & Mood Cookbook*. Indeed, a subset of people sensitive to sugar react quite intensely to something sweet, which can send them emotionally reeling.

Experts vary in their estimates as to what percentage of the population feels downcast and depressed after eating sweets because of their sugar sensitivity. Dr. Christensen estimates that "about 20 percent of people with depression are sugar sensitive," but other experts believe that the figure could be 50 percent or higher.

The Mood-Lifting Serotonin Factor

It's almost impossible to live in America today without hearing about the importance of serotonin, one of the first neurotransmitters scientists linked to depression. Experts believe that serotonin elevates mood and suppresses appetite. In fact, many antidepressant drugs such as Prozac and Zoloft work by raising levels of serotonin and other mood-related neurotransmitters in your brain.

"When serotonin levels are low, you tend to be grumpy, crabby, or downright depressed," says Somer. "You tend not to tolerate pain very well and not to sleep very well."

In the 1970s, Massachusetts Institute of Technology scientists Richard Wurtman, M.D., and Judith Wurtman, Ph.D., developed a serotonin theory. (Dr. Richard Wurtman is a neuroscience professor and former director of MIT's Clinical Research Center, and Dr. Judith Wurtman is a research scientist, director of the women's health program at the MIT Clinical Research Center, and author of *The Serotonin Solution* and *Managing Your Mind and Mood Through Food*.)

As we'll explore further in chapter 15, the Wurtmans suggested that people seek out these carbohydrates when their depressed brains need the amino acid tryptophan (found in such foods such as turkey, fish, beef, dairy products, chicken, oats, bananas, eggs, and peanuts), which is necessary for serotonin production.

CONFESSIONS OF A SUGAR KICKER

"A couple of hours after I have sugar, I become irritable and crabby. My family thought I was just moody until I realized that I had a sugar problem. Now, they're seeing the sugar connection, too."

—Kathy M., 40, St. Charles, Illinois

Mood expert Julia Ross amplifies. "Serotonin deficiency is far and away the most common mood problem we see at our clinic. It inflicts a dark cloud of misery on people of all ages, sexes, and walks of life," Ross says, noting that America's rate of depression has climbed as tryptophan, serotonin's building block, has been diminishing from our food supply over the last century.

Although scientists believe that some people have lower levels of serotonin than others simply because of genetics, serotonin levels can actually be diminished if you drink too much caffeinated soda, diet pop, or coffee, if you don't get enough protein or healthy fats, and as a result of stress or lack of exercise.

The Pleasure-Producing Beta-Endorphins

Dr. Christensen, who has conducted numerous studies examining the link between food and depression, speculates that in addition to serotonin, another group of neurotransmitters collectively called endogenous opioids (which the body produces naturally when consuming foods) could come into play. Specifically, Dr. Christensen cites beta-endorphins (also known as endorphins) as important in influencing our moods. Beta-endorphins, which can enhance feelings of euphoria, self-esteem, and confidence, are chemically similar to morphine and act like opiates (drugs), dulling the pain of both physical and emotional wounds.

Experiments with animals show that eating sweets can raise endorphin levels and provide an almost immediate boost to low moods. Interestingly, scientists have discovered that just tasting sugar can trigger an endorphin rush, but when it is administered so that it bypasses the tongue (by a tube going directly into the stomach, for example), no subsequent endorphin burst occurs. This suggests that simply the pleasurable experience of gobbling cakes, pies, cookies, donuts, and candy is enough to release endorphins in the brain.

In fact, a growing number of scientists now believe that *any* palatable food—the "goodies" that really tickle your taste buds—will lead to that endorphin release. This is what's happening when sensitive individuals crave sugar, believes University of Wales in Swansea psychologist David Benton, Ph.D., who theorizes that it's "more plausible that stress or low mood induces eating . . . palatable foods."

Blood Sugar's Role in Bringing on the Blues

At the same time that sugar and much-like-sugar carbs are affecting our brain chemicals, they're also affecting our blood sugar levels. So neurotransmitters and blood sugar rise in tandem, creating a temporary euphoria, but then they also drop simultaneously—and drop us into depression.

But that depression doesn't occur with everyone, points out Dr. Christensen. "The dropping of blood sugar levels does trigger depression in some people," explains Dr. Christensen, who conducted numerous studies on the mood-food relationship. "And, since some people are very sensitive to sugar, it takes a very little bit to start triggering a reaction such as mood swings."

Hypoglycemia or low blood sugar is one blood sugar disorder that can definitely put a damper on your mood. You'll learn much more about hypoglycemia in chapter 13, but this condition, as noted earlier, can leave you feeling negative, bad-tempered, anxious, afraid, and depressed. Some people even become suicidal as their blood sugar levels plummet.

Those despondent feelings could easily send you looking for the temporary lift that sugar provides. But then, the inevitable occurs: Your blood sugar will drop, leaving you just as hopeless, grouchy, and dejected as you were before you ate it, so you're repeatedly spiraling in and out of SUGAR SHOCK!

People who don't properly manage their blood sugar are, in fact, more likely to be depressed. Thus concludes Patrick Joseph Lustman, Ph.D., a professor in the psychiatry department at Washington University School of

CONFESSIONS OF A SUGAR KICKER

"My husband tells me I used to be really moody at times and bitchy. We thought it was PMS. But, after my hysterectomy, I was still moody, and I blamed it on hormones. Finally, an internist diagnosed hypoglycemia and told me that eating sugar was causing my mood shifts."

—Ann J., 64, Manson, North Carolina

Medicine, in a review study he conducted of all the research into blood sugar control and depression.

Can Sugar Make You Hostile or Aggressive?

For years, scientists have wondered if diets—specifically those high in sugar and processed carbs—could make people hostile, aggressive, or antisocial, and if avoiding those foods could improve their dispositions. During the 1980s, researchers began looking at more than 8,000 inmates in 14 juvenile penal facilities across the United States.

According to psychologist Alex Schauss, Ph.D.—who has conducted studies on the relationship between crime, sugar, and delinquent behavior—the research showed that if prisoners reduced their consumption of refined sugars, their antisocial behavior was reduced by an average of 50 percent.

Dr. Schauss's interest in the sugar–hostility connection began while he was working with a 15-year-old boy with a long rap sheet. "This child craved sugar to the point that he was eating half a pound a day, and he'd been arrested about 45 times," recalls Dr. Schauss, noting that a psychiatrist did *not* diagnose a psychiatric disorder. About three weeks after the youth began a sugar-restricted diet, he became "really polite," his psychological tests improved, he wasn't arrested during the three years Dr. Schauss tracked him, and he didn't relapse into criminal behavior.

Stunned by the dramatic effects of eliminating sugar from the boy's diet, Dr. Schauss began collecting similar case histories throughout the country, and at the request of chemist and Nobel Prize–winner Dr. Linus Pauling, he summarized his findings in his then-controversial book *Diet, Crime and Delinquency*. This led to further research around the world, including double-blind, placebo-controlled trials in juvenile and adult facilities, which confirmed Dr. Schauss's initial results.

"All the studies unquestionably showed the benefit of restricting refined sugar and low-density 'junk foods.' They found significant declines in antisocial behavior. The scientists revealed, as I have, that sugar and refined foods taken in disproportionate amounts could contribute to antisocial behavior," explains Dr. Schauss, now lead scientist at AIBMR Life Sciences, Inc., in Washington State.

Former Ohio probation officer Barbara Reed Stitt, Ph.D., also used to work with bitter, depressed, angry delinquents, who lived on donuts, pastries, white breads, pasta, canned goods, candy, gallons of coffee, and other junk food carbs. Usually upon a judge's order, she began putting the prisoners on a diet that banned sugar, white-flour products, chemical additives, caffeine, and alcohol, and stressed fresh vegetables, fruits, water, healthy fats, lean meats, and fish.

"The results were astounding," she says. "Their behavior completely changed." A whopping 80 percent of probationers went on to become "productive members of society"—a complete reversal of the typical 70 to 85 percent recidivism rates.

It seems then that for certain people, aggression and blood sugar abnormalities go hand in hand. For example, further research from Finland revealed that the blood sugar levels of violent offenders and aggressive students tended to drop quickly after eating carbohydrates. This made them "more likely to make aggressive comments when faced with a frustrating situation," explains Welsh psychologist Dr. David Benton.

"A similar study with young women revealed that the lower their blood sugar level fell, the more aggressive the women got," Dr. Benton continues. "Even moderate dips in blood sugar levels—those not low enough to be officially deemed hypoglycemic—were linked to irritability and aggression," Dr. Benton found.

Meanwhile, further research in the *American Journal of Psychiatry* shows that children with certain nutritional deficiencies become more aggressive as they grow older—they manifest a 41 percent increase in aggression at age 8 and a 51 percent increase in violent and antisocial behaviors at age 17. Indeed, malnourished children weren't getting crucial minerals like zinc and iron, B vitamins, and protein, which are needed to develop a healthy nervous system and are required for mental and emotional health and stability.

Sugar Could Make You Blue by Robbing Your Body of Chromium and More

Most people mistakenly assume that if they eat sugar and take vitamins at the same time they won't be harmed. "As long as you eat refined sugars, many essential nutrients will be depleted from the body," says Nancy Appleton, Ph.D., author of *Lick the Sugar Habit* and *Stopping Inflammation: Relieving the Cause of Degenerative Diseases*.

"Even *minor* nutritional deficiencies can affect your mood," Dr. Appleton asserts, noting that among their many offenses, excess sweeteners can provoke deficiencies of chromium, copper, and other minerals, and interfere with the absorption of calcium, magnesium, and protein.

Chromium, in particular, is affected by consumption of desserts and processed carbs. "The more sugar and refined carbs you eat, the more likely it is that your diet will be low in essential nutrients such as chromium," says nutritionist Sally Rockwell, Ph.D.

But despite the fact that chromium is available in such diverse foods as liver, oysters, egg yolks, mushrooms, and meat, "90 percent of Americans consume less than 40 micrograms of chromium daily, and the safe dose is thought to be between 50 and 200 micrograms," according to nutritionist Robert Ronzio, Ph.D., C.N.S., F.A.I.C., author of *The Encyclopedia of Nutrition and Good Health*.

As Dr. Rockwell explains, "if you don't have enough chromium in the system, your body can't get enough sugar into the cells. Instead, it gets diverted into fat cells. This means that you'll still want more food even if you're full, so you're eating more sugars, which release more insulin, and then suddenly, your blood sugar drops, and you're in a terrible mood. Some people get violent; some get tired. No two people are the same."

Meanwhile, beginning in the early 1990s, psychiatrists Robert Golden, M.D., and Malcolm McLeod, M.D., both of the University of North Carolina Medical School, found that giving depressed, carb-craving patients chromium supplements improved both their glucose tolerance and their mood. In addition, notes Dr. McLeod, author of *Lifting Depression: The Chromium Connection*, chromium picolinate could have a "dramatic impact on normalizing appetite" and reducing carb cravings.

If You Overeat Carbs, You're Likely Low on Fats, Which Also Affect Mood

If you're loading up on sweets and other fast-acting carbs, you're also probably not getting enough of the valuable omega-3 fatty acids that can lift your spirits. (This beneficial fat is found in such sources as salmon, lake trout, herring, and sardines, as well as olive oil, avocados, walnuts, macadamia nuts, and flaxseed.)

In fact, a four-month pilot study at Baylor College of Medicine and Harvard's Brigham and Women's Hospital in Boston found that depressed patients who took omega-3 fatty acid supplements in addition to antidepressants were four times less likely to suffer recurrent mood symptoms than those who took the medication alone.

"Omega-3 fatty acids play an important role in enhancing mood and easing depression," asserts Andrew Stoll, M.D., one of the study's authors. "Unfortunately, omega-3 fatty acids have been depleted by our Western diet since the early twentieth century. At the same time, the rate of depression in the United States has been increasing, and the age of onset has been decreasing," adds Dr. Stoll, noting that in Japan and other countries where fish consumption is high, both depression and heart disease rates are low.

Biotechnology pioneer Barry Sears, Ph.D., author of the bestselling *Zone* books, also extols fish oil as "the best drug to elevate mood. If you're eating a lot of simple carbohydrates, you're probably not eating much fish. Americans consume only about five percent the amount of fish they did at the turn of the century."

Going Sugar Free Could Wipe Away Emotional Malaise

The bottom line is that, if you become depressed, anxious, or hostile after eating sweets, you could be helped considerably by paying close attention to what you eat. "When sugar-sensitive people eliminate sugar, they experience a lift in mood and feel more energy, less anxiety, and more optimism about the future," Dr. Christensen contends. "They'll just have a better outlook on life."

"It is quite possible to improve your disposition, increase your efficiency, and change your personality for the better," wrote the late endocrinologist John W. Tintera, M.D. "The way to do it is to avoid cane and beet sugar in all forms and guises," added the physician, who alerted people to sugar's potential ill effects as far back as the 1950s.

Of course, not every depressed person can be cured by avoiding sugar and eating healthy fats, but Dr. Christensen estimates that at least 20 percent of people with depression could benefit by eliminating sweets.

Ultimately, many people worldwide are convinced of the need to steer clear of sweets.

"Sugar makes me a completely different person," bemoans Tom J., 41, of Portland, Oregon. "They say sugar is a comfort food. But there's no comfort in it."

12

A Sweet Tooth Could Trash Your Relationships and Sex Life

According to some medical experts and researchers, anywhere from 20 to 50 percent of the U.S. population—59 to 147 million Americans—have volatile blood sugar fluctuations, which could lead to off-putting personality transformations.

Renowned endocrinologist Diana Schwarzbein, M.D., author of *The Schwarzbein Principle* and two follow-up books, is one of many astute physicians anxious to get out the truth that people who are sensitive to sugar can become emotionally unpredictable. "You can get irritable, irrational, and almost paranoid. And you tend to take it out on the person you love the most," Dr. Schwarzbein explains.

Kathleen DesMaisons, Ph.D., a pioneer in the field of addictive nutrition, also observes how sweets can transform certain personalities. "Sugar sensitivity turns a person into Dr. Jekyll and Mr. Hyde," she writes in her bestselling book, *Potatoes, Not Prozac.*

"It's like having two different people live in your body. From one moment to the next, your fine sensitivity and openness turn into moodiness and irritability. Your confidence and creativity dry up, only to be replaced by low self-esteem and hopelessness."

Not only that but "the highs and lows of a sugar addict can make the person seem like an alcoholic," adds nutritionist Dr. Sally Rockwell. "Often, sugar addicts get overwhelmed by a sense of impending doom. They feel miserable, hopeless, and unhappy. And they can eventually destroy their relationships," Dr. Rockwell asserts.

Integrative medical practitioner Elson Haas, M.D., author of *The New Detox Diet*, agrees. "Any sugar overload can lead to anger, emotional outbursts, and overall moodiness. But when people get off sugar, their moods and energy levels are more even keeled, and their relationships improve."

Meanwhile, Dr. Nancy Appleton, author of *Lick the Sugar Habit*, points out that not all sugar junkies respond with anger.

"Sugar upsets your body chemistry and negatively affects *all* your hormones, but every person reacts differently to it," she says. "Some people don't experience mood shifts at all, but they develop physical problems instead. Some become angry and lash out, and still others become depressed and withdraw."

In particular, experts say, those with either low blood sugar (hypoglycemia) or high blood sugar (diabetes and prediabetes) are at risk for wreaking havoc on their relationships. (You'll learn more about both of these conditions in the next two chapters.)

In fact, Roberta Ruggiero, founder and president of the Hypoglycemia Support Foundation, Inc., whose website (www.hypoglycemia.org) receives a million visitors a year, told me she gets deluged with pleas from people around the world to help shed some light on why they lost relationships or how to stop jeopardizing them because of their off-putting hypoglycemic reactions.

"She'll call crying, saying, 'My husband walked out on me because I have constant mood swings and chronic crying spells.' He'll complain, 'My fiancée broke up with me because I fly into irrational rages for no reason.'"

What worries such people is that they just don't know why they're so angry, anxious, and depressed, and they find it shocking to finally learn that what they eat is responsible. "Most people just can't understand that eating a lot of sugar or simple carbs and/or having hypoglycemia can cause all that turmoil and erratic behavior," says Ruggiero, who often provides the impetus for a loved one to seek medical treatment, cut out sweets, and try to salvage his or her relationship.

Recognizing and Stopping Sugar-Influenced Outbursts Improves Relationships

Perhaps the best way to dramatize how the SUGAR SHOCK! epidemic could hamper relationships is to tell hopeful tales of those who feel fortunate to have finally learned, after years of embarrassment, that their sugar habit and subsequent poor-blood-sugar swings could have been to blame for their bizarre behavior.

In my free, online KickSugar group, which I founded in November 2002 to support sugar sufferers worldwide, members regularly experience such "eureka moments" when they finally hit upon their sugar truth and learn that the best way to get their moods under control is to get their blood sugar under control. This means removing quickie carbs, eating better, exercising often, and, if necessary, taking medication.

Take Jo N., 41, of San Francisco, who was in a strained marriage for more than a decade until she found out that she had low blood sugar. Once she made that discovery, she quit sugar, joined a support group, and put an end to her mood swings. "Without my rages, my husband and I get along better, and we communicate more effectively."

Likewise, Michele A., 40, of Plantation, Florida, now has perspective on the sudden, seesawing spurts of anger that used to plague her. The now-happily married health food store manager is far removed from the times she would blow up out of the blue at her ex-boyfriend. She now realizes that, for years, she'd been in a catch-22 situation. "Being in bad relationships made me eat more chocolate to make me happy, but then eating all that chocolate messed up me and my relationships."

Happily for him, Aaron R., 25, of Culver City, California, also had such an epiphany. He now realizes that he must avoid sweets or sugary beverages, because whenever he had them, he became "angry, argumentative, and out of control."

Lest you think that sugar addicts such as Jo, Michele, and Aaron are overstating their Jekyll–Hyde transformations, let's turn to three people who are close to sugar sufferers. Indeed, their versions jibe with those of their loved ones.

For instance, Peter B., 57, of Sausalito, California, says that when his wife, Heidi S., 40, used to eat sweets or much-like-sugar carbs, "she wasn't nearly as even tempered as she is now. She became withdrawn and worried about things."

Tom, 52, similarly describes Steve, 48, his partner of 22 years. "When he was under the spell of sweets, everything would take a backseat to sugar. It was frightening, pronounced, and sinister to see this new person enter his body after he binged on sugar."

Robyn also offers a compelling before-and-after portrait of her dad, Robert F., 43, of Longmont, Colorado, who used to eat a lot of sugar.

"A cloud has lifted off him since he quit sweets," she told me in a phone interview. "He's more charismatic, personable, relaxed, energetic, and funny. And he's much more interested in living life."

Inevitably, wherever you go, you can hear many stories such as these. But most don't end as happily, simply because people don't realize they're in SUGAR SHOCK!

Can Unmanaged Blood Sugar Conditions Lead to Marital Discord?

Experts and sugar sufferers are convinced that one possible reason (of many, of course) for discord and disputes among couples is unrecognized, misdiagnosed, and therefore unmanaged high or low blood sugar.

Cindy*, 51, believes this factor led to her divorce from Carl, 46.

"Whenever he consumed sweets and soft drinks, he got completely out of control. He never hit me, but he would shove me, pull my hair, and scream loudly," recalls Cindy, who is also hypoglycemic.

After Carl nearly passed out twice, his doctor ordered a Glucose Tolerance Test, diagnosed hypoglycemia, and told him to cut out sweets. But he never did quit. "At the time, the doctor told me that hypoglycemia can cause verbal and physical abuse."

Too Many Sweets Could Screw Up Your Sex Life

Naturally, becoming moody, bitchy, detached, or violent won't encourage emotional intimacy with your partner. But that's not all. Some experts believe that eating too many sweets and quickie carbs also could create problems that hinder physical intimacy. In short, your sex life could suffer if you're often in SUGAR SHOCK!—especially for years on end.

For example, Marianne, 33, used to polish off a three-pound bag of red

---

*Henceforth I use pseudonyms in this chapter due to the sensitive nature of the topic: The Sex–Sugar Connection.

licorice in a day or two, often replacing the sweet snacks she sneaked so her husband wouldn't know what she'd done. Then, while consumed by her sugar habit, Marianne admits, she had "zero sex drive." Becoming amorous was the *last* thing on her mind.

"All I wanted to do was sit around and eat candy, not make love. I tried to keep our sex life up enough so that he wasn't miserable and insecure, but I just didn't have much interest."

Soon after stopping her sugar sprees, however, Marianne discovered a surprise benefit—a big rise in libido. "My sex drive improved a lot. I also began to have more energy and fewer headaches. I just felt better all around."

Steve (mentioned above) also found that when he was "in the sugar, sex was the farthest thing" from his mind. "I would even be angry if my partner brought it up. But when I'm not eating sweets, I'm interested in making love."

Marianne and Steve have a lot of company. Indeed, a number of experts speculate that the more some people say *yes* to sweets and processed carbs, the more inclined they are to say *no* to sex. Naturally, I can't promise that your situation will improve if you cut your sugar intake, but this simple change just might help restore your libido.

The Intricate Sugar-Sex Brain Connection

What is it that ties sex and sweets so closely together? Is it merely coincidental that dessert foods provide not only terms of endearment but also euphemisms for sexual partners and sex? Some folks like to call their partners "sugar," "honey," "cupcake," "muffin," and "cookie." In some circles, people talk about getting a "sugar donut" or "a jelly roll" when they're headed for the bed, not the bakery.

It turns out that science supports this sugar-sex link. Highly palatable foods and potent sexual stimuli have something in common. According to neuroscientist and Princeton University professor Bartley G. Hoebel, Ph.D., they both activate our brain's reward pathways and the dopamine system, triggering the release of motivating chemicals.

Small wonder, then, that sugar-seeking folks report that when they gave in to their sugar cravings, their sex drive takes a nosedive. They've already gotten a neurochemical high from chocolate or cake that they would otherwise have received from sex.

"If you ask some women if they'd rather have sex or chocolate, they'll ask you, 'What kind of chocolate?' " half jokingly remarks osteopath Alan Goldhamer, D.O., coauthor of *The Pleasure Trap*.

All That Sugar Can Make It Harder to Get Turned On

Given the pervasiveness and acceptability of sweet foods in our culture, it may be tough to conceive of a connection between eating a bunch of cookies and a soda and losing interest in sex, but some experts insist that it can, indeed, happen.

"When you put an overdose of sugar into your body, glucose just burns the system out, overtaking the adrenal glands, stressing the kidneys, and leading to low glucose, which can affect the brain," says integrative physician Keith DeOrio, M.D.

"The brain is really the commanding general for the whole body: It controls sex drive, desire, and orgasm, as well as blood flow. So if it's not being properly fed, it can lead to low libido, inability to achieve orgasm, low sperm count, and infertility."

Cardiologist Patrick Fratellone, M.D., executive medical director of Fratellone Medical Associates, agrees that eating a lot of sweets can lower your sex drive. Diabetics are particularly prone to problems, says the former executive medical director of the Atkins Center for Complementary Medicine.

Reproductive endocrinologist Deborah Metzger, M.D., Ph.D., a leading expert in the field of fertility and reproductive health, also believes that eliminating or cutting back on sweets could help resolve sexual dysfunction problems for both women and men.

"I'd say 60 percent of the women I see exist on sugar and caffeine, and they all complain of fatigue and lack of sex drive," observes the medical director of Los Altos, California–based Harmony Women's Health.

"When you're not feeling good, your sex drive is one of the first things to go. But there's hope. When these women go on a diet that's low in sugar and simple carbs, their fatigue fades away and their sex drive improves," adds Dr. Metzger, medical advisor to the book *Stay Fertile Longer*.

Meanwhile, internist Steven Lamm, M.D., a clinical assistant professor in internal medicine at New York University and author of *The Hardness*

Factor, points to another problem tied to excessive consumption of sugar and much-like-sugar carbs.

"The long-term effects of becoming overweight or obese certainly will have a negative effect on sexuality," asserts Dr. Lamm. "Men need to understand that if they want to be harder, they have to be healthier."

Let's say a man has gained 10 to 20 pounds over time because of his sugar or carb habit and he's headed toward insulin resistance or metabolic syndrome. How would that affect him in the bedroom?

"His ability to perform at the highest efficiency is going to start to diminish over time," explains Dr. Lamm in a phone interview. "He will have performance issues. It'll be more difficult for him to get an erection, to maintain one, and there will be longer times between erections. Excessive weight is a major contributor to decreased sexual performance.

"Ultimately, obesity and disorders such as metabolic syndrome affect the erection quality by promoting decrease in blood flow or circulation and affecting hormone level," says Dr. Lamm, who advises his patients to cut down on their intake of sugar and fast-acting carbs.

James Chow, M.D., coauthor of *Hypoglycemia for Dummies*, however, sees the sugar-sex connection as more indirect.

"As far as I know, there are no studies to suggest that eating too much sugar can trigger sexual dysfunction," explains Dr. Chow, chief medical officer for the Nippon Clinic, which has offices in New York, Chicago, Atlanta, and San Diego.

"But diabetes is known to lead to impotence and sexual dysfunction. So if eating excess sugar is one of the many factors that can lead to diabetes (and this seems to be a possibility in people who have a family history of diabetes), then sugar may be implicated in sexual dysfunction, albeit in a roundabout way."

Doesn't Sugar Sometimes *Increase* Libido Rather Than Decrease It? Only Briefly.

If you're in your teens or twenties and you're a huge soda drinker or cookie muncher, it may be hard to imagine that your sugar habit could put a damper on your sex life. Ironically, eating lots of sweets might actually appear to benefit your bedroom life.

"Initially, sugar can increase sexual desire," explains Dr. Schwarzbein. "In the early phases of sugar addiction, you're not going to complain of sexual problems, but later on, down the road, in, say, 10 to 15 years, sugar can burn out your system so you have sexual problems."

Naura Hayden, author of eight books, including the number-one *New York Times* bestseller *How to Satisfy a Woman Every Time . . . and Have Her Beg for More!,* is also convinced that as sugar intake increases, sexual desire and satisfaction decrease. A hypoglycemic herself, Hayden kicked sugar and found that after doing so, she overcame her tension, anxiety, and depression and achieved greater sexual pleasure.

"Eating a lot of sugar affects every cell in your body, particularly your brain," she told me. "If your brain doesn't function properly, then your sex organs won't function well, either," contends Hayden, referring to the fact that our brain cells need consistently managed blood sugar levels for nourishment.

"A lot of sweets will make you more tense and anxious, then depressed and more on edge with your beloved," she adds. "If you're tense, that's not conducive to a really loving, warm, close relationship, and you won't be receptive. Great sex is best in a relaxed, receptive, loving body. When you're calm, it's much easier to have an orgasm."

Diabetes and Sexual Problems

As Dr. Chow, Dr. Lamm, Hayden, and others have noted, decreased libido isn't the only way wildly swinging blood sugar levels can screw up your sex life. Particularly for men, the sexual organs work best when blood glucose stays within a normal range. When those levels are either too high or too low, your body may lose its ability to perform up to snuff.

The dilemma of male diabetics is best illustrated by an intimate incident described by Nancy. "I was getting involved with a guy, and the first (and last) time we went to bed together, he couldn't get it up. Of course, I tried to be supportive and nonchalant, but by the way he acted, I could tell that this problem was old hat to him. He offhandedly told me that his diabetes made it tough for him to get an erection. But if that's the case, then why did he eat so poorly?"

Actually, it's well known among physicians and sufferers themselves that both men and women with diabetes have a much greater chance than healthy people of developing sexual dysfunction. It's been extensively documented that diabetic men have a higher-than-normal risk of developing erectile dysfunction (ED).

In fact, diabetes is one of the greatest risk factors for ED, which is the inability to attain or maintain an erection sufficient for sexual intercourse. Data show that *complete* erectile dysfunction affects about one-third of men with type 2 diabetes—three to four times the nondiabetic male population. In addition, about 50 percent of men with diabetes experience *some* degree of sexual dysfunction, according to Kenneth Snow, M.D., director of the Sexual Function Clinic at the Joslin Diabetes Center in Boston. The National Institute of Diabetes and Digestive and Kidney Diseases (NIDDK) and the National Diabetes Information Clearinghouse put their estimate at between 35 and 50 percent, and other experts say the number could go as high as 75 percent.

When diabetes is uncontrolled, the high levels of blood sugar can damage the tiny capillaries that carry blood to the spongy cylinders of penile tissue that need to become turgid with blood for an erection to occur, so no blood, no erection. High blood glucose also causes nerve damage that can not only trigger numbness in the feet and hands but can also affect the penis, interfering with the nerve signals that help orchestrate male sexual arousal.

For a healthy male, some stimulation—by sight, touch, sound, or something else—activates the nerves and causes muscles to relax and blood to flow into the penis, which then becomes erect. But a man with diabetes who isn't properly managing his disease can't have an erection or maintain it long enough for satisfactory sex. Finally, male diabetics may experience a reduction in testosterone levels, which also affects their ability to have an erection.

So where does excess sugar intake fit into this equation? In order for diabetic men to have a satisfying sex life, they must keep their blood glucose at normal levels. But while cutting out sweets and refined processed sugars might help, "no one should make the leap that if you eat a good diet, you can control diabetes," Dr. Snow says.

"A therapeutic regimen is much more than a diet. Exercise, diet, insulin levels, and medication when appropriate all need to be in balance to control diabetes," he adds, noting that for men who monitor well, the rate of impotence falls to 30 percent. On the flip side, however, the risk of erectile dysfunction dramatically *increases* if a man with diabetes doesn't tightly control glucose levels.

But it's not just diabetic men who are at risk for sexual dysfunction. Up to

35 percent of women with diabetes also experience sexual dysfunction, according to the Joslin Diabetes Center. In females, as with males, high blood glucose is often to blame, as well as damage to the nerves and the small capillaries that feed the vagina. According to one Swedish study, women with diabetes reported difficulties feeling desire, experiencing arousal, and achieving orgasm, and also reported pain during intercourse. One common complaint is decreased vaginal lubrication, which can lead to sexual discomfort. In addition, female diabetics also have frequent bouts of vaginitis (inflammation of the vagina) and yeast infections, both of which can affect their ability to have sex.

You'll learn more about diabetes and the "chronic big killers" in chapter 14, but it's especially important for people at risk—those who are overweight or obese and who have a family history of diabetes—to quit or cut back on quickie carbs and exercise regularly.

Sex Problems Plague Many with Hypoglycemia

Hypoglycemics also cope with an increase in sexual dysfunction. In fact, most books about low blood sugar cite "impotence" and "lack of sex drive" as common symptoms. One study of thousands of hypoglycemics conducted by Stephen Gyland, M.D., whose work is discussed in chapter 13, found that 44 percent of female hypoglycemics lose their libido and 29 percent of males have impotency problems.

"Women who are hypoglycemic could have an inability to have an orgasm," says Richard Ash, M.D., who has treated thousands of hypoglycemics at the Ash Center for Comprehensive Medicine in New York City.

Intimacy can be especially problematic when both partners are hypoglycemic, as was the case with Cindy and Carl, whom we met earlier. Before finding out that she was hypoglycemic, Cindy would eat a cupcake or donut for breakfast, a cheeseburger and French fries for lunch, a milkshake or hot fudge sundae in midafternoon, fried chicken with high-starch foods for dinner, and dry cereal or lots of chocolate after dinner. "At the time, I couldn't care less if I ever had sex," she recalls.

Now that she's off sugar and eating more healthily, Cindy is more interested in making love—but she's now divorced. "Before, I didn't want sex; now I think about it every day. It surprises me that getting off sugar could make that kind of difference."

When they were married, Carl also was rarely in the mood for sex. "He'd eat lots of starches for dinner, and then by seven that evening, he'd conk out. He didn't want to make love after he ate. Then, he'd wake up by one or two in the morning when I was asleep, and he'd grab a sweet roll or an oatmeal cake.

"Occasionally, when he was interested in making love, he wanted to do it in the morning, but he wouldn't last more than two to three minutes. I suspect that his hypoglycemia had something to do with it," confides Cindy, who, before the divorce, was too embarrassed to discuss the couple's sexual problems with a doctor.

Like Cindy, Katarina, 30, of Perth, Australia, also experienced a huge increase in her libido after she pulled the plug on her sugar habit because of her hypoglycemia.

"I think it's mainly because I have more energy and don't feel like an unattractive whale," she confesses. "I'm not overweight, but when I eat sugar, it puffs me up and makes me look like I'm pregnant. I feel irritable and grumpy, and sex even becomes painful due to all the bloating in my abdomen.

"Normally, we didn't even get to the sex part since we both knew it wasn't worth it, and it would just end up frustrating both of us. Also, when I used to overindulge in sugar, I suffered a lot from thrush [yeast infection], so that put a damper on things, too." Now that she's no longer eating sweets, Katarina reports, she's "a much more confident, happy person and more interested in making love."

Experts say that hypoglycemics often don't have the energy for sex because when their blood sugar is low, they're left with an adrenal insufficiency, their fight-or-flight response has been quelled, and they're simply too weak to do it.

But take a tip from Meghan: "I find the best time for sex is after a meal—maybe not right after—but within an hour for sure. I have the most energy during this time and don't have to worry about my blood sugar falling."

Hypoglycemia for Dummies author Dr. Chow also thinks it's better to eat a healthy meal before jumping into bed with a partner. "For blood-sugar-sensitive people, I would recommend not doing it on an empty stomach," he advises.

Since people with prediabetes, diabetes, and hypoglycemia may be prone to sexual dysfunction problems, experts insist that they should closely monitor their blood sugar levels. To have great sex, they advise, folks with blood sugar issues should closely monitor their diet, exercise regularly, and take proper medication when appropriate.

If you're still reluctant to give up sweets for the sake of your love life, then perhaps sex author Naura Hayden can convince you. "Believe me, the moment's ecstasy of eating a creamy chocolate bar is nothing compared to the longer-lasting ecstasy you get from great sex when you're *not* eating sugar—and the even longer happiness of a calm and relaxed body."

The Link between Sugar, Obesity, Self-Image, and Loss of Libido

All sexual problems related to sugar and quickie carbs aren't, however, caused by mood swings or organic malfunctions. Indeed, because overindulging can lead to obesity, both poor self-image and accompanying loss of libido may also keep a woman or man from enjoying sexual intimacy.

"When I was heavier, I felt self-conscious and unattractive and didn't enjoy sex," confesses Patricia, a now-slim former sugar addict, who enjoys intimacy with her boyfriend. "I had no interest in it, and I couldn't see why anyone would be interested in me."

Meanwhile, 36-year-old Arlene, who used to binge on pork rinds, chocolate, pasta, and breads, sums up the sexual dilemma facing obese people: "I mean, who wants to be rolling around in a bed and feel chunks of fat rolling around with her or him?

"You don't like the way you look, and you're afraid the other person is not going to like the way you look, and even if he does, you still feel that way yourself," says the five-foot, eight-inch woman, whose weight once climbed to a high of 270.

Now divorced, Arlene has lost a great deal of weight, has begun to feel good about herself again, and has started to miss sex. "I have the desire all right—even more so since I lost weight."

For Many, Keeping Happy Relationships Motivates Them to Kick Sweets

Many former sugar addicts such as those you've heard from here wish they'd treated their loved ones better during the times they were hooked on sweets.

Certainly, they could have if they'd known that sugar was to blame for their blues and belligerence.

Now that you've heard from experts and sugar-sensitive people who link mood plunges and loss of libido to their intake of quickie carbs, I invite you to explore this connection. Does eating sweets (a little or a lot) turn you or your significant other into a Sugar Shrew, Sugar Monster, Sugar Zombie, or Sugar Crybaby?

Even if you're unsure about the link, I urge you to set your sights on a loving outcome. If you lower your intake of quickie carbs, your relationships could become more harmonious, and you could build a better bedroom life. What better offer is there than that?

PART 5

HOW EXCESS SWEETS CAN SABOTAGE YOUR HEALTH

It Might *Not* Be "All in Your Head": What Your Doctor Doesn't Know or Believe about Hypoglycemia

"Bipolar II with psychotic episodes." That's the diagnosis a psychiatrist handed Stephanie B. of Chico, California, when she was 23 years old.

By the time a psychiatric hospital rendered the "bipolar" verdict, Stephanie had spent a decade trying to pinpoint the cause of her depression, mania, panic attacks, anxiety, fatigue, temper outbursts, excitability, psychotic-like episodes, confusion, concentration problems, and headaches. These symptoms disabled her so thoroughly that at times she couldn't get out of bed and she had to drop out of school four times.

Physicians, psychologists, and psychiatrists were particularly mystified by Stephanie's strange, scary panic attacks—like the time when, after skipping a meal and rushing to a physics class, her legs wouldn't budge and she felt stuck in the deep end of a swimming hole. Or the incident when she started to hyperventilate while driving down a six-lane highway, developed "extreme tunnel vision," and had to pull over to avoid a collision with an oncoming car.

Doctors prescribed medications to help her cope—a litany of drugs that reads like a pharmacology manual: Zoloft, Depakote, Risperidol, Imipramine, Klonopin, BuSpar, Paxil, Trazodone, Ativan, and Ambien. But the meds helped to bring about another problem. In a year and a half, the 5-foot, 10-inch Stephanie ballooned from "anorexic looking" to 215 pounds.

Curiously, not one in the succession of doctors she saw *ever* asked Stephanie about her diet, which included many inferior, fiber-stripped, nutrient-poor, empty-calorie dessert foods and processed carbs and starches such as pasta, corn tortillas, corn chips, blueberry muffins, sweet rolls, cookies, smoothies, croissants, pizza, and bagels.

On several occasions, she even asked her doctors if she had a blood sugar problem. "I'd explain that if I didn't eat at crucial moments in my day, I'd turn irritable and get a devastating headache. But the doctors paid no attention," she recalls. "Once in a while, they'd give me a blood test right then—when I wasn't having any symptoms—and, of course, my results would come back normal."

Meanwhile, as her twenties slipped by, Stephanie's distress continued, especially near that time of month. "I was putting everything down to PMS," she says. "I'd have horrible mood swings, cramps, bloating, and migraines for a week out of every cycle. One day, I got so upset with my husband that I slapped him across the face for no reason." Her new gynecologist's startling answer to her mood woes? "He kneeled down, took my hand in his, pressed it against his forehead, and prayed for me," she recalls with disbelief.

Finally, in 2002, just before her 31st birthday, after some 20 years of anguish and agony, Stephanie learned the cause of her problems, but not from a medical doctor. Instead, a nutritionally savvy acupuncturist who'd been treating her for a dog bite suspected that Stephanie might have reactive hypoglycemia or low blood sugar caused by her diet high in sugars and refined carbs.

Almost immediately, Stephanie stopped eating processed carbs and desserts. Instead she had meals and snacks with protein, healthy fats, vegetables, some low-sugar fruits, and whole grains. Within days, her health dramatically improved.

"Eating right banished all my symptoms including depression and mood swings," she marvels. "It even helped me get rid of my constant hunger and excess weight. And I've discovered a whole new world of tasty, healthy foods."

Hypoglycemia: "The Great Imitator"

Stephanie's story is not so unusual. Quite the opposite.

In fact, I believe, as do a number of experts, that reactive hypoglycemia is one of the most common and most misunderstood disorders in America today. For starters, many physicians assume that ailments such as mood swings, fatigue, and anxiety are manifestations of psychological problems.

Moreover, hypoglycemia has been called the "Great Imitator" because its strange, startling symptoms—some experts list as many as 125 of them—can mimic a frightening array of diseases and conditions, including bipolar disorder, schizophrenia, neurosis, migraines, Parkinson's syndrome, chronic bronchial asthma, paroxysmal tachycardia (rapid heartbeat), rheumatoid arthritis, cerebral arteriosclerosis (hardening of the brain's arteries), menopause, mental retardation, alcoholism, hyperactive disorder, and senility.

Given the vast array of symptoms and the confusion they can generate, doctors often shrug away patients' complaints as the imaginings of a hypochondriac in dire need of psychiatric help.

"Every time I went to the doctor for any reason, he or she would do a few tests and then tell me that it was 'all in my head,'" laments Linda K. of Gatesville, Texas. "The doctors would say that I was extremely healthy and then try to get me to set up an appointment with a psychologist or psychiatrist. I would get very mad and hardly ever go to the doctor, because I knew they would find nothing, and then I'd just feel really stupid.

"I must have had hypoglycemia all my life, but I wasn't diagnosed until I was 34. And then my doctor *never* told me about my diagnosis until *after* I called to tell him I'd had a major anxiety attack and had no clue what in the world was happening to me."

Stephanie's, Linda's, and my stories are typical of many people with reactive hypoglycemia: We get misdiagnosed again and again in a cycle that could continue for decades unless we're lucky enough to find a knowledgeable, open-minded health practitioner.

Obviously, not all patients with anxiety, depression, heart palpitations, migraines, and other symptoms have hypoglycemia—they could have other very real conditions—but if they do have low blood sugar, it can be a revelation and relief to learn about it.

So what exactly is this medical condition that fools so many doctors so easily and leaves agonized patients without relief for years? First of all, remember that our bodies—and especially our brains—need glucose to survive. Low blood sugar or "hypoglycemia" ("hypo" meaning low and "glycemia" meaning blood sugar) means that your blood glucose drops too low for you to be able to go about your daily activities.

This can happen because your body uses up glucose too rapidly, releases it into the bloodstream too slowly, or calls upon your pancreas to manufacture too much insulin. (Remember that insulin is the vital hormone that removes sugar from your bloodstream.) When any of these things happen, your blood glucose becomes abnormally low, and you become confused, irritable, spacey, lightheaded, and more.

This glucose deprivation also causes many people to become *famished*. But it doesn't stop at hunger. "Perhaps most importantly, low blood sugar triggers an outpouring of counterregulatory hormones, mostly from the adrenals," observes Ronald Hoffman, M.D., founder of the Hoffman Center in New York City, host of the nationally syndicated radio program *Health Talk*, and author of *Tired All the Time?*

"These hormones oppose the action of insulin and push blood sugar back up. Unfortunately for the hypoglycemic, these 'rescue' hormones are the very same ones that produce the adrenaline rush of a fight-or-flight reaction. The results are symptoms like heart palpitations, sweaty palms, nervousness, tremor, and sometimes even full-blown panic attacks," Dr. Hoffman explains.

Hypoglycemia's Historical Highlights

To help you better understand this condition, a quick historical look is in order. Hypoglycemia was discovered in 1924 by Seale Harris, M.D., a year after the Canadian physician Frederick Banting, M.D., received a Nobel Prize for finding a way to extract the hormone insulin, which could help diabetics control the abnormal amounts of sugar in their blood.

Dr. Harris, a professor of medicine at the University of Alabama, observed that many people who were *not* diabetic and *not* taking insulin were also experiencing symptoms of insulin shock, which was at the time believed to be only caused by an insulin overdose. But he found that these nondiabetic people also were having an insulin overdose, which sent their blood sugar plummeting, leading to low levels of glucose in their blood.

In other words, Dr. Harris discovered that a diabetic's dilemma (underproduction of insulin) has a complementary problem: hyperinsulinism (excessive insulin in the blood). He officially reported his discovery, declaring low levels of glucose in the blood to be symptoms of hyperinsulinism (now more commonly referred to as hypoglycemia). He also found that patients with low-blood-sugar symptoms had been wrongly treated for such diverse conditions as hysteria, brain tumor, coronary thrombosis, epilepsy, mental disorders, gall bladder disease, appendicitis, asthma, allergies, ulcers, and alcoholism.

"Dr. Harris pointed out that the cure for low blood glucose or *hyperinsulinism* . . . was something so simple that nobody—not even the medical practitioners—could make any money out of it," William Dufty recounts in *Sugar Blues*.

"The remedy was self-government of the body. The patient with low blood glucose must be prepared to give up refined sugar, candy, coffee, and soft drinks—these items had caused the troubles. Patients with hyperinsulinism could never be made dependent for a lifetime on anybody else," Dufty writes. "They had to fend for themselves. A doctor could merely teach them what to do. Hyperinsulinism or low blood glucose therapy was a do-it-yourself proposition."

"The medical profession landed on Dr. Harris like a ton of bricks. When his findings were not attacked, they were ignored," Dufty goes on. "His discoveries, if allowed to leak out, might make trouble for surgeons, psychoanalysts, and other medical specialists. To this day, hyperinsulinism or low blood glucose is a stepchild of the disease establishment," he concludes.

The Medical Community Brands Hypoglycemia a Nondisease

Here's where hypoglycemia's history becomes even more baffling. In 1949, the AMA finally honored Dr. Harris with the Distinguished Service Medal, its highest scientific award, for the research that led to his discovery of hypoglycemia. "But then in 1973, the American Medical Association did a complete 180-degree turnaround and labeled hypoglycemia a nondisease," points out Roberta Ruggiero, founder and president of the Hypoglycemia Support Foundation, Inc.

Apparently, this dismissive attitude toward low blood sugar came about, at least in part, because in the late 1960s and 1970s, hypoglycemia hit the limelight, Ruggiero recalls.

"It was considered the 'in' health condition, but the problem was that hypoglycemia was used to explain away some of humanity's worst ills, with little or no scientific backing. Many people proclaimed themselves hypoglycemic without bothering to consult a doctor or get a Glucose Tolerance Test. The backlash in the medical establishment was swift."

So a mere 25 years after paying tribute to Dr. Harris for his contributions to medicine by identifying hyperinsulinism or hypoglycemia, the AMA, along with the American Diabetes Association and the Endocrine Society, sent an alarmist "Statement on Hypoglycemia" to the prestigious *Journal of the American Medical Association* to rectify "possible widespread misunderstanding."

The letter announced: "Recent publicity in the popular press has led the public to believe that there is a widespread and unrecognized occurrence of hypoglycemia in this country. Furthermore, it has been suggested repeatedly that the condition is causing many of the common symptoms that affect the American population. These claims are not supported by medical evidence.

"Hypoglycemia means low blood sugar," the letter continued. "When it occurs, it is often attended by symptoms of sweating, shakiness, trembling, anxiety, fast heart action, headache, hunger sensations, brief feelings of weakness, and, occasionally, seizures and coma. However, the majority of people with these kinds of symptoms do not have hypoglycemia."

After that damning, formal "hypoglycemia-is-rare" verdict reached the ears of medical doctors nationwide, they became more closed to the possibility that the condition even existed. Therefore, when patients approached mainstream physicians with suspicions of hypoglycemia, they were often dismissed as misguided and silly.

But a number of open-minded doctors have been standing up for suffering hypoglycemics worldwide. For one, the late Harvey Ross, M.D., the psychiatrist who cowrote *Hypoglycemia: The Classic Healthcare Handbook*, was outraged, dismayed, and troubled by his profession's disdainful attitude.

"For some obscure reasons, which I am unable to understand, a number of physicians refuse to admit that there is such a thing as hypoglycemia," Dr. Ross laments in his book, *Fighting Depression: How to Lift the Cloud That Darkens Millions of Lives.*

Hypoglycemics, he further bemoans, "are sent to psychiatrists after their own physicians have listened to all the varied complaints and have found no other reason for the symptoms than that the patient must be a hypochondriac."

The Doctors of Disbelief

Now, more than eight decades after hypoglycemia's discovery, many—if not most—physicians still think it *unlikely* that your symptoms and your habit of eating sweets and inferior carbs are linked to low blood sugar. *The American Medical Association Family Medical Guide* (Third Edition, 1994) sums up the attitude of many mainstream doctors in one brief sentence: "[Hypoglycemia] occurs most exclusively in people with diabetes mellitus."

Why are physicians so reluctant to identify this condition? "We haven't been teaching our physicians correctly," explains endocrinologist Diana Schwarzbein, M.D. "They're used to identifying diseases with known causes," she points out. "Doctors have no problem believing in hypoglycemia when it's 'disease related'—say, liver or kidney failure, or tumors in the pancreas.

"Here is what usually happens: You go to see your doctor, and you have symptoms while in the doctor's office. Even if you have your blood sugar level drawn *during your low-blood-sugar episode*, it will be normal because the symptoms are caused by your body's response to your dropping blood sugar levels, not the low levels themselves," Dr. Schwarzbein continues.

"You have to understand that if your sugar really were to drop critically low, that would cause seizures and incompatibility with life. That is why your body goes into emergency mode and counters the drop in blood sugar levels by secreting your stress hormones. That is what causes the symptoms of hypoglycemia. So most doctors' ideas of hypoglycemia are about people going into comas and having seizures, and then being able to document it by saying, 'Look, the blood sugar was 30.'

"When a patient with reactive hypoglycemia consults a doctor, the only evidence he can present is a *syndrome*—a collection of symptoms that often occur together but for which there is no known cause. And many things," Dr. Schwarzbein adds, "can trigger those symptoms—skipping meals, eating too much sugar, overexercising, or becoming very, very stressed."

When asked why doctors discount reactive hypoglycemia's existence, Dr. James Chow, coauthor of *Hypoglycemia for Dummies*, notes that "part of the reason is that there are no viruses or anything concrete that one can point to, and the symptoms are too general and nonspecific.

"Also, hypoglycemia is *not a disease* per se, but a *condition* that is managed through dietary and lifestyle changes—*not* something doctors are taught in medical school. If it's not a disease entity for which they can write a prescription, then they don't think it exists," he observes.

Paltry Nutrition Education for Physicians

Interestingly, critics claim that one of the main reasons physicians aren't adept at identifying hypoglycemia, malnutrition, or other nutrition-related illnesses is because the nutrition education they receive in medical school is quite lacking.

"Nutrition training in medical schools is almost nonexistent to substandard," decries renowned alternative medicine practitioner Andrew Weil, M.D., author of the national bestsellers *Spontaneous Healing* and *8 Weeks to Optimum Health*, and other books.

"I've looked at what they teach. Most of the nutrition is buried in biochemistry courses. Students memorize the information and then forget it as soon as the exams are over. The training still lasts just a few hours," says Dr. Weil, who admits that he himself "received essentially no education in nutrition in four years of Harvard Medical School and an internship" but pursued further nutrition training on his own. "It's fair to say that the majority of physicians are functionally [nutritionally] illiterate," he concludes.

Physician Fred Pescatore, M.D., who, in addition to his medical degree, received training to become a certified clinical nutritionist (C.C.N.), also decries the nutrition training would-be doctors get, calling it "completely inadequate and quite appalling."

"Most physicians are nutritionally unbalanced themselves," contends Dr. Pescatore, who is president of the International and American Association of Clinical Nutritionists, an organization that believes nutrition plays a major role in health.

"When you go to a physician who's not properly trained and expect to get expert nutritional advice, you're only fooling yourself."

In fact, for the 1979–1980 academic year, only 12 of 126 medical schools in the United States had required nutrition courses, according to the Association of American Medical Colleges (AAMC). By the 2004–2005 school year, 123 of 125 medical schools offered at least one *required* nutrition course, and 67 schools offered separate *elective* courses, the AAMC found. In addition, some nutrition is couched in other school courses.

While at first glance it appears that tremendous progress has been made, a closer look reveals that the amount of nutritional training is quite minimal and usually not enough for doctors to easily diagnose certain nutrition-related conditions such as hypoglycemia. What's more, the quality of the courses are suspect, according to experts such as Dr. Weil and Dr. Pescatore.

"Even though medical schools have started to offer courses, the ones that they give are inadequate at best," Dr. Pescatore maintains. "They're still tied to [the] dogma of the USDA, which is not meant to make humans healthy but meant to increase the bottom lines of businesses that supply unhealthy food to the population.

"For example, there's a $2 billion subsidized sugar industry. Everywhere along that food chain, people are getting rich, because sugar sells for so cheap. But while sugar has a high profit margin, there's not a high profit margin in organic foods."

The Tragedy of Misdiagnosis: Two Tales of Unnecessary Suffering

One of the saddest and biggest tragedies of modern medicine is that many people suffering from typical symptoms of hypoglycemia are dismissed by their doctors as hypochondriacs or mentally unhinged. Worse yet, they're given diagnoses that are erroneous, if not ludicrous. You'll better grasp the full extent of the situation by learning about two such unnecessary nightmares.

The first horrific tale involves the late Stephen Gyland, M.D., who, in the early 1950s, suffered from anxiety, dizziness, memory loss, weakness, concentration difficulties, tremors, and rapid heartbeat, among other symptoms. For three years, he consulted 14 specialists at three nationally known clinics, who labeled his ailments multiple sclerosis, neurosis, brain tumor, diabetes, and cerebral arteriosclerosis.

One physician even had the audacity to tell Dr. Gyland that "he was neurotic and ought to retire for the good of the profession," writes William Dufty in *Sugar Blues*. Another doctor issued the *correct* diagnosis but the *wrong* prescription: He recommended candy bars, which only worsened Dr. Gyland's symptoms.

When Dr. Gyland happened upon Dr. Harris's original 1924 medical paper about hypoglycemia and subsequently took a Glucose Tolerance Test, he learned that he had low blood sugar—*not* those other diseases. He banished refined sugar and processed carbs from his diet, and his symptoms quickly faded away.

Angered by his unnecessary suffering and that of others like him, Dr. Gyland blasted off a letter to the *Journal of the American Medical Association* in 1953, reproaching his colleagues for overlooking Dr. Harris's pioneering discovery.

Dr. Gyland then went on to treat more than 1,000 hypoglycemic patients and compile an exhaustive study. (His oft-cited list of symptoms is included at the end of this chapter.) But his groundbreaking discoveries went unnoticed. Although he was allowed to read his study before an AMA-associated medical society, it never appeared in any AMA publication and landed instead in a Brazilian medical journal—written in Portuguese.

The second misdiagnosis illustrates that false, misleading medical labels can not only cause delays in proper treatment, but can also result in prescriptions for the wrong drugs and treatment, and even lead to downright dangerous outcomes.

Roberta Ruggiero spent a decade consulting many physicians to find out why she had anxiety, fatigue, crying spells, heart palpitations, headaches, depression, cold hands and feet, and a host of other scary symptoms.

"I was very embarrassed and ashamed because I thought I might be going crazy," says Ruggiero, who submitted to a battery of medical exams, including spinal taps and brain-wave tests. "The doctors kept saying, 'There's nothing wrong with you. All the tests are negative.'"

Over the years, Ruggiero saw a string of psychiatrists who recommended Valium, Mellaril, and Thorazine. Finally, in 1969, when meds didn't help, one doctor suggested another type of treatment.

"I didn't even ask what it was. I was willing to try anything," says Ruggiero, who had no idea that she'd soon be having horrific hospital experiences to rival those in *One Flew Over the Cuckoo's Nest*. Indeed, she was so overcome by frightening ailments that she unknowingly committed herself to a psychiatric facility.

"You'd hear screams, and all these people would come out with a dazed, almost-ghostlike look on their faces. I didn't think I belonged there, but then I began to wonder if I did," recalls Ruggiero, who was injected with muscle relaxants and anesthetics, strapped down by her ankles and hands, and administered electroshock therapy. Nowadays, she calls the dreadful, frightening, unnecessary experience "barbaric." Not surprisingly, electroshock didn't help her low-blood-sugar symptoms one bit.

Although Ruggiero's experiences were extreme, it's not uncommon for hypoglycemics, before being diagnosed, to have been deemed mentally unhinged. Then, once they remove the offending sweets, their personalities often return to normal.

Meanwhile, as is the experience of so many misdiagnosed hypoglycemics, *none* of Ruggiero's doctors *ever* asked her what she was eating, which was "every sugary thing you could think of—hot fudge sundaes, apple pies, chocolate Yankee Doodles, Devil Dogs, you name it." While taking care of her two babies, she also often skipped breakfast and lunch.

Finally, in 1971, after passing out in church, Ruggiero reluctantly saw yet another doctor, who ordered a Glucose Tolerance Test and subsequently identified severe reactive hypoglycemia. "But all he did was give me one sheet of paper with very [few] instructions. It said, 'Cut out junk food and eat properly.' I was like, 'What do I do now?' I had to go educate myself.

"I thought he was crazy to tell me that all I needed to do was change my diet," Ruggiero recalls. "Who knew? I didn't know what a protein was. I'd never heard of a carbohydrate, much less that there were 'good' or 'bad' carbs. 'Nutrition' wasn't even in my vocabulary. Now I realize that I was addicted to sugar and fast-acting carbs due to convenience and ignorance."

For years after her diagnosis, Ruggiero sought out "every bit of information" she could find about low blood sugar. Finally, in 1980, a decade after her diagnosis, she founded the nonprofit Hypoglycemia Support Foundation to help, encourage, and educate hypoglycemics.

"I'm tired of hearing that hypoglycemia doesn't exist. It is real. My goal is to bring knowledge of low blood sugar to the forefront of medicine, where

AN EXPERT'S TAKE ON LOW BLOOD SUGAR

"I have seen so many unhappy, distressed, and miserable individuals whose lives have been wrecked—virtually destroyed—by hypoglycemia."
—Paavo Airola, N.D., Ph.D., author, *Hypoglycemia: A Better Approach*

it belongs," says Ruggiero, whose popular www.hypoglycemia.org website annually draws about a million visitors from around the world.

Those of us who've pointlessly agonized for years, like Ruggiero, Dr. Gyland, and myself, are aghast, dumbstruck, and horrified by the traditional medical profession's dismissive stance toward reactive hypoglycemia.

Dr. Harvey Ross, coauthor of *Hypoglycemia: The Classic Healthcare Handbook*, aptly sums up the sad situation: "How much needless suffering could be relieved but goes on because some physicians will not consider alternatives?"

To This Day, Misdiagnosis Often Occurs

Nowadays, if you ask most doctors, they'll tell you that hypoglycemic symptoms mainly strike diabetics who take too much insulin or other diabetes medications, skip meals, don't eat enough, exercise too much, or drink excessive alcohol. But what you've been reading about here is non-diabetes-related *reactive* or *functional* hypoglycemia. The condition is also called *postprandial* (or after meals) hypoglycemia and *idiopathic reactive* hypoglycemia—the last meaning that doctors don't know what causes it.

Other kinds of hypoglycemia include *fasting* (postabsorptive) hypoglycemia, which could be due to underlying pathological conditions such as certain tumors, liver disease, critical illnesses, hormonal deficiencies, organ failure, genetic conditions, too much alcohol, or certain medications, and *relative* hypoglycemia, a rare condition that infants can get and that can be treated in the hospital.

Reactive hypoglycemia, however, is not usually related to an underlying disease. In fact, many experts argue that when it occurs with no related pathology, it almost always results from eating too many sweets or inferior muchlike-sugar carbs.

More Sugar *Cannot* Resolve Low Blood Sugar or SUGAR SHOCK!

Most people—and many in the medical profession—erroneously believe that the logical approach to treating reactive hypoglycemia or low blood sugar is to advise a patient who starts feeling the wretched symptoms to eat more sugar and more quickie carbs. Of course, you're now hip to the fact that this is *wrong*. Even though diabetics need handy glucose tablets or sweet snack foods to take at the first sign of insulin shock, you must understand that hypoglycemics require different treatment.

In fact, astute experts shrink in horror when hypoglycemics dash for sweets to resolve their strange symptoms.

"Anyone who advises a person with hypoglycemia to eat more sugar is not working with the correct premise," observed Dr. Harvey Ross and coauthor Jeraldine Saunders in their book, *Hypoglycemia: The Classic Healthcare Handbook* (previously more aptly titled *Hypoglycemia: The Disease Your Doctor Won't Treat*).

"Low blood sugar is not caused by a lack of sugar in the diet," the authors point out. "It is caused by the failure of the body's sugar-regulating mechanism, which results in a lowered sugar level in the blood after the person has eaten sugar. The obvious treatment would be to not eat sugar."

People "have been bamboozled into thinking of their bodies the way they think of their checking accounts," bemoans William Dufty in *Sugar Blues*.

"If they suspect they have low blood sugar, they are programmed to snack on vending machine candies and sodas in order to raise their blood sugar level. Get it up. Actually this is the worst thing to do."

What people don't realize is that their hypoglycemic symptoms can be alleviated *only temporarily* by eating sweets. "The underlying condition won't go away until you get off sugary foods," explains Dr. Pescatore. "That's the best way to get rid of your symptoms."

Ann Louise Gittleman, Ph.D., C.N.S., author of *Get the Sugar Out: 501 Simple Ways to Cut the Sugar Out of Any Diet*, also warns of the dire consequences that result from downing enticing desserts year after year.

"Since almost all Americans eat too much sugar, many nutritionists think that most Americans are on an almost certain collision course with hypoglycemia," she cautions.

And Nancy Appleton, Ph.D., author of *Lick the Sugar Habit* and *Stopping Inflammation*, also insists that the average person, who consumes about one-third of his or her calories from refined sugars and carbs, is creating big trouble for his or her poor overworked pancreas.

"Your pancreas is the first organ of the endocrine system to come into contact with foods or chemicals and the one most susceptible to damage by excess sweeteners," Dr. Appleton explains.

"Years and years of overstimulating your pancreas could make your blood sugar drop below normal, and hypoglycemia could develop. But when you remove the allergy-provoking substance of refined sugar, your blood sugar returns to normal," she concludes.

Hypoglycemia Is Rampant, Not Rare

Just how many Americans suffer from reactive hypoglycemia? Experts' opinions vary widely. In fact, medical authorities are as fervently divided and heated about this issue as some people are about religion or politics. Generally, there are two opposing camps—the insistent doubters from the traditional medical establishment and the ardent believers from the integrative or alternative medical community.

"If you ask a conventional physician, hypoglycemia is a rare, practically nonexistent malady," Dr. Ronald Hoffman observes.

"The next time you go to a doctor, try asking him or her if the symptoms you experience are due to hypoglycemia. You will, undoubtedly, evoke a bemused look, perhaps an angry one, and even a referral to a psychiatrist. But the truth is that hypoglycemia is far more prevalent than we're led to believe."

Internist and integrative physician Richard N. Ash, M.D., agrees. "Low blood sugar is *not rare*. It's probably *rampant*," says the physician, who has treated thousands of hypoglycemics at the Ash Center for Comprehensive Medicine in New York City.

"I would say that *many* people have hypoglycemia, but they don't know it," Dr. Ash speculates. "Hypoglycemia is basically triggering the obesity epidemic in this country, because people are overeating after their blood sugar drops and they can't stop."

Arriving at exact statistics for hypoglycemia is difficult, if not virtually impossible, especially if you try to obtain them from a skeptical governmental agency or health-care organization. For example, the website of the Centers for Disease Control and Prevention (www.cdc.gov) flat-out ignores hypoglycemia's existence, with no listing in its extensive A–Z index of health topics, although definitions do exist for bird flu, chronic fatigue syndrome, dog bites, dry cleaning, iron overload, lockjaw, mold, plaque, sex education, and swimmer's itch. When asked about the omission, a CDC health communications specialist explained that the agency just "looks at hypoglycemia as it relates to diabetes."

Meanwhile, *MedlinePlus Medical Encyclopedia*, a service of the U.S. National Library of Medicine and the National Institutes of Health, states (on its website) that hypoglycemia only affects "approximately 1 out of every 1,000 people." If that is true, only 291,000 Americans are suffering from hypoglycemia. Many medical experts, however, deem that figure ludicrously low and laughable, especially given our nation's skyrocketing obesity and overconsumption of sweets and refined carbs.

"Low blood sugar probably affects 50 percent of the U.S. population, if not more," insists integrative physician Keith DeOrio, M.D., who has diagnosed thousands of hypoglycemics. Interestingly, Ross and Saunders cite the same 50 percent figure as Dr. DeOrio. Back in 1966 to 1967, the U.S. government's Department of Health, Education and Welfare compiled almost those exact same percentages, finding that 49.2 percent of people interviewed had hypoglycemic symptoms, a fascinating fact that Dufty cites in *Sugar Blues*. In fact, some experts suspect that the figures are still the same, if not higher, with about half of all Americans suffering from low blood sugar.

Low Blood Sugar Strikes Our Nation's Young in Increasing Numbers

Perhaps the group now most at risk for hypoglycemia is the younger set. If you're a parent, you might want to start carefully observing your soda-guzzling, candy-downing children and teenagers. As we well know, diabetes is striking our nation's young with frightening frequency. This also holds true for hypoglycemia.

Teens, in particular, who flock with their pals to the mall or fast-food eateries for donuts, candy bars, cookies, corn chips, French fries, and other much-like-sugar carbs, can develop low blood sugar, which could potentially hurt their social life, hinder their school performance, and, of course, harm their health over the long term. Indeed, Roberta Ruggiero of the Hypoglycemia Support Foundation is alarmed by the increase in requests she receives from parents whose kids were diagnosed as hypoglycemic after they passed out, fell down the stairs, or had a temper tantrum.

Jessica S., a 19-year-old college student from Ames, Iowa, is one of those young people whose carb habit caught up with her when she developed hypoglycemia.

"I'd never heard of it before," confesses Jessica, who spent a year befuddling doctors before an endocrinologist hit upon the diagnosis.

Nowadays, Jessica sticks to a healthy diet despite peer pressure to eat junk food. "It's not easy," she concedes, noting that when she's out with friends, someone might make a disparaging remark about her "strange diet. I've learned to ignore it. If you want to be healthy, you have to be strong."

Imbibing Booze: A Fast Track to SUGAR SHOCK!

Eating too many sweets isn't the only way to trigger or exacerbate hypoglycemia. Ever wonder why when alcoholics give up drinking, they clamor after sweets with something approaching obsession and fanaticism?

Indeed, many alcoholics have hypoglycemia as an underlying condition. Nutritionist Joan Mathews Larson, Ph.D., who has successfully treated thousands of alcoholics at the Health Recovery Center in Minneapolis, Minnesota, found that 88 of 100 randomly selected clients were hypoglycemic. "Some doctors now believe that blood sugar imbalances are a causal factor in alcoholism," says Dr. Larson, author of the best-selling *Seven Weeks to Sobriety* and *Depression-Free Naturally*.

A number of studies confirm Dr. Larson's observations about the high incidence of hypoglycemia among alcoholics. One study found that of 100 alcoholics, 96 were hypoglycemic; another showed that 95 percent of alcoholics had low blood sugar. This research confirms the findings of the late endocrinologist, Dr. John Tintera, who discovered that even recovered alcoholics who have been sober for many years continue to suffer hypoglycemia's effects.

To effectively treat alcoholism, you must focus on controlling diet, maintained Dr. Tintera, who insisted that "by far the most important part of the physiological treatment of alcoholics is the complete restriction of easily absorbed carbohydrates." He warned that until their severe blood sugar fluctuations are stabilized, alcoholics will be predisposed to depression and what appears to be "deep-rooted emotional or psychiatric disorders."

Meanwhile, bear in mind that "drinking, especially binge drinking, also can cause low blood sugar because your body's breakdown of alcohol interferes with your liver's efforts to raise blood glucose," according to the National Diabetes Information Clearinghouse (NDIC) website. What's more, hypoglycemia "caused by excessive drinking can be very serious and even fatal."

But you don't have to consume massive amounts of alcohol to be adversely affected. "Even one or two glasses of wine are enough to trigger reactive hypoglycemic reactions in some sensitive people," says Dr. Pescatore. "There's a lot of sugar in two glasses of wine. This condition is not strictly limited to alcoholics."

Hypoglycemia: A Potential Prelude to Diabetes

Although it's not universally acknowledged, clinical evidence suggests that people with long-term hypoglycemia are headed toward diabetes. In fact, endocrinologist Dr. Schwarzbein, who has treated many diabetics, found that most of her patients were hypoglycemic for years before coming down with the more serious disease.

This shouldn't be too surprising, since both hypoglycemia and diabetes are related to blood sugar problems. Whether you're suffering from low blood sugar (hypoglycemia) or diabetes (high blood sugar), you can't properly assimilate or tolerate sugars or starches because of underlying blood sugar imbalances.

"Both diabetics and hypoglycemics have a glitch in their insulin functioning," observe James Chow, M.D., and Cheryl Chow, coauthors of *Hypoglycemia for Dummies*. "Although it's still a point of discussion, many researchers believe that hypoglycemia can be seen as a prediabetic form of glucose intolerance, which can eventually develop into full-blown diabetes in people who are genetically disposed to diabetes. In other words, diabetes and hypoglycemia may fall on the continuum of the same degenerative disease."

The Chows point to a possible progression of syndromes that includes hypoglycemia, glucose intolerance (or impaired glucose tolerance), insulin resistance, Syndrome X (also called insulin resistance syndrome), and finally type 2 diabetes.

Cynthia Geyer, M.D., who sees thousands of patients as Director of Women's Health at Canyon Ranch health resort in Lenox, Massachusetts, puts it another way. "Hypoglycemia can be one of the manifestations of insulin resistance," she explains, "which may reflect an 'overshoot' phenomenon characterized by a large spike in insulin, followed by a drop in blood sugar. Over time, repeated insulin spikes may lead to a decrease in pancreatic reserve, or more insulin resistance."

Dr. DeOrio further describes the sequence that could lead to type 2 diabetes. "The brain craves more glucose so you consume more simple carbs to get your blood sugar back up again," he says. "You get into this vicious cycle of low sugar, high sugar, low sugar, high sugar, low sugar, high sugar. And that taxes your pancreas, which then leads to either insulin deficiency or to greater insulin resistance and, therefore, type 2 diabetes. Diabetes really is chronic hypoglycemia."

To learn if a link exists between hypoglycemia and diabetes, the Hypoglycemia Support Foundation (HSF) conducted an extensive online survey, receiving more than 5,500 responses, 3,752 of them from diagnosed hypoglycemics from 25 countries. Although the survey was not a double-blind, scientific study, it nonetheless revealed that 64 percent of hypoglycemics (diagnosed by a doctor with a Glucose Tolerance Test) had one or more family members diagnosed with diabetes.

Interestingly, only 59 percent reported changing their diet, including cutting back on sweets, after being diagnosed with hypoglycemia, despite having symptoms such as heart palpitations (80 percent), dizziness (79 percent), mood swings (77 percent), headaches (74 percent), depression (67 percent), addiction to sweets (62 percent), and extreme fatigue (52 percent).

"Unfortunately 23 percent wrongly considered candy the cure-all for their low-blood-sugar problems," reported Roberta Ruggiero, founder and president of the Hypoglycemia Support Foundation.

The HSF survey came about because over the years, Ruggiero has received thousands of e-mails and letters from people wanting to know if there's any kind of connection between low blood sugar (hypoglycemia) and high blood sugar (diabetes).

"For instance, I recieved e-mails and letters from upset people who had been originally diagnosed as having low blood sugar and then developed high blood sugar or diabetes a few years later. When they first received their hypoglycemia diagnosis, their doctors gave them no diet advice, no direction, and told them not to worry, because they just had borderline or mild hypoglycemia. So not being concerned, they continued with their poor diet and then a few later they developed diabetes."

DR. GYLAND'S LIST OF SYMPTOMS OF HYPOGLYCEMIA OR LOW BLOOD SUGAR

Experienced by over 90 percent of hypoglycemics:

Nervousness

Experienced by over 80 percent:

Irritability & mood swings (Dr. Jekyll & Mr. Hyde)

Exhaustion & unexplained tiredness

Faintness

Tremors

Dizziness

Cold sweats

Weak spells

Depression

Experienced by over 70 percent:

Vertigo

Drowsiness

Headaches

Experienced by over 60 percent:

Digestive disturbances

Forgetfulness

Insomnia

Constant worrying

Anxieties

Experienced by over 50 percent:

Mental confusion ("brain fog")

Heart palpitations (tachycardia), rapid pulse

Obesity

Muscle pains

Indecisiveness

Numbness

Internal trembling

Experienced by over 40 percent:

Crying spells

Asthma

Unsocial, asocial, or antisocial behavior

Lack of sex drive (females)

Allergies

Respiratory problems (shallow breathing)

Lack of coordination

Leg cramps

Lack of concentration

Blurred vision

Twitching and jerking muscles

Experienced by over 30 percent:

Itching and crawling sensations on the skin

Gasping for breath

Smothering spells

Staggering

Sighing and yawning

Experienced by over 20 percent:

Impotence (males)

Night terrors, nightmares

Arthritis

Phobias

Fears

Skin conditions, neurodermatitis

Suicidal impulses

Unconsciousness

Rheumatoid arthritis

Experienced by 17 percent:

Nervous breakdown

Experienced by 2 percent:

Convulsions

A Few of Many Other
Hypoglycemic Ailments
Often Cited (Other Sources)

Alcoholism

Bizarre behavior

Blackouts

Brittle hair and nails

Candidiasis (Candida Albicans)

Craving for sweets, salt, alcohol,
   and coffee

Difficulties handling stress

Family history of diabetes or low blood
   sugar

Feeling of "going crazy"

Hot flashes

Hyperactivity in children

Immune system disorders

Joint pain

Learning disabilities

Limited attention span

"Motor Mouth" (constant
   talking)

Negative thoughts and attitudes

Ringing in ears

Sensitivity to light or noise

Severe PMS and bad menstrual
   cramps

The shakes (when hungry)

Uncontrollable weight gain,
   abnormal weight (too high or
   low)

Waking up with a feeling like a
   "hangover"

In addition, Ruggiero says, "I kept getting e-mails asking me, 'If type 2 diabetes runs in my family, will I get it?' Or they'd want to know, 'I have hypoglycemia. Is there a correlation? Will I become diabetic?'"

Ruggiero insists that the HSF survey clearly demonstrates that bona fide medical research examining this link is badly needed. "Of course, this survey cannot take the place of well-structured clinical trials. But it gives us the questions that need answering so that we can encourage scientific research into this condition, which is so often not taken seriously.

"Our survey results, as well as the thousands of e-mails and letters I've received, suggest that hypoglycemia can lead to diabetes," she contends.

"We need to alert hypoglycemics to the seriousness of their condition. If low blood sugar is left untreated, diabetes could become the next stage."

Experts agree, including, Seale Harris, M.D., who discovered hypoglycemia. "The low blood sugar of today is the diabetes of tomorrow," he concluded.

GETTING A VALID HYPOGLYCEMIA DIAGNOSIS

Although it's not easy to get a valid diagnosis of hypoglycemia, a traditional standard of testing has been to administer an extended five- or six-hour Oral Glucose Tolerance Test (GTT), which requires the patient to fast overnight or for about 12 hours.

The next morning, the patient's blood will be drawn to check for glucose levels. Some labs also check insulin levels. Then he or she drinks a disgustingly sweet glucose solution (containing 100 grams of glucose). Although not all diagnostic companies adhere to the same protocol, ideally, the patient's blood is drawn to check glucose and insulin levels half an hour after drinking the sugary liquid and then again at the one-hour mark, and again after two, three, three and half, four, five, and six hours.

If you suspect you're hypoglycemic, you need to know that the five- or six-hour Glucose Tolerance Test is much more preferable to the three-hour one. Even so, a number of doctors tend to order the shorter test anyhow, because they're used to ordering the three-hour GTT to help diagnose diabetes. However, if the patient has hypoglycemia, this three-hour Glucose Tolerance Test can provide inaccurate, misleading results, because the test results often miss the low-blood sugar condition that can occur in the last two hours of a five- or six-hour test.

If your blood glucose levels drop to below 70, 60, or 50 milligrams per one-tenth of a liter (milligram/deciliter) of blood, you could have hypoglycemia. But experts disagree on what number is the exact cutoff point to determine low blood sugar. "What's so-called normal and what provokes symptoms may not correlate," says Dr. Geyer. "In other words, you might have hypoglycemic symptoms even though your blood sugar falls within what's considered a normal range."

In addition, test results aren't always reliable and can be tricky to interpret. "For example, 1 out of 5 normal people tested has *low* blood sugar, with symptoms, *during* the Glucose Tolerance Test, and some people with low-blood-sugar symptoms demonstrate *normal* blood glucose levels during the exam," explains clinical endocrinologist Barrett Chapin, M.D., of Laconia, New Hampshire. Either way, he gives the same sugar-shunning dietary advice.

Moreover, some doctors are reluctant to order the GTT for their patients, because it can be grueling and traumatic for a hypoglycemic, whose blood sugar levels are jerked around with the glucose solution and for whom it can be tough to not eat for hours without getting the shakes, headaches, dizziness, and so on. In fact, if a patient becomes ill, the test may have to be cut short.

Physicians who won't order the GTT for their patients prefer to rely on symptoms to make their diagnosis. "The test is meaningless. Once you have 10 symptoms and you're consuming a lot of sugar, it's obvious you have hypoglycemia," contends Dr. DeOrio. "In medical school, they taught us that 90 percent of the diagnosis should come from the medical history and 10 percent from lab work. The test results are there to support the history, but many physicians overemphasize lab work and de-emphasize symptoms. They may end up ignoring the facts. The problem is weighing clinical symptoms against a lab diagnosis. The patient may have symptoms, but they may not be picked up in a lab test, because results aren't always accurate."

But the GTT can be a valuable tool for someone who doesn't improve after making dietary changes. This could be a sign that an underlying health condition is causing the hypoglycemia. "I need to do all these tests to see if the patient has a tumor," Dr. Chapin says.

Still another method used to diagnose hypoglycemia is the "Whipple triad." According to this exam, a person must have three criteria to be considered hypoglycemic. (1) He or she must show hypoglycemic symptoms; (2) he or she must have a documented blood glucose level of less than 50 milligram/deciliter of blood while symptoms are occurring, and (3) symptoms must improve or disappear when glucose or carbs are injected or eaten. But again, experts find that this test, too, has its limitations.

One caution for people who think they may have hypoglycemia: You may be tempted to test glucose levels yourselves on a drugstore-bought glucometer. This isn't a good idea. In fact, it could be both unsafe and inaccurate. You should always see a doctor to get an accurate diagnosis.

Catch Hypoglycemia Now and Ward Off SUGAR SHOCK! to Change Your Life

If you've been vigorously nodding your head in recognition while reading this chapter, it would be wise to consult a knowledgeable physician as soon as possible to learn if your symptoms are due to hypoglycemia or another blood sugar condition. (Visit my www.SugarShockBlog.com for a list of ways to find a nutritionally savvy doctor.)

Unless you have an underlying disease, reactive hypoglycemia is relatively easy to treat with some simple dietary changes, which you'll learn about shortly.

Now that you've learned about the condition that "rarely exists"—at least according to many in the medical profession—you may have been marveling in disbelief at the multiple agonies of misdiagnosed sufferers who've spent years searching for answers to their problems. But you've also been privy to inspirational tales of those who've kicked sugar and transformed their lifestyles, only to find that their ailments almost magically disappeared.

Jeraldine Saunders, coauthor of *Hypoglycemia: The Classic Healthcare Handbook*, offers testimony to the multiple benefits of making these diet and lifestyle changes.

"It's totally worth it to do without sweets," declares Saunders, a hypoglycemic who has been sugar free for more than four decades. "I'm 83, but I feel much better than I ever have, and I have more energy now than I did when I was 23. And believe it or not, I still have the same slim figure that I had when I was a professional model years ago."

14

Sugar's Role in "The Chronic Big Killers": Diabetes, Cancer, Heart Disease, and Obesity

Even though Ivan Strausz is a physician and a self-proclaimed "sugar lover," he was taken totally by surprise when he found out in 2003 that he was on the fast track to spending the rest of his life with diabetes.

"My internist put his foot down and gave me the speech about how I needed to lose weight, exercise more, and pass up desserts," recalls the 70-year-old gynecologist, who, at the time, carried 168 pounds on his five-foot, six-inch frame, which most would consider close to normal weight.

As a physician, Dr. Strausz was well aware of the risks associated with diabetes, but, as a native Hungarian raised on rich pastries and poppy-seed strudel, he didn't think it was going to be easy for him to follow his doctor's instructions to cut down on sugary foods and refined carbs.

The "borderline diabetes" diagnosis, however, turned out to be just the wake-up call he needed. "I cut sweets, breads, and pasta down to almost nothing, and I actually got used to not having them," says the New York City–based Strausz, author of *You Don't Need a Hysterectomy* and *Women's Symptoms*. He also began eating more fish, fresh vegetables, and fruits, and began exercising at least four times a week.

Within three months, Dr. Strausz dropped 15 pounds. More importantly, his blood sugar, cholesterol levels, and glycohemoglobin (the average level of glucose in the blood over a period of two to three months) had dropped to normal levels. It was a health report card that postponed his date with diabetes—he hopes forever. "I was astonished by how easily things changed for me, and I'm not an easily astonished guy," he says.

It's no surprise that even a physician like Dr. Strausz had no idea he was prediabetic. Like high blood pressure, the most infamous "silent killer," diabetes gives little warning in its early stages, and what symptoms there are can be so subtle that they're often overlooked. Known in medical circles as "the three polys," the most typical of these symptoms are *polyuria*, excess water in the tissues, which causes frequent urination; *polydipsia*, excess thirst; and *polyphagia*, excess hunger.

Culprit Carbs Can Lead to the Chronic Big Killers

If Dr. Strausz hadn't gone for a physical and taken the blood sugar tests that identified his borderline diabetes, he might not have been tipped off early enough to prevent it from progressing into the full-blown form of the disease. But researchers are discovering that if you change the quality of your carbs, you could prevent the onset of diabetes and other deadly diseases.

Mounting medical research now links excess sweets and refined carbs to a number of chronic, debilitating, potentially life-threatening diseases or conditions—or what I call the Chronic Big Killers. Indeed, habitually overconsuming low-quality carbs—which most Americans do—could play a role in the development of heart disease (the nation's number one killer), cancer (number two cause of death), stroke (number three), and diabetes (number six). Bear in mind that all those quickie culprit carbs also could trigger obesity and Syndrome X (metabolic syndrome), which could lead to heart disease and diabetes.

(In case you're wondering, chronic lower respiratory conditions such as bronchitis, emphysema, and asthma rank as the fourth biggest killer, and accidents comprise the number five cause for death in the United States, although the *Journal of the American Medical Association* ranked iatrogenic causes, resulting from doctors' therapy or activity, as the third leading cause of death. Still other experts blame doctors as the leading cause of death.)

Acclaimed physician Mark Hyman, M.D., author of *UltraMetabolism* and former co–medical director of Canyon Ranch health resort in Lenox, Massachusetts, puts it succinctly: "All the diseases that kill us in our society are related to refined carbohydrates and sugars—cancer, heart disease, obesity, diabetes, stroke, and Alzheimer's."

Shortly, I'll discuss some compelling research that uncovers this sugar-chronic disease connection, but it's helpful to know first that, in early 2006, as I was completing final editing on this book, a landmark, seven-year, government-sponsored study, the Women's Health Initiative, found, as reported in the prestigious *Journal of the American Medical Association*, that the low-fat diet *did not* prevent breast cancer, colon cancer, or heart disease, as the USDA, the American Heart Association, and other groups had been predicting since the 1970s.

The $415 million federal study, which looked at nearly 49,000 women, also found that a low-fat regime doesn't necessarily lead to weight loss. In fact, as Barry Sears, Ph.D., creator of *The Zone* diet, pointed out, women in the low-fat group actually gained waist circumference even though they were consuming 361 fewer calories per day.

Unfortunately, many media reports drew incorrect conclusions and took information out of context about the study. Harvard's Dr. Walter Willett gave some much-needed perspective.

"The Women's Health Initiative basically debunks what the USDA has been recommending for three decades," he says. "Besides, you can't just look at fats and carbs. The *types* of fats and carbs that you eat are what's important," adds the renowned physician and nutritionist, who has spearheaded considerable research (which you'll soon learn about) showing that eating refined, fiber-lacking carbs can trigger chronic diseases.

Reproductive endocrinologist Gil Wilshire, M.D., contends that for the past three decades, "the low-fat advice wasn't based on 'level-one evidence.' The whole low-fat dogma was built on a house of cards, which falls apart once you realize that the effect of dietary fat and cholesterol depends upon the context in which they're eaten.

"When you restrict carbohydrates, especially refined ones, all diseases improve," adds Dr. Wilshire, founder and chief scientific officer of the nonprofit Carbohydrate Awareness Council, which advocates evidence-based nutrition advice.

"Once you stop being afraid of fat and get off the fat-is-bad-for-you kick, then you can see everything clearly and carbohydrate restriction makes complete sense," he explains. "My hope is that people will now start basing nutritional recommendations on level-one evidence from properly done research studies."

So now we'll focus on some of this convincing research corroboration.

Cancer Feeds on Sugar: Facts Already Known in the 1930s

Back in the early 1900s, cancer was known as the "white man's disease" among Eskimos living in the Arctic Circle, because there were no known or reported fatalities from it. Their cancer-free lives were documented by Harvard-trained anthropologist Vilhjalmur Stefansson, who lived for 10 winters among the Eskimos between 1906 and 1918. During his time among them, Stefansson shared the typical Eskimo diet of almost-raw fish and blubber supplemented by an occasional chunk of meat, but no quickie carbs, no vegetables, no grains, and no sugar. He, like the Eskimos, remained lean, active, healthy, and cancer-free.

But by the 1920s, the Eskimos had begun to adopt Western ways and a Western diet, Stefansson noted in his 1960 report *Cancer: A Disease of Civilization?* And so it began: In 1933, an Eskimo died of liver cancer in Alaska. Two years later, a second Eskimo passed away of colon cancer in Labrador. And from that time on, death rates from cancer have risen steadily in the frozen north.

Actually, the cancer-sugar connection was discovered even earlier, points out Joseph Mercola, D.O., founder of www.mercola.com. "In fact, already in 1931, the German scientist Dr. Otto Warburg became a Nobel Laureate for discovering that cancer cells use glucose as fuel," Dr. Mercola points out.

Finally, more than 70 years after Dr. Warburg's discovery, a growing number of scientists are citing a high sugar intake as a factor in the development of cancers of the breast, gallbladder, prostate, colon, uterus, and pancreas. In fact, researchers suspect that high sugar and insulin levels *encourage* tumor growth.

Internationally recognized integrative cancer-care specialist Keith I. Block, M.D., points out: "A major ingredient in the recipe for getting cancer is a diet high in refined sugar, and high in unhealthy fats, particularly omega-6 fatty acids and saturated fats," contends Dr. Block, medical director of the Block Center for Integrative Cancer Care in Evanston, Illinois, and a clinical assistant professor at the College of Medicine at the University of Illinois at Chicago.

"Reducing or eliminating refined and simple sugars can provide many benefits, including reducing and containing cancer growth.

EXPERT VIEWPOINT

"It puzzles me why the simple concept 'sugar feeds cancer' can be so dramatically overlooked as part of a comprehensive cancer treatment plan. Of the 4 million cancer patients being treated in America today, hardly any are offered any scientifically guided nutrition therapy beyond being told to 'just eat good foods.' I believe many cancer patients would have a major improvement in their outcome if they controlled the supply of cancer's preferred fuel, glucose."

—The Alternative Research Foundation (from www.mercola.com)

"We know that tumors are glucose guzzlers. If you strangulate the supply of sugar to a tumor, it may actually trigger a form of biological suicide among the malignant cells.

"Very few cancers can survive without a steady supply of glucose," adds Dr. Block, who is also a medical research consultant to the National Center for Complementary and Alternative Medicine, the National Institutes of Health (NIH), and editor-in-chief of the peer-reviewed medical journal *Integrative Cancer Therapies*.

Ultimately, what it comes down to is this: somehow in the midst of all our concern about fat intake, physicians and patients alike have often ignored sugar's role in developing major killer diseases such as cancer.

That opinion is confirmed by the ongoing, 10-year Nurses' Health Study of more than 120,000 women, which has found that sedentary, overweight women who follow a diet high in refined carbs and sweets have a greater risk of type 2 diabetes, heart disease, cancer, and other potentially life-threatening conditions than those who don't.

Compelling Cancer Research Fingers Quickie-Carb Consumption

Scientists have amassed considerable compelling research that connects eating culprit carbs with developing cancer. Let's take a look at some of the results regarding breast cancer. Consider the following:

- Research conducted jointly by scientists at the Harvard School of Public Health, Harvard Medical School, the Instituto de Salud Publica in Cuernavaca, Mexico, and Brigham and Women's Hospital in Boston showed that of 1,866 women aged 20 to 75 in Mexico, those who ate the most carbohydrates, particularly sugary foods, had more than twice (2.2 times higher) the risk of breast cancer than women on more balanced diets. As reported in *Cancer Epidemiology, Biomarkers & Prevention*, of the carbohydrates consumed, sucrose and fructose demonstrated the strongest association with breast-cancer risk. "This study raises important questions about high-carbohydrate diets, particularly among populations or individuals prone to insulin resistance, and more work on this topic is urgently needed," points out one of the authors, renowned obesity researcher Walter C. Willett, M.D., noting that Mexican people tend to be prone to insulin resistance.

- Another study following 512 nondiabetic women with early-stage breast cancer found a correlation between high blood levels of sugar and progression of the disease. As a result, the researchers recommended that patients with cancer of all types "stay on the safe side with a naturally based, insulin-controlling diet."

- Additional researchers looking at 2,500 women in Italy in the early stages of breast cancer found that they ate more refined carbohydrates than an equal number of healthy women.

- In addition, more scientists from Albert Einstein College of Medicine in New York, the University of Toronto, and Columbia University reported in the *International Journal of Cancer* that consuming diets "with high GI [glycemic-index] values may be associated with increased risk of breast cancer among postmenopausal women."

More convincing research shows similar links between eating refined carbs and developing colon cancer. For instance:

- One study looking at more than 1,500 Chinese American men and women found that the 500 participants who eventually developed colon cancer ate the most refined foods and sweets.

■ Another study, which followed the eating habits of 38,451 women over a period of eight years, found that "a diet with a high dietary glycemic load may increase the risk of colorectal cancer in women," according to head researcher and epidemiologist Susan Higginbotham, Ph.D., of the School of Public Health at the University of Southern California. More specifically, as the researchers pointed out in the *Journal of the National Cancer Institute*, women with higher-glycemic-load diets were found nearly three times more likely to develop colon cancer.

■ And scientists at Colorado State University who reviewed a series of population studies concluded that 12 out of the 14 studies they examined showed that excessive sugar intake was tied to colon cancer.

Still more research examined carbohydrate's link to other types of cancer:

■ Researchers from Italy, France, and Canada who studied 1,000 women in Italy and Switzerland for 10 years found that the more high-glycemic foods participants ate, the higher their risks of endometrial cancer (cancer of the uterus).

■ And scientists from the Johns Hopkins University School of Medicine; the National Heart, Lung, and Blood Institute; the Centers for Disease Control and Prevention; and Johns Hopkins Bloomberg School of Public Health found an association between those who died of cancer and those with high blood sugar levels. After looking at data of more than 3,054 adults aged 30 to 74 from the second

CELEBRITY FIGHTS SUGAR SHOCK!

"Diabetes saved my life. I'm actually healthier now than before I took ill. Now I eat so much better: lots of chicken, fish, no red meat, some pasta, and loads of fresh vegetables. I don't eat many fruits because of the sugar content. I need to pay attention to everything that can affect my blood sugar levels, including diet, stress, and exercise."

—actress Halle Berry in *Diabetes*, 2003

National Health and Nutrition Examination Survey and the second National Health and Nutrition Examination Survey Mortality Study, they found that those participants with impaired glucose tolerance were nearly twice as likely to die from *any type of cancer* than those with normal blood sugar levels. Writing in the *American Journal of Epidemiology*, the researchers noted these people with elevated blood sugar levels had more than quadruple the chance of developing the condition than folks who didn't have the condition. Their findings, they concluded, suggest that, "in the United States, impaired glucose tolerance is an independent predictor for cancer mortality."

A Closer Look at the Sugar-Diabetes Connection

Diabetes, as I said previously, is the sixth leading cause of death in the United States. (It is also the fifth leading cause of death by disease.) Nearly 21 million people, or 7 percent of the population, already have diabetes, and another 41 million Americans have prediabetes, meaning that their blood glucose levels are higher than normal but not yet high enough to be diagnosed as diabetes.

Of that, 14.6 million are diagnosed and another 6.2 million are undiagnosed. The total cost for this disease to Americans is a whopping $132 billion, with $92 billion in direct medical costs.

In this book, Dr. Sinatra and I are focusing on type 2 diabetes, which accounts for about 90 to 95 percent of all diagnosed cases of diabetes, because this is the type that can be prevented or reversed by cutting inferior carbs and exercising. As you have read here and elsewhere, if left uncontrolled, diabetes can lead to heart disease, stroke, high blood pressure, kidney disease, nervous system disorders, and impaired circulation, which can, in turn, result in blindness and/or loss of limbs.

We are heartened to witness an increasing number of experts now coming to the conclusion that eating too many refined, fiber-stripped carbs could play a pivotal role in the increased incidence of type 2 diabetes.

"The findings are consistent. A high-glycemic-level diet is consistently related to type 2 diabetes," says renowned Harvard researcher, physician, and nutritionist Dr. Walter Willett, citing three groundbreaking, much-acclaimed, long-term studies: the Nurses' Health Study I (which studied the dietary habits of 121,700 people), the Health Professionals Follow-Up Study (52,000 participants), and the Nurses' Health Study II (116,000 folks), all of which followed their participants for years.

"All three studies showed that people with a higher intake of refined starches and sugars had approximately twice of risk of diabetes compared to those with a low intake," adds Dr. Willett, noting that these studies, which looked at people's intake of high-glycemic-index and high-glycemic-load foods, generated hundreds of different papers.

Let's focus on one recent study, written about in the prestigious *Journal of the American Medical Association*. For the Nurses' Health Study II, researchers from the Harvard School of Public Health, Brigham and Women's Hospital, and Children's Hospital Boston analyzed data on more than 91,000 female nurses between 1991 and 1999 and found that those women who reported having more than one soft drink per day showed an *80 percent* increased risk for type 2 diabetes compared to those who drank less than one soda a month. This increase was *independent* of other lifestyle factors such as smoking, drinking alcohol, physical activity, and other dietary habits. In addition, the nurses who drank more than one fruit punch a day (rather than soda) nearly *doubled* their risk of diabetes as opposed to those who had punch less than once a month.

Not only that, but the study participants who stepped up their intake of soft drinks and drank one or more per day over the eight years of the study gained, on average, more than 17 pounds. But their counterparts—those who cut back on soda to one soft drink or less per week—gained only six pounds on average. Interestingly, those women who increased their soda intake also took in about 360 more calories per day, were less physically active, smoked more, and took in less protein and fiber than the low-soda-drinking subjects.

Frank Hu, Ph.D., senior author of the study and associate professor of nutrition and epidemiology at the Harvard School of Public Health, notes that "the study suggests that limiting these sweet beverages, especially soft drinks, is an important public health strategy to curb the epidemic of obesity and type 2 diabetes.

"We know that people are not satisfied with liquid calories so that's why they consume so many of them, and that leads to more weight gain and obesity. But high amounts of sugars in sodas can have an independent effect

THE PIMA INDIANS TEACH US ABOUT DIABETES

Much of what we know about the link between diabetes and obesity comes from research conducted over the past 30 years on the Pima Indians of Arizona by the National Institute of Diabetes and Digestive and Kidney Diseases (NIDDK). In fact, studies of these people have helped scientists prove that obesity is a major risk factor in the development of diabetes.

The Pima Indians are among the most obese in the world, and they also have the highest rates of diabetes anywhere—one-half of adult Pima Indians have diabetes, and 95 percent of those with diabetes are overweight or obese. Nowadays, it's common to find 300-pound adults.

The Pima Indians weren't always obese. "We have photographs of the Pimas more than 100 years earlier, and they were slender," observes Eric Ravussin, Ph.D., professor at Pennington Biomedical Research Center in Baton Rouge, Louisiana, and a past visiting NIDDK scientist, who has studied the Pimas since 1984.

In the early 1900s, the traditional Pima diet was high in superior starches and fiber and included about 15 percent fat. In fact, according to Dr. Ravussin, until after World War II, the Pima Indians maintained a traditional way of life and economy until their water supply was diverted by American farmers who settled upstream. Then, the Pimas began to eat lard, sugar, and white flour that the U.S. government gave them to survive. Apparently, these sugary, processed foods, especially deep-fried bread—a combination of flour and lard—contributed to their weight gain.

Some experts speculate that when confronted with famine, the Pimas who survived were those whose "thrifty gene" led them to store as much fat as possible. They theorize that this genetic predisposition—along with other genetic traits and their poor, processed diet—could have eventually led, generations later, to an obese, often-diabetic population. Interestingly, other indigenous populations such as the Pueblo and Navajo Indians, the South Sea islanders, and Central and South Americans, seem equally susceptible to developing diabetes.

However, some promising plans are under way to try to halt diabetes in the Native American population, as correspondent Vicki Mabrey of

60 Minutes II reported. For example, at St. Peter Indian Mission School, where 200 students are overweight and at risk for diabetes, the principal, Sister Martha Mary Carpenter, is trying to buck the trend. While the kids are allowed ham, potatoes, green beans, watermelon, and fat-free milk, they can't have sugar. "That's the rule, and we really observe it religiously," says Carpenter, who adds that it works. "None of our children are diabetic. None."

on diabetes," Dr. Hu theorizes. "The large amounts of sugars can increase the demand of beta cells in the pancreas to secrete more insulin. In the long run, this can lead to exhaustion or burnout of the beta cells and lead to diabetes."

The link between sugar and diabetes appears to be twofold: On the one hand, "overconsumption of sugar and other rapidly absorbed carbohydrates can cause excessive demand for insulin and ultimately lead to failure of the pancreas to secrete adequate amounts of insulin," Dr. Willett explains. At the same time, all those extra quickie carbs can lead to obesity, which is indisputably linked to an increased risk of type 2 diabetes.

Studies Show Rewards of Changing Your Lifestyle to Halt Diabetes

If you're at high risk for type 2 diabetes, don't be discouraged. Research suggests at least 10 million Americans who appear to be headed toward the disease can sharply lower their chances of getting diabetes simply through dietary changes and exercise. For instance, the Diabetes Prevention Program (DPP), which examined 3,234 people at high risk for diabetes for three years, found that participants were able to reduce their risk of developing the disease by 58 percent by losing weight and exercising regularly.

"We were floored with how big an impact diet and exercise made in reversing the slide into diabetes and that a weight loss of, say, 10 or 15 pounds could make such a difference in health," says Mary Hoskin, R.D., M.S., coordinator of the study, which was written up in the prestigious *New England Journal of Medicine.*

"This research conveys a powerful message of hope to people at risk for type 2 diabetes," pronounced then Health and Human Services Secretary Tommy G. Thompson. "By adopting a moderate, consistent diet and exercise program, many people with one or more of the risk factors for type 2 diabetes can stop the disease before it becomes irreversible."

Meanwhile, another study from Australian researchers, written about in *Diabetes Care*, followed 36,787 men and women aged 40 to 69 without diabetes and followed up on them four years later. Their results, too, were promising.

"We found that the people who had high-quality, low-glycemic-index carbohydrates in their diet had a *lower risk* of getting type 2 diabetes," says epidemiologist Allison Hodge, who led a group of scientists from the Cancer Epidemiology Centre of the Cancer Council Victoria in Melbourne, Australia.

"This suggests that people could reduce their risk of type 2 diabetes by cutting back on foods high on the glycemic index while maintaining a high-carbohydrate intake from healthy sources such as vegetables, fruits, and whole grains. For example, substituting white bread with low-GI, wholegrain bread could be a step in the right direction," Hodge said, speaking by phone from Australia.

Repeatedly, researchers and experts espouse the benefits of eating right and exercising. "Up to 80 percent of type 2 diabetes is preventable by changing diet, increasing physical activity, and improving the living environment," reports the International Diabetes Federation (IDF), a Brussels, Belgium–based, umbrella organization with more than 190 member associations in more than 150 countries.

Research Shows You Can Manage Type 2 Diabetes by Cutting Culprit Carbs

Even if you do get type 2 diabetes, you don't have to resign yourself to always being reliant on insulin or oral agents. Indeed, Mary C. Gannon, Ph.D., and Frank Q. Nuttall, M.D., Ph.D., both at the Minneapolis V.A. Medical Center and the University of Minnesota in Minneapolis, have been conducting groundbreaking, but sadly, little-reported, research showing absolutely dramatic results. They've found that people with type 2 diabetes could improve their blood glucose level just by altering their diet: decreasing highly refined or starchy foods such as fiber-stripped white rice, processed cereal and cookies; increasing protein; and upping the intake of monounsaturated and polyunsaturated fats. Not only that, but apparently you don't even have to lose weight or take insulin or other medications to experience such benefits.

"We were shocked that you could lower the blood glucose as much as the patients did just by changing their diet," says Dr. Nuttall, chief of the Endocrine, Metabolic and Nutrition Section at the Minneapolis V.A. Medical Center and a professor of medicine at the University of Minnesota.

"We thought they'd be improved, but we didn't think it would be improved as much as it was. The results were better than you get when you put patients on oral agents," adds Dr. Nuttall, who's been studying type 2 diabetes treatment since the 1980s.

"Altering your diet composition could be a patient-empowering method of improving type 2 diabetes for patients without pills or insulin," Dr. Nuttall said in an interview, noting that he and coresearcher Dr. Gannon have arrived at similar results three different times, with one study published in *Diabetes*, another in *Nutrition and Metabolism*, and one more to come out sometime in the future.

In the study published in *Diabetes*, eight male participants followed a low-fat diet for five weeks (comprising 55 percent carbohydrates, 15 percent protein, and 30 percent fat, such as that recommended by the USDA and the American Heart Association), then took five weeks off (called a "washout"), and then came back and ate a low-carb diet (20 percent carbs, 30 percent protein, and 50 percent fat) for another five weeks. (Or they started with the low-carb diet first and finished with the low-fat diet.) Whatever the order in which they followed the diets, "when they switched to the low-carb diet, their blood glucose decreased dramatically and was approaching the normal range," Dr. Nuttall explains, adding that he and Dr. Gannon call this low-carb diet a low-biologically-available-glucose diet or "LoBAG diet."

"Our focus was on lowering the glucose content of the diet," says Dr. Nuttall, a former chairman of the Council on Nutritional Sciences and Metabolism at the American Diabetes Association and former president of the American College of Nutrition.

Dr. Nuttall's colleague, Dr. Gannon, is a professor of food sciences and nutrition and associate professor of medicine at the University of Minnesota and past chair of the Council of Nutritional Sciences and Metabolism for the American Diabetes Association.

CELEBRITY FIGHTS SUGAR SHOCK!

"You know, having diabetes is like having to treat your body like a temple, not an amusement park. . . . Diabetes is no joke. It is a silent killer. You don't feel sick. You don't feel anything. You think you're all that and think you can eat a Snickers bar—but it will kick you in the butt the next morning. You really have to check yourself before you wreck yourself."

—singer Patti LaBelle, ADA spokesperson and author of *Patti's Pearls*

Their thesis, based on previous work, was that it is largely the glucose content of the diet that raises blood glucose. Starches are 100 percent glucose whereas fruit sugar and milk sugar are only 50 percent glucose.

In the course of doing this research, Dr. Gannon and Dr. Nuttall witnessed that fats don't raise blood glucose, something many patients don't realize; protein in low-carb diets aids the production of insulin and can lower the blood glucose; and highly refined starch foods strongly raise blood sugar and do so quickly (something that you, of course, now know).

Frankly, Dr. Sinatra and I are mystified as to why this study, which was supported by grants from the American Diabetes Association and the Minnesota, Colorado, and Nebraska Beef Councils, didn't hit front pages all across America when first published in 2004.

Meanwhile, in January 2006, the ADA released its new position statement regarding "Standards of Medical Care in Diabetes—2006," which stated that low-carbohydrate diets (restricted to less than 130 grams a day) aren't recommended to manage diabetes. (The LoBAG diet suggests a daily diet of 20 percent carbs, 30 percent protein, and 50 percent fat.)

A mere two months later, Dr. Gannon and Dr. Nuttall released another cutting-edge study in *Nutrition and Metabolism*, which also found that diabetics can manage and control their disease simply by eating ample protein and fats, and restricting those culprit carbs, without needing to lose weight or taking insulin medications.

Dr. Nuttall and Dr. Gannon consider their data to be preliminary and "proof of concept" type studies, and they plan to conduct additional, longer-term studies with people of all ages and ethnic groups and varying duration of diabetes.

Diabetics Want to Know: Is It Safe for Them to Eat Sugar?

Given the many studies linking consumption of fast-acting carbs (as well as lack of exercise) to diabetes, you may wonder whether it's a good idea for diabetics to consume any sugar at all.

This is, in fact, a hotly debated topic among some experts, especially since 1999, when the American Diabetes Association reversed its earlier position and released a statement stating that "sugar and sugar-containing foods can be a part of a diet for someone with diabetes." Prior to that, the ADA had recommended that diabetics avoid sugar.

This sugar-is-okay announcement, which came as a surprise and disappointment to many nutrition-minded doctors and experts, also stated that "these [sugar-containing] foods shouldn't be simply added to the diet; rather, they should be substituted for other carbohydrates already in the diet."

The ADA also contended that "research studies show that, gram for gram, sugars, like table sugar, do not raise blood glucose any more quickly than do other carbohydrates, like potatoes, rice, or pasta."

That may be true, but we believe that, although the ADA has an important goal to help people prevent, treat, and diagnose diabetes, the organization should be warning people with this disease to stay away from *all* processed, potentially dangerous, fast-acting carbs, because they're rapidly released into the bloodstream, giving the person an undesired quick sugar "rush" and subsequent insulin blast.

Vague as the ADA directive was, the statement did at least recommend that people should heed the message for all Americans—to choose "a diet moderate in sugar."

But this last caveat notwithstanding, we—along with a number of forward-looking physicians interviewed for this book—wish that the American Diabetes Association would go even further in its recommendations. For example, the organization's official stand (at least, at press time) was that it didn't recognize distinct differences between inferior, fiber-stripped, nutrient-deprived quickie carbs and superior, fiber-rich, nutrient-dense, slower-acting quality carbs.

We're concerned that many of the group's fans may misinterpret the ADA's dietary advice to their detriment and wrongly assume that it's fine to consume an abundance of refined carbs instead of wholesome, intact carbs. Despite our disappointment, we're hopeful that this very needed, influential, and inspiring organization will, at some point soon, change its recommendations.

Renowned endocrinologist Diana Schwarzbein, M.D., who has helped many diabetics at her Endocrinology Institute of Santa Barbara, is one physician who finds the American Diabetes Association position insupportable. When the statement came out, Dr. Schwarzbein was president of her local ADA chapter.

"I quit that day," Dr. Schwarzbein recalls. "I refused to have myself quoted saying that refined carbs and sweets were okay. The ADA is saying that it doesn't matter what kind of sugar you eat. They're saying that sugar, simple carbs, complex carbs are all the same. They're *not* all the same.

"If you eat refined sugar, you get *nothing*, no nutrients, no vitamins, nothing," Dr. Schwarzbein explains. "It's already predigested into sugar. It's just a disaccharide—two sugar molecules put together. It goes right through your system, right into your portal vein, and your insulin levels get really high. So you get a big, big spike of insulin by eating refined sugars.

"Complex carbohydrates take longer to digest," Dr. Schwarzbein continues. "So even though eventually they're going to end up as sugar, most carbohydrates also contain vitamins, minerals, and small amounts of fats and proteins. You're getting some nutrients, not just a big sugar hit."

Likewise, esteemed researcher Dr. Walter Willett of Harvard believes that "the ADA is way behind the science on this issue. They fail to recognize the advantages of high-fiber, low-glycemic carbohydrates compared to refined starches."

The facts are obvious, Dr. Willett insists. "Sweets and high-glycemic carbs, including white bread, white rice, and potatoes, have adverse metabolic effects on blood insulin and lipids. As would be expected, they contribute to excess risks of type 2 diabetes and coronary heart disease. Moreover," he points out, "they contribute plenty of calories and excess weight, our number one nutritional problem."

Reproductive endocrinologist Dr. Gil Wilshire agrees. "It's a dangerous statement to say that it's okay for diabetics to eat sugar. They're just trying to placate everybody," says Dr. Wilshire, who, as you may recall, founded and serves as chief scientific officer for the Carbohydrate Awareness Council, which advocates evidence-based nutrition recommendations.

Besides, points out University of Connecticut professor Jeff Volek, Ph.D., R.D., "sugar causes disruption in insulin function. How can you recommend sugar—even in moderation—to diabetics? It doesn't make metabolic sense, and it's unscientific."

Internist and alternative medicine specialist Richard N. Ash, M.D., is another expert who can't fathom the American Diabetes Association's position.

"It's simply archaic and not relevant to the problems that exist today," he says. "It demonstrates their lack of understanding about the true reality of the problem. It shows a certain level of superficiality without any true understanding of the nature of the sugar problem today."

What Leads to Heart Disease: Bad Fat, Sugar, or Both?

Although a high-fat diet has been shown to be a major factor in heart disease, we must now finger another more dangerous suspect—sugar. Indeed, as Dr. Sinatra wrote in chapter 2, people worry way too much about their cholesterol levels and their consumption of fats and not nearly enough about their sugar intake.

Inevitably, as new research has been disproving previous low-fat-is-good theories, experts are now wondering which is the greater evil—a diet high in unhealthy fats or one high in sugar?

"You mean which poison is worse?" remarks renowned cancer expert Dr. Block. "I used to call this the 'SnackWell generation.' Many people, particularly those watching their weight, quit high-fat consumption, and they traded it for products loaded with refined sugars. Although cookies were marketed as no-fat or low-fat, they were loaded with sugar. They were essentially trading excessive estrogens for excessive insulin. So the answer to 'Which poses the greater health threat?' is *both*," he insists. "It just depends on your biology and which pathway is more vulnerable. We know that *both* unhealthy fats and sugars are associated with inflammation, and this has the potential to both cause and accelerate the big killer diseases."

Metabolic diseases expert Victor Zammit, Ph.D., director of the Clinical Sciences Research Institute and a professor of experimental diabetes at Warwick Medical School in Coventry, Great Britain, sums it up well: "For too long, we've been concerned about the risks of a diet high in bad fats when one high in sugars can be just as dangerous."

"A diet very high in sugars, not complex carbs, ends up making your liver secrete more triglycerides," continues Dr. Zammit, former head of cell biochemistry at the internationally known Hannah Research Institute in Ayr, Scotland.

"You arrive at the same endpoint as if you took in fat," he adds, also noting that people do tend to eat foods that are high in both sugar and saturated fats at the same time.

Already, in the 1960s, renowned English physician, biochemist, and nutrition researcher John Yudkin, M.D., Ph.D.—who at the time was chairman of the department of nutrition at Queen Elizabeth College in London—hypothesized that eating large quantities of sugar and carbohydrates could be a major contributor to coronary heart disease. "He was noticing that the tremendous rise in heart disease coincided with the increased intake of refined carbohydrates," explains Dr. Zammit.

In fact, his studies showed that when rats were fed sugar, they developed dangerously high levels of both bad cholesterol and triglycerides. Your "chances of developing [heart disease] would be significantly reduced if you reduced your sugar consumption," Dr. Yudkin asserted in his landmark 1972 book *Sweet and Dangerous*.

Now, decades later, Dr. Yudkin's theories are being backed by new research. For instance, the Nurses Health Study, mentioned earlier, found that overweight, sedentary subjects who consumed a diet heavy in dessert foods and processed starches had approximately double the risk of coronary heart disease than people in the study who ate less of those foods.

"Thus, refined starches and sugars are one of the most powerful predictors of heart disease," Harvard's Dr. Willett explains. "Replacing those foods with whole-grain, high-fiber forms of carbs, in turn, will actually reduce the risk of heart disease."

Let's look now at more compelling research showing the sugar–heart-disease link:

■ The nation's largest, ongoing nutrition-related survey, NHANES, found that high dietary glycemic index and high glycemic load (i.e., diets high in refined carbohydrates) are associated with lower HDL ("good" cholesterol) levels. So reported researchers from the CDC's

National Center for Chronic Disease Prevention and Health Promotion in the *Archives of Internal Medicine.*

- As described in London's *New Scientist*, scientists in Ayr, Scotland, under metabolic diseases expert Dr. Zammit found that metabolic syndrome (insulin resistance syndrome or Syndrome X) may be linked to consumption of high-energy, sugary snacks and drinks, and that the continually elevated insulin and insulin resistance can, in turn, raise triglyceride levels, increasing the risk of heart disease. (Shortly, we'll discuss this syndrome further.)

- Researchers from Northwestern University Medical School's Department of Preventive Medicine wrote in the *Annals of Epidemiology* that diets low in sugar were associated with an increase in HDL ("good" cholesterol) levels.

- Increased intake of highly processed carbohydrates has a complex and mostly unfavorable effect on blood lipids, reducing HDL and raising triglycerides, report researchers from the University of Massachusetts in the *Journal of the American College of Nutrition.*

- Sugars, particularly sucrose and fructose, elevate serum triglyceride levels by 60 percent more than do starches, reported Rutgers University researchers in the *American Journal of Clinical Nutrition.* They also noticed that diets high in sugary foods are associated with higher triglyceride concentration and greater risk of heart disease in women.

- The heart-damaging effects of a diet high in refined carbohydrates may be worst in women who are overweight (BMI > 25), because these women tend to experience the greatest increase in serum triglyceride levels, according to Harvard Medical School researchers writing in the *American Journal of Clinical Nutrition.*

- A team of scientists at UCLA and Cedars-Sinai Medical Center in Los Angeles found that men with cardiovascular disease may be at considerably increased risk for death even when their blood sugar is in a "normal" range. "Our findings suggest that for men with cardiovascular disease, there is apparently no 'normal' blood sugar level," said Sidney Port, UCLA professor emeritus of mathematics and statistics and lead author of the study, published in the *American Journal of Epidemiology*. "For these men across the normal range, the lower their blood sugar, the better."

To date, the American Heart Association still doesn't accept theories linking the rise in heart disease to our escalating consumption of sugars. Although regrettably the organization allows its endorsement to be emblazoned on packages of low-fat, sugary, processed foods such as Cocoa Puffs, Cookie Crisp, Lucky Charms, Pop-Tarts, and Frosted Mini-Wheats, the AHA does concede that studies suggest that "high sugar intake should be avoided," and it recommends that carb intake come mainly from complex carbohydrates.

But, as far back as 1998, the AHA's peer-reviewed journal, *Circulation*, published a medical study noting that in middle-aged and elderly white men, a high level of fasting triglycerides is "a strong risk factor" for heart disease that's "independent of other major risk factors, including HDL cholesterol." Other studies have suggested that diets high in fructose are, in fact, linked to high triglyceride levels.

Now, a growing group of cardiologists, including Dr. Sinatra, are working hard to spread the word about this convincing theory: Too much sugar and refined carbs can harm your heart.

For instance, Dr. Patrick Fratellone, who runs a cardiology, infectious-diseases, and internal medicine practice in New York City, also insists that "stabilizing blood glucose is essential to help heart patients heal."

Like many cardiologists, Dr. Fratellone hears "horror stories" from patients flirting with disastrous dietary behavior—cereal, white bread, or bagel for breakfast, fast food for lunch, and maybe a few vegetables and protein for dinner.

"The higher the carbohydrate intake, the higher your triglycerides will be. When your triglycerides go up, your HDL or 'good' cholesterol goes down. Not enough people know that high triglycerides are an even bigger risk factor for a heart attack than high cholesterol," says Dr. Fratellone, former executive medical director of the Atkins Center for Complementary Medicine.

"People are walking around with normal cholesterol, normal LDL, normal HDL, and high triglycerides, and that's why they have a heart attack. The only way to decrease your triglycerides is through diet: You need to restrict refined carbohydrates and sugar."

Halt Diseases Early by Identifying and Treating Metabolic Syndrome

In recent years, the medical community has become increasingly aware of a cluster of symptoms now known as metabolic syndrome (alternately called Syndrome X and insulin resistance syndrome), which could significantly increase a person's risk of heart attack, stroke, and diabetes. Increasingly, experts are realizing that identifying this condition is an effective way to catch diseases while they are still in the developmental stage. Although Syndrome X doesn't show up in the blood tests normally given in the course of a routine medical checkup, a physician can order a series of specific tests to identify its six classic symptoms, any three of which are enough to classify you as having Syndrome X. According to the American Heart Association and leading metabolic-syndrome researcher Dr. Victor Zammit, this cluster of symptoms includes:

- *Excess abdominal fat*—For men, your abdomen is greater than 40 inches; for women, your abdomen is larger than 35 inches.

- *Insulin resistance or glucose intolerance (elevated levels of glucose)*— Your body can't properly use insulin or blood sugar.

- *Hyperlipidemia*—Blood fat disorders, mainly high triglycerides (fats that circulate in the blood), and low levels of the "good" HDL (high-density lipoprotein) cholesterol, which can clean out your coronary arteries and prevent plaque buildup. If you have high triglycerides and low HDL, you are at risk for plaque building up in your artery walls.

- *Hypertension (high blood pressure)*—Your blood pressure reads 130/85 mmHg (millimeters of mercury) or higher.

- *Prothrombotic state*—You have an increased tendency for blood to clot.

- *Proinflammatory state*—The lining of your blood vessels is inflamed. This is one of the first steps to forming plaque in your arteries.

According to recent estimates, some 47 to 95 million adults now have metabolic syndrome (Syndrome X). In fact, it is so prevalent that in October

2000, the American Heart Association officially recognized the syndrome in its dietary guidelines, which call for avoiding high-carb and very low-fat foods and emphasizing unsaturated fats. Whatever the incidence, the syndrome can lead to such potentially fatal diseases as diabetes and coronary heart disease.

For instance, men with metabolic syndrome are shown to have a 78 percent greater risk of stroke (the nation's third biggest killer) than males without the condition, and women have more than twice the risk, according to data from the Framingham Offspring Study, which looked at children of the original participants in the landmark Framingham Heart Study. (The Framingham Heart Study, which began in 1948, has involved two generations of study participants, as well as researchers from the National Heart, Lung, and Blood Institute and Boston University. The study has produced more than 1,000 scientific papers, has identified major risk factors associated with heart disease, stroke, and other diseases, and has paved the way for researchers to undertake further investigations based on the Framingham findings.)

How Sugar Plays into Metabolic Syndrome (Syndrome X)

For two decades, experts have been seeking reasons for Syndrome X, which some have called "sugar-overload disorder." Now, "there's wide agreement that a prolonged, high-sugar diet is a leading suspect," says metabolic-syndrome expert Dr. Victor Zammit, who, for the past decade, has been investigating its causes.

"If sugar is eaten often enough, tissues are exposed to high insulin and glucose levels for prolonged periods of time, and this damages tissues. A diet high in sugar is bad enough. But people tend to have chocolate bars and biscuits and soft drinks throughout the day. The system is continuously stimulated with no resting periods between peaks of insulin and glucose," explains Dr. Zammit, speaking by phone from Great Britain, where he is director of the Clinical Sciences Research Institute and a professor of experimental diabetes at Warwick Medical School in Coventry.

"If excess insulin is present for long periods as a result of eating all those refined carbs, the liver is prompted to pump out even more dangerous triglycerides. This process can then snowball to the point where excess triglycerides cause insulin resistance in the muscle cells, which stops them from removing glucose from the blood. As time goes by, more insulin is secreted. The blood becomes flooded with fatty acids, which start destroying the pancreatic cells that produce insulin, causing insulin levels to plummet. The result is type 2 diabetes."

Dr. Zammit further explains: "Ultimately, all those symptoms of metabolic syndrome are related to the development of insulin resistance in the various tissues. If your cells become resistant to insulin, then they give you the syndrome.

"You could have symptoms for 10 to 15 years before being diagnosed as a diabetic. Syndrome X is a silent, insidious disease, with slow onset."

Loren Cordain, Ph.D., a professor at Colorado State University who has conducted groundbreaking research over the past two decades that dramatically links our modern, high-refined-carb diet to various diseases, believes that insulin resistance isn't only a problem for developing Syndrome X.

"Diseases of insulin resistance," he contends, "represent far and away the major health problem, not just in the United States, but in virtually all of Western civilization." In fact, Dr. Cordain believes, as do other researchers, that Syndrome X and the underlying blood sugar disorder may also be inextricably connected to our nation's worst chronic diseases such as heart disease, cancer, and diabetes—all of which, he's convinced, are related to diets high in sugar and processed grains.

Researchers Find Cutting Carbs Helps Metabolic Syndrome

Like Dr. Zammit and Dr. Cordain, researchers from the University of Connecticut and SUNY Downstate in New York also arrived at the same conclusion. Indeed, after reviewing medical literature about low-carb diets, they discovered "every single aspect of metabolic syndrome could be improved just by restricting carbs," according to biochemist Richard Feinman, Ph.D., a professor at SUNY Downstate and founder/director of the Nutrition and Metabolism Society.

Jeff Volek, Ph.D., R.D., lead researcher for the review paper *Nutrition & Metabolism*, expounded. "Make a list of the features of metabolic syndrome;

PASTA- AND SUGAR-LOVING HEALTH REPORTER NIPS SYNDROME X IN THE BUD

Veteran Arizona nutrition columnist Jack Challem, author of *The Nutrition Reporter* (www.nutritionreporter.com), was often tired and stressed, had a "spare tire" around his middle, and frequently ate pasta-centered meals. He also ate a lot of refined breads, cereals, and sweets, especially "health food desserts" such as energy bars, which, of course, contained lots of "natural sugars."

But the five-foot, seven-inch journalist, whose weight climbed to 170 pounds, was clueless as to the state of his health. Then, while Challem was working on a story about the Bright Spot for Health in Wichita, Kansas, the center's director Hugh Riordan, M.D., suggested doing a medical workup. To Challem's astonishment, a blood test showed that he had a fasting blood sugar of 111—just four points short of prediabetes. What's more, his cholesterol was high, and his chromium level (important in glucose metabolism) was low.

The diagnosis? Syndrome X. This was rather ironic: At the time, the medical reporter was trying to sell a book about the very medical condition with which he'd been diagnosed.

To reverse the onslaught of Syndrome X, Challem created new, positive habits. The pasta bowl became a salad bowl. He stopped eating desserts and breads. And he began taking long walks and going cycling three to four times a week.

Six months later, Challem's bulging gut was history (he lost 22 pounds); his blood sugar, insulin, and cholesterol levels had dropped significantly; and his energy had improved—enough for him to coauthor *Syndrome X: The Complete Nutritional Program to Prevent and Reverse Insulin Resistance*.

Nowadays, the medical writer, who has since written a follow-up book, *Feed Your Genes Right*, eats a diet of fish, chicken, high-fiber veggies, and low-sugar fruits. And he enjoys one big plus: "I'm at the same weight I was 16 years ago," Challem happily reports, and now relishes his 34-inch waist. "How nice it is to get back your old body!"

then, make a list of the things that carbohydrate restriction is good at fixing. They're the same list," says the nutrition expert and University of Connecticut professor.

"When you restrict carbs, your triglycerides go down, your HDL ('good' cholesterol) increases, the quality of your LDL improves, you lose fat in your midsection, and your blood pressure, insulin, glucose, and inflammatory markers all improve. Those have been the consistent findings from at least eight separate studies," Dr. Volek observes.

"We know that the cause of metabolic syndrome is often linked to disruption of insulin," he explains. "Thus, the key to treating metabolic syndrome is to control insulin, and carbohydrates are the major stimulus for insulin."

Interestingly, the researchers also found that if you reduce carbohydrates, you can be less concerned about your fat intake. "Carbohydrates are much more deleterious for you than saturated fat," Dr. Feinman observes, echoing conclusions Dr. Sinatra made in chapter 2.

Quality Carbs Contribute to Weight Loss

While recent research suggests that you might be able to avoid heart disease and cancer by consuming more quality, unprocessed, slow-release carbs, eating in this manner also is proving to be an effective tool to achieve short- and long-term weight loss. Bear in mind that we're not talking about diets that drastically restrict carbs although, as you've no doubt heard, low-carb diets also can lead to weight loss.

For example, a groundbreaking study conducted by researchers at the Children's Hospital Boston, Brigham and Women's Hospital, the Joslin Diabetes Center, and the University of Minnesota and published in the *Journal of the American Medical Association* in 2004 shows that weight-loss diets reducing glycemic load (the degree to which blood glucose rises after a meal) may be more effective over the short and long term than limiting fat intake for "the prevention and treatment of obesity, cardiovascular disease, and diabetes mellitus."

"Our data suggest that the type of calories consumed—independent of the amount—can alter metabolic rate," observes David Ludwig, M.D.,

SUGAR SHOCKER! CARBS BLAMED FOR WEIGHT GAIN IN 1825!

"I know what causes obesity. Just talk to fat people. They eat too much starches and sugars. I have 500 conversations over the year with stout people, and each one, they're telling me, 'I love the potatoes. I love the rice. I love the bread.'"

—Jean Anthelme Brillat-Savarin, *The Physiology of Taste*, published in 1825

Ph.D., director of the Optimal Weight for Life (OWL) obesity program at Children's Hospital Boston and the study's senior investigator. "That hasn't been shown before. The idea that 'a calorie is a calorie is a calorie' doesn't really explain why conventional weight-loss diets usually don't work for more than a few months."

For the study, Dr. Ludwig and his colleagues looked at 46 overweight or obese adults aged 18 to 40 who consumed either a standard low-fat diet or a low-glycemic-load (GL) diet. Both diets provided about 1,500 calories a day, but the low-GL group ate more fat and superior carbs, consuming, for instance, steel-cut oats instead of instant oatmeal, blueberries instead of raisins, and cracked-wheat bread instead of tortilla chips. The 39 subjects who remained in the study lost about 10 percent of their body weight, but the low-GL dieters had smaller decreases in their resting energy expenditure than the low-fat dieters—meaning their metabolism didn't slow as much. They also reported less hunger.

In addition, Dr. Ludwig conducted another experiment in which rats were fed a diet consisting of 69 percent carbohydrates, and those fed a high-glycemic diet had 71 percent more body fat and 8 percent less lean muscle mass than rats on a low-GI diet.

"These findings suggest that low-glycemic diets might help prevent or treat obesity, diabetes, and heart disease," Dr. Ludwig says. "A low-GI diet is the perfect compromise between a low-fat diet and an Atkins-type, very low-carbohydrate diet."

And it appears that eating fewer fast-acting carbs also can help a person to keep the weight off. Scientists believe that each of us has a "setpoint," Dr. Ludwig explains, and "when you diet, internal mechanisms work to restore your weight to that setpoint. But a low-GL diet," he theorizes, "may work better with these internal biological responses to create the greatest likelihood of long-term weight loss."

Dr. Ludwig's team also confirmed other research by finding that the low-glycemic-load group had significantly greater improvements in insulin resistance (a risk factor for diabetes), as well as levels of serum triglyceride and C-reactive protein (both heart disease risk factors).

Curbing Quickie Carbs Can Ward Off the Chronic Big Killers

Given space constraints, I've mentioned only a few of the many cutting-edge studies that illustrate just how debilitating and potentially deadly overeating processed carbs could be. I would, however, like to look at what I believe is one of the most dramatic examples of the kind of damage that can result from eating fast-acting carbs.

Researchers from Children's Hospital Boston and Harvard Medical School's Department of Pediatrics examined a number of rats and mice while giving them either a high- or low-glycemic diet over an 18-week period. When the scientists examined slides of the pancreases of the biopsied animals, the implications were astounding.

"A high proportion of animals on a high-GI diet had damaged or scarred islet cells in the pancreas," explained Dr. Ludwig, who spearheaded the project. "If the damage had progressed, I'd expect type 2 diabetes would develop."

On the other hand, the group eating the healthier carbs didn't have those problems. "The low-GI group had normal-appearing pancreases," Dr. Ludwig observes.

I hope that you've received ample information so that you'll consider kicking culprit carbs to avoid the chronic big killers. Let's close with thoughts from two experts.

In discussing current sugar/cancer research, Melanie Polk, director of nutritional education at the American Institute for Cancer Research, concludes: "The studies tell us that diet does [have an] impact on health. By choosing the right foods—staying away from refined sugar products—we can make ourselves healthier."

"Bottom line," says Harvard's Dr. Willett, is that "greatly reducing or eliminating refined starches and sugar is one of most important steps you can take toward a better diet and long-term well-being."

15

FOR WOMEN ONLY: TOO MUCH SUGAR

CAN AFFECT FERTILITY, PMS,

AND MENOPAUSE

When it comes to loving sweets, we women take the cake. Simply put, many of us ladies do indeed have a troubling, tempestuous, and passionate relationship with sugary foods.

Sure, the men in our lives often love the sugary stuff, too, but there's just no question about it: Sweets exert considerably more power over us females. In fact, many of us can predict our periods by the wild wave of chocolate lust that hits us each month.

Sadly, however, as scrumptious as those sweet snacks taste, indulging too much and too often could contribute to a number of serious female problems, including infertility, miscarriage, birth defects, polycystic ovary syndrome (PCOS), and even fibromyalgia (a chronic disorder involving musculoskeletal pain, fatigue, and tenderness in areas such as the neck, spine, shoulders, and hips).

What's more, a high-sugar diet also could be connected to chronic fatigue, stubborn yeast infections, severe premenstrual syndrome (PMS), excessive menopausal symptoms, and pelvic pain, according to a number of experts including reproductive endocrinologist and gynecologist Deborah Metzger, Ph.D., M.D., medical director of Harmony Women's Health in Los Altos, California.

The Connection between Cravings and Carbs

Those of us who've found ourselves beelining to a donut shop, piling on the pasta, or knocking off a pint of ice cream right before our periods find it easy to blame our hormones for our behavior, but in the backs of our minds, let's face it, we still might wonder, "Are we really just making excuses?"

Take heart. Science shows that there are valid reasons for craving sugar when we're premenstrual. In fact, Louise Dye, Ph.D., a senior lecturer in biopsychology at the University of Leeds in England and an expert on female-related cravings, has studied more than 5,000 women and found that 74 percent of them had cravings before that time of the month. Of those, 56 percent reported that their cravings were reduced at the start of their period, and only 27 percent observed cravings when they neared midcycle.

In short, three-quarters of the women studied had cravings that could be tied in to their menstrual cycle. "The predominant pattern that emerges from all the literature to date is an increase in both the *frequency* and the *severity* of food cravings for women in the premenstrual phase," Dr. Dye concludes.

And guess what most women crave just before their periods? You got it: nearly 80 percent of the women Dr. Dye surveyed wanted those tantalizing sweets. (Thank goodness, when I kicked sugar, all my PMS-related cravings disappeared.)

Anyhow, at least four other medical studies also reveal that before their period, women consume more sweets, carbs, and calories. Not surprisingly, they also gain weight.

Jean Endicott, Ph.D., director of the premenstrual evaluation unit at Columbia Medical Center in New York City, also notices that "women most frequently crave sweets. But some also like salty foods."

We females also prefer the combination of sweet and fat. Michele Mercer, Ph.D., a psychology professor and food-mood expert at Memorial University of Newfoundland, found that women long for "comfort foods" when premenstrual, in part because during this time the pain threshold goes down. That gives females a biological "predisposition" for foods that trigger the release of opioids (morphinelike substances) that help them endure premenstrual cramps and irritability. In fact, the "female" hormones estrogen and progesterone stimulate the release of the opioid beta-endorphin around that time of the month.

The dilemma is that our cravings for sweets and fast-acting carbs can, unfortunately, also lead to further premenstrual dilemmas. In fact, nutritionist Elizabeth Somer, author of *Food & Mood*, contends that premenstrual women tend to overeat quickie carbs to boost their moods, but doing so *aggravates* PMS.

And Cynthia Geyer, M.D., who sees hundreds of women as director of women's health at Canyon Ranch health resort in Lenox, Massachusetts, also observes that "very often, women with severe PMS have a lot of refined carbohydrates in their diets."

According to the American College of Obstetricians and Gynecologists, 85 percent of women who menstruate report one or more symptoms of PMS. But, as many have already discovered, managing your sugar intake could be one of the most powerful and effective ways to curtail PMS-triggered symptoms.

Of Sugar, Serotonin, PMS, and Cravings

As I previously discussed, serotonin is a potent brain chemical that regulates emotional states and influences when and how much we eat. For women, this is particularly important because our reproductive hormones modulate our body's sensitivity to serotonin. In short, when we are premenstrual, our serotonin levels drop.

As a result, Dr. Endicott of Columbia Medical Center theorizes, "a lower availability of serotonin might be related to carbohydrate cravings during PMS. The serotonin is there, but it's not as accessible to the brain as it normally would be, bringing on the blues and possibly the cravings."

Dr. Judith Wurtman—who has spent nearly three decades doing research on the relationship between carb cravings and mood swings—also believes that serotonin levels are low in women who have chocolate cravings or a sweet tooth when they have PMS. She suggests that women who feel depressed premenstrually may be overeating sweets and other carbs to raise their serotonin levels.

"Our research shows that women suffering from mood swings of PMS eat carbohydrates to improve their mood and try to relieve their anger, depression, fatigue, irritability, confusion, or memory lapses," she says.

"Eating these foods eventually triggers the manufacture of serotonin, which has a beneficial effect on mood. Insulin, which is released when you eat carbohydrates, suppresses the circulating levels of most amino acids except that of tryptophan, the amino acid from which serotonin is made," Dr. Wurtman contends. "About 20 to 30 minutes after you eat carbohydrates, the serotonin is made by the brain and starts its work at restoring good moods.

"All carbohydrates will do it except fruit, but, of course, from a nutritional standpoint, it's obviously better to eat healthy carbohydrates such as whole grains and sweet potatoes. The *correct* types of carbohydrates can boost serotonin and take the edge off of PMS symptoms."

Although Dr. Wurtman's theories are convincing, other experts such as Dr. Sinatra believe that it's better to eat some protein and fat at the same time to offset blood-sugar swings. And Julia Ross, author of *The Mood Cure* and *The Diet Cure*, contends that, "Increasing dietary protein and adding serotonin-boosting supplements such as 5-HTP is a more direct, effective, healthier strategy to improve PMS symptoms."

Outsmart Your Hormone-Related Cravings

As frustrating as our hormone-induced cravings may be, we can control them by understanding our triggers. "It's actually empowering if you know when your weaker times are to indulge, because then you can actually make some kind of behavioral changes to reduce the effects," says cravings expert Dr. Dye, who recommends planning "environmental intervention" to prevent us from pigging out.

In other words, if you know you're about to menstruate and you're craving chocolate-covered peanuts or pretzels, make sure to eat a well-balanced meal before going to the movies. When you're "hormonal" or PMSing, make social plans that revolve around nonfood activities. For example, meet a friend for a walk in the park rather than at your favorite restaurant.

Such tactics do, indeed, work well, as many of us have discovered. (For more helpful tips on how to beat sugar cravings, which can work any time of the month, see chapter 22, which addresses frequently asked questions from Sugar Kickers in KickSugar, my free, online international support group.)

Whatever you do, keep in mind that we ladies are *not* "bad" for eating more at this time of the month. We're just doing what our bodies are programmed to do. In fact, numerous studies document that mammals such as baboons, rhesus monkeys, and pigtail monkeys experience cyclic changes in their food intake, too. Like us humans, they consume the most food in the premenstrual phase of their cycle. And, when ovulating (midcycle), baboons, sheep, goats, rats, and even guinea pigs also eat markedly less.

Tame the Sneaky Yeast Beast to Restore Vitality and Comfort

Take one female body, add sugar, mix with fluctuating hormone levels and some other ingredients such as frequent antibiotics, and you have the recipe for a very pesky yeast infection. A yeast infection, also known as candidiasis, is caused by the overgrowth of a fungus called *Candida albicans*.

Normally, *Candida* is present everywhere on the skin, in your mucous membranes, in the vagina and the bowel, and it lives in the body in harmony with hundreds of other beneficial bacteria. "It's when there's an imbalance— that can be caused by such disruptors as a chronic sugar diet, stress, and antibiotics—that *Candida* can become opportunistic," explains reproductive endocrinologist and gynecologist Dr. Metzger. "But sugar is the number one contributor to *Candida*. Because the sugar feeds the yeast, *Candida* starts to grow where the good bacteria can no longer keep it under control."

You have problems when the *Candida* proliferates to the point where it starts to outnumber the rest of the beneficial bacteria. By the time it overruns the vagina, it's likely also lurking in other mucous membranes throughout the body, as well as in the gastrointestinal tract, causing a variety of symptoms including fatigue, rashes, bloating, and "mind fog," according to Jacob Teitelbaum, M.D., medical director of the Annapolis Research Center for Effective Chronic Fatigue Syndrome and Fibromyalgia Therapies and author of *From Fatigued to Fantastic!*

Now reverse the recipe. Take sugar out of the mix, add high-quality nutritional supplements, several weeks of an antifungal remedy, and improved self-care, and in one to four months, a more vibrant woman is likely to emerge—free of many debilitating symptoms.

As any beer maker knows, the fermentation process works by combining yeast with sugar. The warmer and moister the environment (like our gastrointestinal and vaginal tracts), the more robustly the yeast can reproduce, especially when it's fed a lot of sugar. And so, although men can also develop yeast infections, women are at least three times more likely to get them, because female hormone fluctuations make women more hospitable hosts. During each menstrual cycle, a woman undergoes a flood of both estrogen and progesterone, which increases the amount of sugar in the mucous membranes, thus encouraging yeast growth.

"If a woman has *Candida*, she craves sugar to begin with—like those little yeasties are banging their spoons, saying 'Feed me,' " explains nutritionist Dr. Sally Rockwell. "Throw in the premenstrual cravings for sweets, and women get a little nuts."

So the cycle is self-perpetuating. As *Candida* grows, so does the long, irksome list of symptoms it causes. And, at the same time, the imbalance of normal flora in the intestinal tract makes it harder for the body to absorb the nutrients it needs to support the immune system, says Dr. Metzger.

Candida Is Linked to Fibromyalgia and Chronic Fatigue

Excessive sugar consumption also can play a role in the onset of chronic fatigue syndrome (CFS) and fibromyalgia. Experts suspect that if a woman's body is already burdened by stress, lack of sleep, and a compromised immune system, yeast can be the "starter mix" for chronic fatigue syndrome, an underactive thyroid, allergies, chemical sensitivities, and fibromyalgia.

In addition to the lethargy that characterizes candidiasis, both chronic fatigue and fibromyalgia also cause arthritis-like pain and sleep disorders. In fact, these disorders have so much in common that many physicians and researchers believe they are, in fact, part of a single syndrome sometimes referred to as dysregulation spectrum syndrome (DSS) or central sensitivity syndrome (CSS).

Also related to chronic fatigue syndrome and fibromyalgia are hypothyroidism, chemical sensitivities, irritable bowel, and other chronic pain conditions. And according to Dr. Teitelbaum, since poor sleep characterizes all of these conditions, the body produces less growth hormone, which can lead to insulin resistance, which, in turn, causes weight gain.

Approximately 1 to 3 percent of the population or some 3 million to 9 million Americans have fibromyalgia, according to the National Fibromyalgia Association. In addition, according to recent research, 24 percent report fatigue that interferes with their ability to function. And not surprising to many females, fatigue has been found to be "more prevalent in women than men," one study concluded.

In addition, the Chronic Fatigue and Immune Dysfunction Syndrome (CFIDS) Association of America reports that as many as 800,000 people suffer from CFIDS, although Dr. Metzger and other experts consider these figures "a gross underestimate."

Now, a growing number of doctors are noticing that chronic fatigue and fibromyalgia are closely related. "There's so much overlap between chronic fatigue and fibromyalgia that the current consensus among medical professionals is that they're just variants of the same syndrome," Dr. Metzger explains in a phone interview.

Like fatigue, fibromyalgia also is more likely to affect women than men. And, not surprisingly, a number of experts say that cutting sweets is perhaps *the most important* change you can make to reverse either chronic fatigue or fibromyalgia.

"Starve the yeast by cutting out sugar," suggests Dr. Teitelbaum, who finds that 90 percent of his patients with fibromyalgia and CFS get better by following his treatment protocol. In addition to eliminating sweets, he recommends getting 8 to 10 hours of sleep a night, treating adrenal and thyroid hormone deficiencies with supplements and herbs, correcting nutritional deficiencies, drinking plenty of water, and, of course, reducing stress and anxiety.

The Metabolic Trickery of Polycystic Ovary Syndrome (PCOS)

As you now know, eating too many sweets and quickie carbs ultimately forces your body to produce excess insulin, and in the female body, extra insulin spells trouble for reproductive health. All that insulin can overwhelm a woman's ovaries to the point where she stops producing progesterone, the hormone that is required to prepare the uterus for pregnancy and to maintain that pregnancy. What happens is that instead of progesterone, the ovaries begin to turn out excessive amounts of androgens or "masculine hormones." Mind you, we women want a little testosterone in our system to maintain a healthy sex drive, but too much androgen can be, as you might expect, rather unfeminine.

"Androgens and insulin and its counterparts conspire to block the development and monthly release of an egg," says Ron Feinberg, M.D., a reproductive endocrinologist and adjunct associate professor of obstetrics and gynecology at Yale University School of Medicine. This can result in polycystic ovary syndrome (PCOS), which affects an estimated 5 to 10 percent of women of childbearing age and is a leading cause of infertility, according to the International Council on Infertility Information Dissemination. The syndrome is the most common endocrine disorder among reproductive-age women.

Dr. Feinberg describes PCOS (which he refers to as "Syndrome O") as "World War III on a woman's ovaries and many other organs of the body." The ovaries may bubble up with characteristic cysts. The androgens may bring out male characteristics such as excess body and facial hair, balding, and even a lower voice. Acne and darkening of the skin also characterize the disease. With this condition, a woman may not ovulate for months at a time and then have a very heavy period.

"By the time a woman is diagnosed with 'polycystic ovaries' or anovulatory (not ovulating) infertility, it's likely that the harmful consequences of Syndrome O have already seriously affected many organ systems in her body," observes Dr. Feinberg, author of *Healing Syndrome O*.

On the bright side, early symptoms of PCOS may alert women that they have an insulin imbalance *before* it progresses to a life-threatening case of diabetes or heart disease. Dr. Feinberg advises women to see their family doctor or an endocrinologist at *the first sign* of menstrual irregularity, unexplained weight gain, worsening acne, or unusual hair growth. Since a predisposition to PCOS is genetic, a woman may never actually be "cured," but with proper treatment and lifestyle changes, symptoms can become barely noticeable, he assures.

But research shows that even women *without* PCOS can have problems conceiving when insulin levels are elevated. "Even mildly elevated insulin in women contributes to infertility," Dr. Metzger notes.

Experts say that, as with chronic fatigue syndrome, *Candida*, and fibromyalgia, committing to a diet of no sugar or inferior, fast-acting carbs is one of the most important lifestyle changes a person with PCOS can make. This hypothesis was backed up by University of Alabama at Birmingham researchers, who suggest, as they reported in the journal *Fertility and Sterility*, that a low-carb diet may improve fertility problems and hormone profiles of women with PCOS.

PCOS sufferer Bea S., 28, of Nashville, Tennessee, who had tried in vain for three years to get pregnant, is one of many women who've benefited from drastic dietary changes. When her new, blood-sugar-savvy endocrinologist discovered insulin resistance in addition to her PCOS (which another M.D. diagnosed), he instructed her to "quit eating white foods like white sugar, white rice, and white potatoes."

"I asked my doctor, 'How is cutting out all white foods going to help me have a baby?'" recalls Bea, who used to consume large quantities of sugary and carb-filled foods. "He explained that insulin is your master hormone and when you don't use insulin properly, your reproductive system shuts down. He also said my PCOS is a direct result of insulin imbalance."

After cutting out white foods, taking the medication Glucophage, and praying, Bea gave birth to a baby boy and lost a lot of weight. "I've learned the importance of not having refined sugar," she says. "Our bodies just aren't created to process it."

In addition to cutting out culprit carbs, experts such as Dr. Feinberg recommend that instead of eating two or three large meals, it's best to consume five or six lighter meals to prevent overwhelming insulin-resistant cells with too many calories at a time. This is the same diet that works for hypoglycemics and sugar-sensitive people as well.

It's also important for overweight women with PCOS to lose weight. In fact, Dr. Feinberg points out that because excess insulin can cause women's bodies to turn sugar into fat, an estimated 80 to 90 percent of those with PCOS are overweight or obese.

Admittedly, women with the syndrome will have to work against their metabolism to lose weight, but it's worth the hard work, because as they drop the pounds, their hormones will begin to normalize, he explains. Regular exercise will also help to manage weight at the same time that it helps the cells to process insulin.

Why Childbearing and Sugar Don't Mix

It's imperative for both women trying to conceive and those who already have conceived to control their sugar intake. Indeed, consuming too much sugar and having elevated insulin can create or aggravate conception and pregnancy problems for *every* woman, not just those with diabetes or gestational diabetes.

In fact, reproductive endocrinologist and gynecologist Dr. Metzger puts *all* her patients, whether they're trying to conceive or not, on a "white-out diet" free of white flour, white sugar, white pasta, and other much-like-sugar carbs. "Estrogen and progesterone enhance the release of insulin from the pancreas. That can make insulin resistance even worse, and then, you can get gestational diabetes," warns Dr. Metzger, medical advisor to the book *Stay Fertile Longer* by Mary Kittel.

Diabetes, for example, is associated with higher rates of miscarriage and fetal problems. But the good news is that proper blood sugar management can lower these risks. Not only can quitting white-carb foods improve the insulin profiles of infertility patients, but it also helps women with other reproductive health challenges such as endometriosis, a disease that causes an overgrowth of tissue outside the uterine lining.

In fact, Dr. David Ludwig of Children's Hospital Boston warns of the dangers of being pregnant while insulin resistant. The mother delivers nutrients to the fetus across the placenta, and if the mom is insulin resistant, too much sugar goes across so the baby will be born with blood sugar problems, he cautions.

Granted, once a woman is pregnant, it can be a challenge to defeat nagging cravings for sweets, especially chocolate, but giving in to those cravings can cause problems.

Meanwhile, it's important for the mother to think of her baby before overconsuming sweets. For instance, in one cutting-edge study of 1,000 women living in California, researchers found that those who ate the most refined and sugary foods experienced up to a fourfold increase in birth defects compared to women whose diets consisted mainly of unprocessed whole grains, beans, fruits, vegetables, and some dairy products. It appears that the mother's high blood sugar can overwhelm the embryo in the early stages of pregnancy, particularly before its pancreas develops. And experts believe that the hypoglycemia that often accompanies a sugar spike also could cause birth defects.

As you can see, it would be prudent for a pregnant woman to fight sugar and carb cravings, not just for her own sake, but also for the health of her unborn baby.

Kick Sugar for a More Peaceful Menopause

While limiting or eliminating those fast-release carbs can help women become pregnant, following the same carb-cutting strategies can help them ease their way through "the change."

Indeed, renowned fitness expert Kathy Smith, author of eight books, including *Kathy Smith's Moving Through Menopause*, noticed that her chocolate habit was hampering her own ability to sail smoothly through menopause.

"It became so apparent to me that *after* I ate rich chocolaty things, I would get very warm, start perspiring, and become crabby and more impatient," she recalls. The symptoms were so intense that she tracked her reactions by keeping a food-symptoms diary and found some compelling data that implicated sugar.

"Sugar was triggering hot flashes, interrupting my sleep, making me spacey and forgetful, and causing volatility in my personality," Smith admits. "I'd go on a talk show, and the menopausal symptoms would get in the way. It became easy for me to say that the chocolate just was not worth it."

Accustomed to a busy lifestyle, Smith cut back on sugar and sought more healthy ways to satisfy her sweet tooth. "High-fiber whole foods like fruits, vegetables, and whole grains are easier to handle than more refined starches and sugars."

Anita Flegg, 43, of Ottawa, Canada, also found that reducing her sugar intake helped her through perimenopause. "I was able to go off the estrogen treatment I had been on for five years, and my symptoms never returned," marvels the electrical engineer, who became so intrigued by the subject that she self-published *Hypoglycemia: The Other Sugar Disease*.

Moreover, Ruth M., 53, of Great Britain, credits her having "come through menopause without hot flashes or insomnia" to cutting out sugar, taking evening primrose oil, eating more nuts and seeds, and adopting an Ayurvedic-type diet.

As a woman moves toward menopause, Dr. Metzger explains, her hormone levels fluctuate. Naturally, this is an oversimplification, but estrogen and progesterone levels begin to drop either rapidly, slowly, or erratically. And, because both these hormones influence a woman's response to insulin, the shift can also affect how sugar is processed by the body.

"That's why women often gain weight in menopause, because their hormones are changing," Dr. Metzger explains. "That, in turn, changes their response to insulin so they need to be even more fastidious about avoiding sugar and refined carbs. Your levels of estrogen and progesterone will still lower, but you become less reactive to the changes when you improve your diet. You'll have more control over your weight, and you won't have as many hot flashes, night sweats, and difficult[ies] sleeping."

On the other hand, "eating a lot of carbs can eventually lead to weight gain, which can put you at risk for insulin resistance," points out epidemiologist Lewis Kuller, M.D., Ph.D., a professor in the University of Pittsburgh's Department of Epidemiology and a principal investigator with the 15-year government-funded Women's Health Initiative. (This is a study that examines the most common causes of death, disability, and poor quality of life in postmenopausal women.)

Like Kathy Smith, Dr. Kuller also stresses to women approaching menopause that "cutting back on simple carbohydrates, reducing sugar, and exercising every day can help you live an enjoyable, pleasurable life."

As you've learned here, the evidence is mounting that reducing or cutting out sweets and much-like-sugar carbs could help us females weather the ups and downs of hormonal shifts from PMS to pregnancy to menopause. Not only that, but eating right also could reduce your risk of yeast infections, chronic fatigue, fibromyalgia, PCOS, infertility, and endometrial cancer.

FOR YOUR BEAUTY: SUGAR GLUTTING COULD GIVE YOU PIMPLES, WRINKLES, AND MORE

For years, we've heard that chocolate and other sweets are bad for our complexion. Of course, many Americans have blithely continued to ingest the stuff. But scientists are now finding a close connection between pigging out on processed carbs and sugar and developing acne, wrinkles, fine lines, brittle nails, dull, lifeless hair, bloating, and skin tags.

The Sugar–Acne Connection

Historically, dermatologists did not believe that diet triggered acne, points out Margaret E. Olsen, M.D., chief of dermatology at St. John's Hospital in Santa Monica, California, and assistant clinical professor of dermatology at UCLA. "Our grandmothers and mothers knew there was a link, but we dermatologists didn't think it was true."

That's exactly what Andria P., 30, was told. "My doctors always insisted that my acne wasn't food related," says the Manhattan-based publicist, who spent years suffering from an agonizing pimple problem that often included "big, blotchy, swollen cysts" on her face—sometimes "as many as ten to twelve in a week."

For Lent, in 2001, Andria gave up chocolate—after an 11-year daily habit that even had her hiding candy bars under her bed or in her closet. "When I quit chocolate and other sweets, my skin cleared up," says an elated Andria. What's more, kicking those dessert foods "worked better than years of incredibly painful anti-inflammatory injections in each cyst and prescription acne medications."

Now, new studies are providing research support for the anecdotal claims of people like Andria who break out after eating chocolate and other sweets. For the past two decades Loren Cordain, Ph.D., a professor in the Department of Health and Exercise Science at Colorado State University, has been spending extended periods of time traveling to different parts of the world not overrun with processed foods to research the effects of various diets. Every single time, he's arrived at the same conclusion: A diet of sugary foods and processed carbohydrates can cause pimples.

"Non-Westernized" Folks Have *No* Pimples!

We can learn a lot from those "less civilized" than we. In one of Dr. Cordain's most dramatic and convincing studies, his research team spent six weeks examining the diets—and the skin—of 1,200 Kitavan Islanders in Papua, New Guinea. The upshot: They found *not a single case of acne* in the entire population, including 300 teens. The natives lived simply, on fish, fruit, coconut, and root vegetables (or tubers). And sure enough, they ate *almost no* cereals or refined sugars.

For another study, Dr. Cordain and his fellow researchers traveled to Paraguay where they examined the eating habits of Ache hunter-gatherers over a two-year period. There, the native population mainly ate wild game, maize, rice, and sweet manioc—a root vegetable from cassava, which is "the staff of life" for people in tropical countries. Sure enough, as in New Guinea, processed foods, grains, and dairy were scarce, constituting only 8 percent of the diet.

And all that good food paid off on the natives' skin. "Again, there wasn't a single case of acne in the 115 people we studied, including 15 people aged 15 to 25," recounts Dr. Cordain, whose book, *The Paleo Diet*, advocates the protein-and-vegetable-rich way of eating followed by our ancestors.

Convincing Conclusions

Dr. Cordain's landmark study, "*Acne vulgaris*: A Disease of Western Civilization," garnered considerable attention when it appeared in the American Medical Association's *Archives of Dermatology*. Certainly, the intriguing results—that acne is less prevalent in non-Westernized countries—support suspicions long held by vegetable-and-protein-consuming health advocates but dismissed by chocolate-and-cookie-eating folks.

In effect, the results of Dr. Cordain's and other researchers' studies contradict the dermatological community's prevailing point of view that diet doesn't cause acne. Indeed, "a large body of evidence," Dr. Cordain contends in a 2005 review article, shows that diet may, in fact, directly or indirectly influence acne.

So why do sugary and processed foods bring out pimples and other unwanted skin conditions?

"Our high-glycemic diet has set us up for a situation that makes us insulin resistant," Dr. Cordain explains. "Refined carbs require torrents of insulin to process them. We believe that this excess insulin sets off a hormonal cascade that promotes unregulated tissue growth such as in acne."

Here's the scenario, according to Dr. Cordain and other experts: Excess sugar and processed carbs trigger high insulin levels. In turn, these high insulin levels bring about an endocrine (hormonal) response that simultaneously promotes unregulated tissue growth, which causes a buildup of pore-clogging skin cells and enhanced androgen (male hormone) secretions.

In other words, chronic high-insulin levels bring about excessive andro-

CONFESSIONS OF A SUGAR KICKER

"I've had skin issues since I was 13. My acne was anywhere from moderate to intense. I found that the key to having good skin is cutting out sugar. After six months off desserts, my skin started to become very radiant, supple, and smooth. People started saying, 'Wow, you look really good. What are you doing?'"

—Lisa J., 44, massage therapist and performance artist, New York City

gen, which leads you to overproduce sebum, a greasy substance that feeds pimple-promoting bacteria. The consequence: a dermatological nightmare.

Even normally clear-skinned Pacific Islanders and South American Indians get acne when they move to urban areas and eat our typical Westernized diet (high in sugar and refined carbs), points out Dr. Cordain, who presented his fascinating findings linking acne to the Western diet at the 2004 annual meeting of the Society for Investigative Dermatology. "The same thing happens when Eskimos start eating Western foods."

Australian Researchers Also Link Pimples to Quickie Carbs

To test the theory that sugary foods and fast-acting carbs could promote acne, an Australian team put 50 pimple-plagued males aged 16 to 23 on a high-protein diet that excluded refined carbohydrates but included higher quality carbohydrates such as vegetables, fruits, nuts, and seeds, as well as lean meat, fish, and low-fat dairy foods.

Neil Mann, Ph.D., associate professor of human nutrition at RMIT University in Melbourne, Australia, and lead author of the study, along with his colleague, George Varigos, M.D., head of dermatology at the Royal Melbourne Hospital, arrived at conclusions similar to Dr. Cordain's when studying 50 males aged 16 to 23 who had moderate to severe acne.

In fact, Dr. Mann says their findings did "confirm their hypothesis that foods high in glycemic impact, which constantly raise blood sugar levels to a high level and hence elevate blood insulin levels, could help trigger acne proliferation."

Conversely, when teens ate less carbs, a minimum amount of high-GI processed foods, and more protein they experienced "lowered acne proliferation and severity" compared with those who had a large intake of high-GI carbs.

When asked for tips to reverse pimple progression, Dr. Mann suggested, "Best advice for acne sufferers would be cut down on processed carb foods and high-GI foods such as potatoes and rice and eat a diet rich in vegetables, fruits, whole grains, and lean meat and fish."

So there you have it. Scientists doing research completely independent of one another in different parts of the world, no less, are arriving at exactly the same advice.

TAKE HEART: SOMETIMES IT'S DARKEST BEFORE THE BLEMISH-FREE SKIN

A quick caution for would-be Sugar Kickers. Although not everyone experiences this reaction, some people who give up sweets or refined carbs apparently find that pimples may *initially* pop up instead of disappearing. But *don't fret,* because the outbreak is temporary and it will probably die down rather quickly. According to Dr. Nancy Appleton, it just means that "your body is detoxing." Think of it as a facial working from the inside out. With facials, there are a few breakouts and redness before the glow.

Medical experts also emphasize the importance to our skin (and overall health) of eating "good fats" (omega-3) and avoiding the "bad fats" (omega-6) often found in processed carbs. "A diet rich in omega-3 fats, found in salmon, fish oil, and flaxseed oil, also seems to underlie prevention of acne," Dr. Cordain observes.

Less Junk Food Could Mean Fewer Wrinkles

Apparently, cutting back on bad carbs could do much more than rid you of acne. Scientists are also finding that low-sugar, nutrient-rich diets actually reduce wrinkling and enable your skin to stay supple longer. This remarkable food/wrinkle link was documented by an Australian study of 453 adults over age 70 who were originally from Greece, Sweden, or Australia.

Published in the *Journal of the American College of Nutrition*, "Skin Wrinkling: Can Food Make a Difference?" reported that study participants who ate vegetables, legumes, and monounsaturated fats such as olive oil and fish, wrinkled less, *even if* they lived in a sunny climate. By contrast, people who gobbled cakes, pastries, soft drinks, milk products, butter, margarine, and red meat were more likely to develop wrinkles. The study, spearheaded by Mark L. Wahlqvist, M.D., a professor at the Asia Pacific Health and Nutrition Centre in Melbourne, also hinted that the old adage—"an apple a day keeps the doctor away"—holds some truth: eating apples and drinking tea was found to reduce skin damage by 34 percent, sunny weather or not.

Actually, dermatologists are already aware that diabetics tend to age more quickly and suffer more skin damage than nondiabetics, points out Frederic Fenig, M.D., a dermatologist in private practice in New York City. "Long-standing diabetics may get all kinds of discolorations and splotches on their legs, forearms, and thighs, as well as reddening of their faces, hands, and feet."

But as experts know, diabetics aren't the only group that tends to age more quickly. Experts believe that having even *mildly* high blood sugar levels (prediabetes) or *low* blood sugar (hypoglycemia) can speed up the aging process. In other words, those blood sugar swings ultimately tax the skin, causing people to look older than they are. As dermatologist Dr. Olsen explains: "Wrinkles are worse in people who have bad nutrition. If you're unwell, you may have more lines."

So how does excess sugar speed up those unwanted lines and wrinkles? Here, in theory, is what happens: When we eat sweets and refined carbs that rapidly convert to sugar in our bloodstream, those sugar molecules attach themselves to proteins in our bloodstream. And in a manner slightly reminiscent of a doomed relationship, once sugar and protein bind together, undesired chemical reactions ensue. Sugar and proteins do something called "cross-linking"—a process that scientists call glycation or glycosylation.

If you absentmindedly snack on a sweet roll and candy bar every day, as well as drink a couple of sodas, you're going to cause browning or glycating of the protein in your tissues, explains dermatologist and best-selling author Dr. Nicholas Perricone, who wrote about this phenomenon in the foreword to this book.

"Glycation is a process known to discolor and toughen food in storage, but it occurs in skin as well," says Dr. Perricone, who paints a distasteful picture: "Sugar is exceptionally damaging to your skin because sugar molecules attach to collagen fibers, ultimately causing them to 'cross-link' and become stiff and inflexible. This extensive cross-linking of collagen and sugar leads to the wrinkling, leathering, and loss of elasticity of your skin." (Incidentally, cross-linking can also lead to a number of other health conditions, including stiffening of the joints and hardening of the arteries.)

Years of eating those captivating, quickie carbs could cause chronically high levels of blood glucose, and when all those sugar molecules cross-link with protein, you end up with a new chemical structure called "AGEs" or advanced glycosylation [or Glycated] end products.

Antiaging expert Ron Rosedale, M.D., cofounder of Advanced Metabolic

Laboratories and author of *The Rosedale Diet*, describes glycation as "a major mechanism of damage that fundamentally affects the aging process. It's on a par with oxidation."

And Oz Garcia, Ph.D., author of *Look and Feel Fabulous Forever*, who's often called "nutritionist to the stars," also drums into the heads of his celebrity and corporate clients the need to steer clear of sugar because "glycation speeds up the aging process."

"I tell them, 'If you don't want to look ragged and want to be in great condition for your next TV show or film, then you're going to have to reduce your exposure to sugar.'

"Then they can begin to use good thoughts to overwhelm bad impulses," says Dr. Garcia, whose clients include Oscar winner Hilary Swank, singer Roberta Flack, and former *Sex and the City* star Kim Cattrall.

Other Ways Too Much Sugar Could Mess Up Our Skin

Acne and glycation aren't the only ways sugar could harm our skin. Preventive medicine specialist Michael Lam, M.D., M.P.H., believes that "sugar, when it's metabolized into the body, leads to the release of free radicals. This damages your tissue's cellular structure, leading to the breakdown of collagen.

"And collagen," Dr. Lam explains, "is the matrix that forms the foundation of the epidermis of the skin. When you have collagen breakdown, that's when wrinkles and fine lines start to appear."

But our bodies are quite miraculous: Collagen can be rebuilt. "The skin goes through a regenerative process every 28 days. It doesn't matter at what age you start," says Dr. Lam, medical education director at the Pasadena, California–based Academy of Anti-Aging Research, a worldwide society of health professionals dedicated to advancing antiaging medicine.

"Of course, the more damage you have to your skin, the harder it is to repair. But as long as you stop feeding it sugar, the free radicals will reduce, and the damage to collagen will reduce. The *best* way to build collagen is from the inside."

Sweets and much-like-sugar carbs damage skin in another way, too. "Eating sugar and processed carbohydrates causes a burst of inflammation in cells throughout your body," explains Dr. Perricone, who presents a pretty scary scenario.

"If we took some skin cells, put them into a culture, and let them grow, and then added a couple of drops of sugar, we could measure inflammatory chemicals going up by 1,000 percent over the baseline within a matter of an hour.

"If you're in a proinflammatory state, your insulin and sugar levels are high, you store body fat, you have a cloudy outlook, you have no energy, your cells aren't functioning, your hormones are thrown off, you get more acne, your sex drive goes down, you feel less pleasure in life, and you get wrinkles," Dr. Perricone continues, speaking in a phone interview.

"The way I describe this whole process is this: You can be fat, dumb, and wrinkled, or you can be beautiful, smart, and energetic. You can choose the one you want to be by what you eat."

Ultimately, the brain and the skin are more intertwined than perhaps many of us think. "Anything that has a beneficial effect on the brain makes the skin look better," Dr. Perricone says. "If sugar is bad for the brain, then it's horrible for the skin. They're derived from the same tissue. I call it the brain-beauty connection. Learning to eat correctly with high-protein foods, essential fatty acids, and low-glycemic carbs is the key to beauty."

Once again, restoring insulin sensitivity is the key. Dr. Rosedale believes that "when you change your diet, you improve your insulin sensitivity within weeks. The rate at which you age is largely determined by how your body reacts to insulin. And when your insulin is regulated, you'll lose excess fluid . . . This will positively impact swollen ankles, varicose veins, and bloating."

Tags and Other Skin Woes

Scientists also link other skin conditions to gorging on sugar and processed carbs. For example, skin tags—those little flaps of skin that crop up in the armpit, neck, or groin area—are "external signs and symptoms of insulin resistance," according to Dr. Cordain, who notes that obese people tend to get them more often than those who maintain a healthy weight.

The good news? You probably won't develop more skin tags if you switch to a healthy, unprocessed diet.

Acanthosis nigricans, a skin disorder involving a velvety thickening of skin around the neck or backs of hands, also tends to occur in people with insulin resistance and/or obesity. The condition affects 7 to 10 percent of the population, primarily people with dark skin, Dr. Cordain estimates. Again, a change in diet can yield wondrous results.

"If you take people with skin tags and put them on a low-glycemic-load diet, their insulin resistance, acne, and acanthosis all subside," Dr. Cordain says. "The closer you are to normal weight and the less insulin resistant you are, the quicker they will fade."

How Quitting Sweets Could Improve Your Hair and Nails

If ridding yourself of wrinkles and pimples and having a smoother, more glowing complexion don't motivate you enough to banish your sugar and quickie-carb habit, rest assured that you get still other beauty benefits from changing to a more healthy diet.

For example, like Lynne C., 59, of Sydney, Australia, you might find that if you kick sugar, your hair and nails will grow more quickly.

"I've been off sugar for four weeks, and a few strange things have been happening," Lynne happily related to my online KickSugar group.

"My acrylic nails usually need to be 'done' every two weeks. This time, after 8 days they were where they should be in 14. I bleach my hair every three weeks, and this time, within two weeks, my black roots grew back so fast that I had to bleach them more often!"

Indeed, experts say that hair and nail deficiencies are diet related, too. For example, Dr. Cordain cites studies in which rats fed biotin-deficient diets (a high-grain way of eating) developed rough, dry, scaly skin; brittle hair; ridges in their nails; and pelts that were dull, lifeless, and brittle.

In fact, Dr. Cordain believes that we humans can improve our nails and hair by cutting back on grains, especially refined ones, which he characterizes as "humanity's double-edged sword," because on the one hand they've allowed us to develop culturally and technologically but, on the other hand, "many of the world's people suffer disease and dysfunction directly attributable to the consumption of these foods."

We Can't Sugarcoat the Facts: The Bottom Line

Ultimately, the evidence is mounting that curbing your sweet tooth will do much more for you than a trip to the beauty parlor. More and more, scientists—and us Sugar Kickers alike—are learning that what you put into your body can affect how you look.

Indeed, I often hear from delighted women and men from around the world who are pleasantly surprised by the tremendous beauty benefits they receive just by kicking sugar and quickie carbs.

"I still remember my shock when my skin became glowing and smooth within weeks of kicking sugar," recalls Roberta Ruggiero, founder and president of the Hypoglycemia Support Foundation. "All the skin creams in the world did nothing compared with removing sweets from my diet."

Former sugar lover Phyllis S., a filmmaker/actress from Los Angeles, puts it cleverly:

"At first I wanted to get off sugar for my vanity. Now I abstain for my sanity."

17

For Parents:

Help Your Young

Sugar Brats End Their Fits

of Fury

Ask almost any mother or father what happens when his or her normally sweet, funny, loving child overdoses on candies, cookies, and sweetened soda, and she or he will very likely complain—for as long as you're willing to listen—about how the kid becomes wild, wired, and weird.

Parents, grandparents, and even family friends are full of tales about how a simply adorable, mild-mannered youngster did a complete turn-around, becoming hyperactive, quarrelsome, confrontational, depressed, irrational, unruly, rowdy, raging, and tantrum throwing—in short, a little monster that I dub a "Sugar Brat."

Perhaps this exasperating, maddening child-on-sweets situation is best illustrated by a wonderful John McPherson "Close to Home" cartoon. In the comic strip, an out-of-control kid hoists an armchair in the air, while a smashed TV and badly bent lamp lie in shambles on the floor nearby. The mom then explains to the dad, "He does not have a discipline problem! He's just had a little too much sugar, that's all."

Parents *Know* There's a Food-Mood Connection, Conflicting Research or Not

So do sweets really turn your child into a hostile, argumentative, cantankerous creature you'd rather not have around? Certainly, parents will tell you with more than 1,000 percent certainty that eating a slice or two of birthday cake and drinking lots of soda lead to all kinds of unseemly conduct.

But not all scientists agree that a sugary diet makes a kid hyperactive and unruly. In fact, this alleged link between sugar and children's behavior is one of the most hotly debated issues among pediatricians, parents, researchers, the medical community, and activists. Interestingly, ample arguments exist to support either point of view.

"Researchers have been unable to document a causal relationship, because this is a difficult study to scientifically predict and reproduce," says Carden Johnston, M.D., former president of the American Academy of Pediatrics, a national organization with 57,000 members. "But, when you talk to parents, there's no doubt that sugar leads to hyperactivity."

Mother Kathy M., 39, of St. Charles, Illinois, for example, notices changes within two hours of her child's eating sweets or much-like-sugar carbs. "He gets belligerent, defiant, extremely crabby, and impulsive," she observes. "He won't listen, he picks fights, he doesn't get along with his brothers, and he just lashes out. It's not that he's a difficult kid. The sugar makes him that way!"

Adamant naysayers dismiss the theory that sugar revs up kids. "The data doesn't support it," maintains Robin Kanarek, Ph.D., a Tufts University psychology and nutrition professor and dean of the Graduate School of Arts and Sciences.

"There have been hundreds of studies," says Dr. Kanarek, who credits a festive party atmosphere—not sugar—with revving up kids and making them trash toys or wrap a room with toilet paper.

Of course, you, as a parent, know better. So do your kids' physicians. And so do many experts.

"Talk to any mother who's given her kid sugar or food coloring and noticed hyperactivity," observes pediatric allergist Doris Rapp, M.D., who simply can't fathom why the medical community is so reluctant to accept the idea that sweets could make sweet kids outrageously rambunctious, contrary, and rowdy.

"How can doctors deny it? Physicians are losing credibility because parents are picking up this information on their own. Nobody knows a child as well as the parent," says Dr. Rapp, author of *Is This Your Child?*, *Allergies and the Hyperactive Child*, and *Our Toxic World: A Wake-Up Call*.

"Sensitivity to sugar is genetic," asserts Dr. Rapp, who maintains that some 40 to 50 percent of hyperactive kids are sensitive to sugar. "If you have an allergic mom or dad, you would expect sensitivity to develop early in life. Some children get hyperactive in the uterus when the mother eats certain foods," believes Dr. Rapp, who contends that ingesting both sugar and additives can cause learning problems, headaches, and fatigue.

Problems with Studies That Seek to Debunk Hyperactivity Theory

In reviewing hundreds of medical studies, Dr. Nancy Appleton, author of *Lick the Sugar Habit*, found considerable research linking multiple behavioral problems to sweets, including hyperactivity, anxiety, crankiness, and concentration problems.

Like other experts, Dr. Appleton expresses strong reservations about the methodology used by studies seeking to disprove the sugar-makes-kids-hyperactive theory. For example, she notes that in one study children were given *small* amounts of sugar *throughout the day*, including the equivalent of half a can of soda.

"Nobody *ever* drinks *just part of a can of soda*. They didn't give them large amounts at one sitting. It's the *jolt*—how fast and how much—that causes problems," Dr. Appleton maintains. Moreover, she argues, in other research experiments, scientists waited way too long before taking blood sugar samples.

> ## YOUR IRRITABLE, IRRATIONAL CHILD COULD BE SUFFERING BLOOD SUGAR FLUCTUATIONS
>
> If your child grapples with rage, depression, fatigue, insomnia, or other symptoms, watch how he or she eats. If your kid drinks a lot of soda, chomps often on candies or cookies, that could be triggering SUGAR SHOCK! moments. Test your child's behavior by taking away those sweet snacks for a few days. Your kid's behavioral and physical ailments could provide clues indicating that he or she has hypoglycemia, prediabetes, or type 2 diabetes, particularly if diabetes runs in your family. If you think your kid is too young to have diabetes, bear in mind that diabetes is now striking our nation's youth with increasing prevalence. As a parent, you owe it to your kid to do whatever you can to help your child be healthy.

In trying to assess whether sugar makes your child hyperactive, it's important to keep in mind that soda and chocolate contain not only sugar, but also caffeine, because some kids can be sensitive to both. For example, Dr. Appleton cites one research project in which kids showed signs of hyperactivity within 45 to 60 minutes of ingesting a dose of sugar and caffeine equivalent to the amount found in a single 12-ounce can of soda.

What Can a Frustrated Parent Do to Help an Ill-Mannered, Sugar-Hooked Kid?

Parents who want to improve their child's behavior should remember that getting a tot or teen to cut back on sweets provides many positives. "It could help him or her to have more friends, sleep better, or do better in school. The list goes on and on," says Dr. Appleton.

Here, then, are some tips from experts to help aggravated, exasperated parents wean their kids off sweets and/or to pinpoint their blood sugar problems:

- **Look and listen.** "Before you even *think* about putting your kid on Ritalin or any medication to control attention deficit disorder (ADD) or attention deficit hyperactivity disorder (ADHD), evaluate your child's dietary habits and keep a symptom diary to track moods and energy levels," advises Ruggiero, author of *The Do's and Don'ts of Hypoglycemia*: *An Everyday Guide to Low Blood Sugar*. "If your kid skips meals and eats a diet high in sugars, this could contribute to his or her awful behavior. Doing a diet change first could save many years of unnecessary medication."

- **Look out for number one.** "Take care of yourself first. Get yourself solid and stable, and then deal with your kids. If you're a cranky parent, you can't deal with a cranky kid. Put your own oxygen mask on first," suggests Kathleen DesMaisons, Ph.D., a pioneer in the field of addictive nutrition and author of *Little Sugar Addicts*.

- **Set a good example.** "The best way to get your kids to cut back on their sugar intake is to be a good role model by scaling back your own sugar consumption," advises New York–based integrative medicine specialist and stress-management expert Jill Baron, M.D.

- **Offer fresh foods.** Stock your cabinets and refrigerator with fruits and vegetables instead of chips and cookies, recommends Dr. Rapp. Give your children such healthy, tasty snacks as apples, oranges, and nuts, or celery with sugarfree almond butter or peanut butter. "Give them healthy alternatives like sweet potatoes," suggests Dr. Appleton. "Whatever you do, don't resort to nagging or scare tactics, both of which can backfire."

- **Freeze fruit.** "You can actually change your kids' taste buds by not giving them sugary sweet sodas. Try freezing fruit such as strawberries, bananas, and raspberries, and blueberries. You could blend in milk or yogurt, and it comes out like ice cream. You can't tell the difference," recommends nutritionist Shari Lieberman, Ph.D., C.N.S., F.A.C.N., and author of *Dare to Lose*.

- **Involve your kids.** Take your kids with you when you go food shopping and ask them to help you cook dinner or prepare their school lunches, recommends Dr. Appleton. "Their involvement is key," she explains. "They feel more in control this way. And remember to praise and reinforce their good behavior often."

TRICK OR TREAT . . . GIVE KIDS SOMETHING GOOD TO . . . PLAY WITH!

What's Halloween without candy? Just as much fun, according to kids who participated in a Yale University study. Given a choice between lollipops, fruit-flavored chews, and hard candies, or toys like glow-in-the-dark insects, stretch pumpkin men, or Halloween-themed stickers and pencils, *half* the 284 three- to fourteen-year-old trick-or-treater participants picked the toys.

"As a society, we've gotten into the mind-set that *the only way* to celebrate special occasions with children is by serving something sweet," says Marlene Schwartz, Ph.D., principal investigator for the research paper, which was published in the *Journal of Nutrition, Education and Behavior*.

"This study can reassure parents that children will respond favorably to noncandy treats," adds Dr. Schwartz, director of research at Yale University's Rudd Center for Food Policy and Obesity. So, next Halloween, feel free to forgo sweet treats and hand out toys instead.

■ **Cut back slowly.** "Don't try to take your kids off sugar all at once," advises Dr. DesMaisons. Doing so, she says, will put too much stress on their young bodies, and the withdrawal symptoms might be too intense to take.

■ **Share your red-flag findings.** Ask other adults in your child's life such as his or her teacher, child-care provider, and physician, as well as relatives and neighbors, to help you to phase sweets out of your kid's life, advises Ruggiero.

■ **Play whole-grain games.** "Do something innovative with your kids like, 'Guess the grain night' while serving quinoa, millet, or kamut," Dr. Baron suggests.

More Tips to Parents to Help Your Sugar-Addict Kids

■ **Begin with breakfast.** Ample research shows the importance of that first meal of the day. "People who eat [a good] breakfast think better and faster, remember more, react quicker, and are mentally sharper than breakfast skippers. They also miss fewer days of school and work," notes nutritionist Elizabeth Somer, M.A., R.D., author of *Food & Mood*. "Just about every measure of thinking ability improves after eating a good breakfast, from math scores and creative thinking to speed and efficiency in solving problems, concentration, recall, and accuracy in work performance." For example, a study in the *Journal of Nursing Research* reported that healthy-breakfast eaters had higher grades and a higher class rank. But make sure your child, teen, or adolescent understands that a "good" breakfast doesn't mean a monster-sized cinnamon roll, but rather more like a fresh orange, a vegetable omelette, and some steel-cut oats with chopped almonds.

■ **Keep H$_2$O around.** Get a water purifier and always keep pitchers handy so that your kids can drink it instead of soda or other drinks sweetened with sugar or high-fructose corn syrup, says Dr. Baron.

■ **Make your own drinks.** If your kid nags you for soda or juice, make your own together. For example, take half a fresh orange or a full lemon, squeeze it, then add sparkling or purified water.

■ **Urge your kids to get off their butts.** Your best defense against obesity and other diseases is to teach your kids the value and joy of exercising. If they learn at a young age to exercise to replace unhealthy behaviors such as eating too much sugar or watching too much TV, they can create good habits for life.

■ **Get involved.** "Take an active role with parents' groups and other organizations that are fighting to get companies to quit marketing junk food and soda pop in schools," recommends pediatrician Dr. Johnston. "And urge your kids' schools to carry vending machines that stock more healthy foods."

■ **Learn.** Study about the diet-behavior connection. "What your child eats *or doesn't eat* directly relates to how he or she thinks, feels, and acts," Ruggiero says. Put into practice tips from *Little Sugar Addicts* by Dr. DesMaisons, *Allergies and the Hyperactive Child* by Dr. Rapp, *Feed Your Kids Right* by Lendon Smith, M.D., and Ruggiero's *The Do's and Don'ts of Hypoglycemia*.

- **Make TV the exception, not the rule.** Encourage your child to be active instead of watching TV or playing video games. If you can, limit Saturday morning TV, where ads for sugary foods are often aired. Try to get your children hooked on educational TV. Provide some healthy snacks at the same time.

- **Be patient and flexible.** Remember, your child is tempted often by sweets (just as you are), so take time to put changes into effect, Dr. Baron advises. "Aim for progress, not perfection."

Give Your Child a Life of Hope

Ultimately, to be a good parent, you must set a good example for your kids. "Since sugar has been a staple in the household, a new generation can grow up addicted, angry, depressed, overweight, difficult to get along with, and more likely to be sick as adults," Dr. Appleton explains.

"It is a vicious cycle. That's why you need to break it now."

At age eight, Adele B. of Ocean City, New Jersey, was already one of those sugar-driven, angry, troubled, overly rambunctious kids.

"I'd come home from school . . . and go grab 20 cookies. Then I'd switch into a different person—I'd go from being sweet and nice to nasty, disobedient, and antisocial. It took me years to piece this all together," she mournfully recalls.

Adele's situation illustrates the importance of trying to help your kids *now*.

PART 6

PULL THE PLUG ON SUGAR SHOCK! FOR A HAPPIER, HEALTHIER LIFE

18

Trapped by Your Sugar or Carb Habit? Connie's Tips on What to Do Next

If you now suspect that you're in SUGAR SHOCK!, you're probably wondering how to break free. You may be wondering whether you should quit sweets altogether or just cut back. Either way, you can take some positive steps right away to change your relationship with quickie carbs. Here are some tips on how to begin:

1. TURN YOUR DIET AROUND. EAT "MOTHER NATURE'S CARB GIFTS" AND MORE.
Start gravitating more toward rainbow-colored vegetables and low-sugar fruits such as strawberries, apples, and blueberries. Select high-quality protein sources such as fish, chicken, lean cuts of meat, and soy. Enjoy nuts, seeds, and legumes. Judiciously use healthy fats such as olive oil, flaxseed oil, and macadamia nut oil. If you wish, eat modest amounts of whole grains such as quinoa, brown rice, and amaranth.

If, at this point, you still choose to have a dessert food, pick a small, polite portion and eat it *only after* consuming healthy foods such as those listed above. And remember to drink plenty of water to flush out toxins, carry nutrients to your body's cells, metabolize fat, and perform other vital functions. (Most experts suggest consuming half your body weight in ounces. "You need more than 64 ounces if you exercise regularly [an extra 8 ounces per 15 minutes to be exact], live in a hot, dry, or humid environment, or are overweight," says nutritionist and exercise physiologist Jill Vollmuth.

2. TAKE CHARGE OF YOUR MEDICAL TREATMENT.

Consult a physician to find out if you have a blood sugar condition such as prediabetes, diabetes, or hypoglycemia. (Visit my website, www.Sugar Shock.com, for tips on finding an educated, sugar-savvy doctor.) If you're beset by mysterious ailments such as fatigue, headaches, severe PMS, angry outbursts, and/or anxiety, ask your M.D. if he or she thinks a five- or six-hour Glucose Tolerance Test might be useful to learn if you have hypoglycemia.

If you experience frequent urination, excess thirst, and excess hunger, find out if you have prediabetes. If you're inactive, overweight, and hooked on sweets and quickie carbs, it's a good idea to get checked for diabetes, prediabetes, or Syndrome X.

3. DO SOME SUGARY SOUL-SEARCHING.

Look inward and do what I call "Sugary Soul-Searching"—a vital first step to sever the hold that sweets and refined carbs have over you. In other words, face your sugar reality. Pay attention to what, when, where, why, and how you eat or overeat sweets or quickie carbs. Learn what personal and professional situations or emotions trigger you. Identify your patterns. In short, zero in on *why* you turn to those fast-acting carbs. Next, explore how you react, both emotionally and physically, within minutes, hours, and days after indulging. Next, start a journal and jot down how you feel and act within an hour of eating sweets or processed carbs, then after 2 hours, 4 hours, 24 hours, 2 days, and so on. While conducting your enlightening Sugary Soul-Searching, ask yourself questions such as the following. For example, after eating desserts and simple carbs, do you get wired, tired, or argumentative; lose your motivation; feel down and desolate; or get spacey and forgetful?

4. JOIN MY FREE, ONLINE KICKSUGAR SUPPORT GROUP (ON YAHOO!).

You'll find this KickSugar Internet oasis (on Yahoo!) to be a warm, welcoming, nurturing place full of camaraderie and helpful information. Everyone is welcome—no matter what your size, age, sex, or nationality. You'll feel right at home whether you are struggling with excess weight; have just found out you have a blood sugar condition such as hypoglycemia, prediabetes, insulin resistance, or diabetes; are grappling with severe sugar cravings; or are experiencing mystifying symptoms such as mood swings, crying spells, and fuzzy headedness.

I launched my free, international online KickSugar group on Yahoo! in November 2002 to provide encouragement, information, motivation, and inspiration to hooked-on-sweets victims as I once was. To join KickSugar, visit my website (www.SugarShock.com) or blog (www.SugarShockBlog.com), and click on the link that says, "Kick Sugar with Us!" (Just look for the colorful artwork of figures holding hands.)

5. GET LIVE SUPPORT.
In addition to getting support online, you may wish to attend a "live" support group such as Overeaters Anonymous (OA), Food Addicts Anonymous (FAA), Eating Disorders Anonymous, Take Off Pounds Sensibly (TOPS), or another self-help program. Millions find these groups invaluable. If you're not comfortable with the 12-step approach, then find a nurturing group whose approach and philosophy click best with you so you can accomplish your KickSugar goals.

6. CONSIDER PRIVATE OR GROUP THERAPY.
Many people with sugar issues find that seeing a psychiatrist, psychologist, or other mental health professional can help them to discover the underlying emotional causes for their sugar behavior. It's also important to learn if you're 1 of 10 million females or 1 million males struggling with bulimia and/or anorexia nervosa or one of 25 million folks battling binge eating disorder (BED) or compulsive overeating.

If you suspect that you have one of these dangerous disorders, then learn about them and/or find a therapist by contacting the National Eating Disorders Association (www.nationaleatingdisorders.org), the Eating Disorder Referral and Information Center (www.edreferral.com), Help End Eating Disorders (www.heedfoundation.org), the International Association of Eating Disorders Professionals (www.iaedp.com), or the Academy for Eating Disorders (www.aedweb.org).

7. PURSUE YOUR PASSIONS.
Finally, as you explore your relationship with sugar, it's important to find fun, healthy alternatives. "People who are the most successful at conquering

addictions are the ones who make constructive choices," says psychologist Howard J. Shaffer, Ph.D., C.A.S., former director of the Harvard Medical School's Division on Addictions.

"Find things that once made you happy. Take up new hobbies. Learn new skills. Find better substitutes. Exercise," he advises. "Those are the *best* protections against addictions and the best activities to recover from them."

What it comes down to is that "you need to have passions," insists Ira M. Sacker, M.D., an eating disorders specialist and author of *Dying to Be Thin*.

"If you don't know what your passions are, then you've got to find them," he urges. "To get over your sugar habit, you've got to find something positive that fills your needs."

19

Without Sugar, What's Left to Eat? Plenty!

Often, when people find out that I don't eat sweets or quickie carbs, they're stumped. Mystified, they're likely to ask me in amazement, "Well, what the heck can you eat then?" Amused, I often quip, "Well, I can have air and water. Oh, and if I'm really daring, dirt and sand!"

In truth, however, if your dietary mainstays are now pastries, pizza, and other processed carbs, giving them up means you'll have a lot *more* to eat. While it may be tough to imagine leaving behind your favorite "goodies," doing just that will allow you to explore a whole new world of fresh, flavorful foods.

When You Stop the Sugar and Processed Carbs, Foods Taste Better!

Most folks who put their sugarcoated days behind them report that foods they once scorned as "boring" suddenly taste luscious. As they embark upon their sugar-free adventure, they're stunned to discover that vegetables and fruits, nuts and grains such as cherry tomatoes, red peppers, jicama, carrots, yams, fennel, brown rice, almonds, strawberries, and blueberries taste delectably sweet and flavorful. What's more, they're often taken by surprise when, within days to weeks of giving up sugary "treats," their former favorites lose their appeal or even taste overpoweringly sweet.

Such was the case with Jodi D., 36, of Park Hills, Kentucky. "Before it was 'the sweeter, the better.' Now, I've pretty much lost my taste for sugary desserts."

Start Stocking Up on Healthy Foods

Now that you're embarking upon a new, improved, more health-oriented life, you'll want to start stocking up on quality foods that won't cause your blood sugar levels to swing widely. Basically, you'll want to quit eating inferior, speedy sweets and carbs that send you into SUGAR SHOCK!

Ideally, you'll select from a wide variety of wholesome, fiber-filled, intact, high-quality, rainbow-colored, nutritious, preferably organic, low-glycemic, plant-based foods—vegetables and fruits—in their natural state, with no added sugars.

You'll also choose high-quality protein sources, from animal or plant protein sources (it's up to you), such as seafood, poultry, and lean meats, all preferably free range and organic, where animals aren't given antibiotics or hormones, as well as soy sources like tofu and seitan.

In addition, I recommend that you eat beans and legumes, nuts and seeds, and healthy fats. You also may wish to cook whole grains (I suggest gluten-free ones) and dairy products, if you're not allergic or sensitive to them.

For my recommended shopping list, visit my website at www.SugarShock .com.

The Tasty World of Organic Foods

As you quit or cut back on sweets, I recommend joining the growing trend of eating organically. Here are some compelling reasons to switch to organic foods, thanks to the Organic Trade Association (OTA) and the Organic Consumers Association (OCA):

- Organic foods are more nutritious. Mounting evidence shows that organically grown fruits, vegetables, and grains contain more vitamin C, iron, magnesium, and phosphorus than their nonorganic counterparts.

Since sugar-loaded junk foods strip our bodies of such nutrients, we benefit from these extra vitamins and minerals.

■ Organic foods are safer. The soil organic foods are grown in is richer, containing no herbicides or pesticides to destroy or dissolve the natural nutrients in the plants and the fruits. On the other hand, regular crops are contaminated with pesticides, other chemicals, and irradiation, and undergo genetic modification. Organic foods are exposed to fewer nitrates and other harmful residues.

■ Organic foods are healthier for children in their growth years. Some foods that kids favor, such as peanut butter, raisins, and peaches, have among the highest levels of pesticide residue, and these pesticides can cause neurological damage in children.

■ Organic foods taste better, thanks to the better-balanced soils in which they're grown.

■ Organic farming is better for the environment because it protects water resources and the soil.

If you decide to eat a mixture of organic and conventionally grown produce, here are the best vegetables and fruits to buy organic, because otherwise they're found consistently contaminated with pesticides, according to the Environmental Working Group:

■ Apples	■ Peaches
■ Bell peppers	■ Pears
■ Celery	■ Potatoes
■ Cherries	■ Red raspberries
■ Imported grapes	■ Spinach
■ Nectarines	■ Strawberries

Stop SUGAR SHOCK! to Lose Weight

Sugar Kickers around the world say that kicking sweets and refined carbs peeled off pounds like no other diet they've undertaken. If you're shunning sugar to shed unwanted, excess pounds, here are tips to help you reach your weight-loss goals:

- Enjoy quality sources of protein such as soy, fish, and meat. (See my website, www.SugarShock.com, for some vendors.)

- Eat generous amounts of colorful vegetables, preferably organic.

- Enjoy two to three servings of high-fiber fruits such as raspberries, apples, oranges, and blueberries. (Note: If you limit fruits to one serving per day or totally remove them for the first three weeks, you could lose weight more quickly.)

- Consume modest amounts of healthy fats such as flaxseed oil, olive oil, macadamia nut oil, avocado, and raw nuts.

- Stay away completely from *all* refined carbs. That includes cookies, most crackers, and candies (even low-calorie ones); breads and pasta; and alcohol and fruit juices. It's vital, we believe, to quit your quickie-carb habit so you can kick-start your weight loss and break the cravings cycle.

- For the first three weeks, avoid high-glycemic fruits or veggies like corn, potatoes, beets, dates, raisins, bananas, grapes, watermelon, and dried mango. Later, you can introduce fruits (preferably lower-glycemic ones like honeydew, cantaloupe, blueberries, strawberries, raspberries, and blackberries) in small portions, but if your cravings increase or your weight loss slows, you may be sensitive to them. (Symptoms of food sensitivities or allergies include fatigue, bloating, gas, skin disturbances such as rashes and acne, water retention, memory troubles, cravings, stalled weight loss, shortness of breath, and stuffy/runny nose.)

- For the first three weeks, stop eating dairy products and whole-grain products, especially those with wheat or gluten. If you're not too sensitive to them, you may want to add them back in later, but in small portions.

- Totally eliminate artificially sweetened drinks, foods, and products, even if they have no calories or sugar content. We're concerned about potential dangers and the possibility that such products could trigger sugar cravings and overeating and be linked to weight gain, not weight loss. (See chapter 21, which contains a number of answers to Frequently Asked Questions, for more info.)

Bear in mind that your Stop SUGAR SHOCK! Program is a way of life, of which weight loss is just *one* of numerous benefits. Indeed, if you seek to banish or reduce headaches, mood swings, and brain fog, you may find ample enticement to embrace a sugar-free life for good.

And remember, if you yearn for something sweet, you have a wide variety of tasty fruits and veggies from which to choose.

20

Top 10 Food-Label

Misconceptions about

Sweeteners

It's now time to turn you into a Savvy Sugar Sleuth by unmasking the 10 most common food-label misconceptions that may have you fooled. Here's the scoop that it took me years to discover:

1. BOTH "REDUCED SUGAR" AND "NO ADDED SUGAR" MEAN THE PRODUCT HAS NO SUGAR.
WRONG. The U.S. Food and Drug Administration (FDA) allows the term "reduced sugar" on products with "at least 25 percent less sugars" than leading brands. That means a reduced-sugar Coca-Cola must have 25 percent less sugar than the regular Coke. (In other words, the lower-sugar soda can still contain 75 percent of the sugar in the original formula.) Meanwhile, the term "no added sugar" is used for a variety of foods with *naturally occurring sugars* such as jams, jellies, and other preserves; yogurt; milk; some vegetables; and tomato sauce.

2. IF A FOOD IS LABELED "SUGAR FREE," IT CONTAINS NO SUGAR.
NOT NECESSARILY TRUE. So-called sugar-free foods can legally contain *trace* amounts of sugar—less than .5 grams per serving, according to the FDA, which sets labeling guidelines. This means about one-eighth (or less) of a teaspoon of sugar might be in that tomato sauce you're eating. "If you consume only one serving, then you're getting negligible amounts of sugar," points out

Lynn Grieger, R.D., www.ivillage.com's healthy-eating expert, "but if you eat several servings of one food or many 'sugar-free' foods throughout the day, then the amount of sugar you get can add up."

3. "LOW FAT" AND "FAT FREE" MEAN "SUGAR FREE."

FALSE. Low-fat yogurt may seem like a healthy choice, but it's possible that it still contains *as much* or even *more sugar* than its high-fat counterpart. For example, at last look, a 6-ounce container of Stonyfield Farm organic *low-fat* strawberry yogurt contains 22 grams of sugar while the strawberries and cream *whole milk* version has the *exact same amount* of sugar. Meanwhile, the six-ounce *fat-free* strawberry offering has two grams *more* sugar, topping off at 24 grams. Since one teaspoon equals roughly four grams, *that's six teaspoons* of sugar in your fat-free yogurt or *5.5 teaspoons* in your low-fat yogurt. In fact, many low-fat muffins, breads, cookies, and salad dressings contain as much or more sugar than regular products, explains Kelly Stuart, founder of www.DietFacts.com, which offers nutrition information for 18,000-plus restaurant and grocery food items. In addition, low-fat or fat-free products often contain potentially health-harming artificial sweeteners.

4. RAW SUGAR, BROWN RICE SYRUP, BARLEY MALT, AND MAPLE SYRUP ARE BETTER FOR YOU THAN REFINED WHITE SUGAR.

NOT TRUE. This seems to be a universal belief, especially among the "health conscious." "This is a way that manufacturers fool consumers by capitalizing on our desire to buy natural sugars," observes Dr. Ann Louise Gittleman.

"I think people want to believe that some of these products are better for you," adds Lynn Baillif, M.S., L.D., R.D., C.D.E., diabetes nutrition educator at Mercy Medical Center's Diabetes Center in Baltimore. "Even though raw sugar and maple syrup may have different flavors, people have to understand that their nutritional value is *no different* from that of plain table sugar."

In fact, as Dr. Nancy Appleton, author of *Lick the Sugar Habit*, further explains, "Raw sugar, maple syrup, brown rice syrup, and barley malt are all metabolized by our bodies like sucrose, raising our blood sugar levels rapidly, upsetting mineral relationships and suppressing the immune system." Furthermore, the sugar content is high in these sweeteners. For example, one company's farm maple syrup is comprised of "88 to 99 percent sucrose and 1 to 11 percent glucose," according to its website.

5. FRUIT JUICE CONCENTRATES ARE BETTER FOR YOU THAN REFINED SUGARS.

FALSE. Granted, foods containing orange, pineapple, or other fruit concentrates may *look* healthier, but fruit juice concentrates are metabolized in the same way as refined sugars, according to dietician Grieger. "People think fruit juice concentrate is as healthy as fruit, but it's stripped of most of its vitamins, minerals, and fiber," she explains.

6. HONEY IS MUCH BETTER FOR YOU THAN SUGAR, AND WE PROCESS IT DIFFERENTLY.

NOT TRUE. While widely touted as a much safer alternative to sugar, honey is made up of roughly one-third fructose, one-third glucose, and a little maltose, along with nearly 20 percent water. "It's a common misunderstanding that honey is different from other sugars or sweeteners," Dr. Appleton says. "But honey is even more concentrated than table sugar. It has 5 grams of sugar per teaspoon versus 4 grams of sugar per teaspoon for sucrose or table sugar. Some studies even have shown that honey raises your glucose levels *higher* than table sugar and suppresses your white blood cell count more."

7. SUCROSE (SUGAR) IS NATURAL.

NOT SO. This oft-cited assertion strikes me as baffling. In its natural state, sugar would be inside a 10-to-20-foot cane stalk or in a beet in the ground. Natural means you can pick it off a tree or bush or dig out the root.

"White, commercial sugar is highly refined and chemically altered from its origins as cane stalks or sugar beets," explains experienced food and beverage formulator Russ Bianchi. "To make sugar, you first have to take the stalks or beets and do physical processing or crushing, followed by filtering. Then some refiners use an industrial acid and/or chemical enzymatic treatment, which means you're adding hydrochloric acid or sulfuric acid to assist in ridding the product of impurities or foreign matter."

The sugar-making process continues. "Other steps involve centrifuging [rotating in a large, rapidly-spinning apparatus that separates the molasses from the crystals], bleaching, clarifying [to make clear by removing impurities or solid matter], desiccating [drying or dehydrating], boiling, and crystallizing," Bianchi continues. "In addition, sodium nitrate or salt is added, as are other potentially harmful agents such as ground bone or calcium carbonate, silicon dioxide [another chemical drying agent], chlorine [a bleaching agent and class 1 carcinogen], and titanium dioxide [a whitening agent that typically contains arsenic]. By any logical or reasonable definition, sugar is not natural," Bianchi contends, noting that despite these extensive procedures, sugar still can be legitimately called natural. "That's because the FDA has no legal definition for the term 'natural' in food or beverage law [known as the Code of Federal Regulations or CFR]."

But an FDA spokesman says the agency has policy guidelines: "natural" should mean "that nothing artificial or synthetic, including all color additives, regardless of source, has been included in or has been added to a food that would not normally be expected to be in the food." Interestingly, the FDA has "plenty of dialogue with plenty of companies regarding their use of the term 'natural,'" the spokesman reported.

"This claim that 'sucrose is natural' is very troubling," says nutritionist Grieger. "People want to know the truth about the foods they eat."

8. ANYTHING LABELED "ALL NATURAL" IS BETTER THAN ANYTHING REFINED.

I WISH THIS WERE TRUE! Since, as discussed above, there's no legal standard for using the term "natural" under U.S. food law, companies have ample leeway to call foods "natural" even if they aren't. "'Natural' is a misleading term," points out dietitian Baillif. Dr. Gittleman agrees: "The words 'all natural' on a label don't have any real meaning and certainly don't mean that the product is low in sugars. Some sweeteners are made from all-natural ingredients but are highly concentrated sources of sugars."

9. FRUCTOSE COMES *ONLY* FROM FRUIT.

WRONG. This premise stumps most consumers. "Fruit consists of many sugars. Only one of them is fructose—technically known as levulose—and it's only a small portion of sugars found," explains food scientist Bianchi. "Fruit also contains sucrose (which is half fructose), glucose, dextrose, maltose, galactose and other higher saccharides [sugars]."

But while the fructose found in berries, melons, apples, and some root vegetables is naturally occurring and therefore more healthy for you, "the fructose that Americans get from processed foods and beverages, as well as pharmaceuticals, flavors, cosmetics, and dietary supplements, is *not* derived from fruit," Bianchi explains. "Instead, the fructose typically is chemically refined from corn in the United States. The reason people get confused is because fructose sounds like it's from fruit.

"How can a chemically refined and synthesized sweetener whose origin many chemical steps ago was corn be [described as] identical to the fructose that is naturally occurring in fruit, with all its fiber, vitamins, and minerals? That's the moral equivalent of saying that a chocolate bar exists by itself in nature," continues Bianchi, who, like many experts, believes that "fructose may even be more damaging than sucrose if overconsumed."

Jack Challem, writer/editor of *Nutrition Reporter* and author of *Syndrome X,* calls this "fructose-is-fruit-sugar misconception one of the biggest nutritional bait-and-switch ploys in years. Both fructose and high-fructose corn syrup [in processed foods] have been aggressively promoted as natural sugars. But neither of them are."

So how did this misconception arise? "I think most people assume fructose and high-fructose corn syrup are from fruit, because we were all taught in elementary school that fructose is fruit sugar, and that sticks with people," Challem replies. "The makers of high-fructose corn syrup have really exploited this."

Peter J. Havel, D.V.M., Ph.D., a nutrition and endocrinology researcher at the University of California at Davis, says that nowadays "people are getting a lot more fructose from high-fructose corn syrup contained in processed foods and sweetened beverages than from eating fruit."

Moreover, as we noted earlier, scientists have been, as Dr. Havel puts it, "conducting research showing that fructose—which is present in sodas, other sweetened beverages, and many other food products—does not trigger the normal appetite-regulating mechanisms, such as the release of certain hormones (insulin and leptin), which are activated by other types of dietary carbohydrates composed of glucose.

"In addition, fructose is more readily metabolized to a form of fat known as triglycerides in the liver and this can raise triglyceride levels in the blood. Therefore, consumption of a diet high in fructose could not only lead to weight gain, but an increased risk of cardiovascular disease," Dr. Havel theorizes.

And the American Diabetes Association, as cited earlier, now advises diabetics not to use fructose because of worries that it could hurt plasma lipids.

Interestingly, this fructose-is-fruit-sugar misconception leads some people to buy granulated or crystallized fructose, because they erroneously assume that it's made from fruit, food scientist Bianchi observes. "And while refined corn fructose is getting a bad name, several manufacturers are even trying to hide their use of it by adding other sweeteners to a product as well."

So why is fructose so popular? "It's the lowest cost bulking ingredient after air, water, and salt," Bianchi explains. "That financial incentive is what drives these megacompanies to use [it]."

10. EVAPORATED CANE JUICE, CANE-SYRUP SOLIDS, CANE NECTAR, BEET NECTAR, CANE JUICE, BEET JUICE, AND NATURALLY MILLED CANE ARE ALL BETTER FOR YOU THAN SUGAR.

NOT TRUE! For starters, it's illegal and in direct violation of the FDA's Code of Federal Regulations (CFR) to use terms like "evaporated cane juice" and "beet nectar" because they suggest that the food contains no sugar, which is misleading. "Sugar is a strictly defined term by the FDA. You must use the designated term," an FDA spokesman explained.

Explains Bianchi, "All these falsely labeled sugars are metabolized 100 percent identically to white refined sugar."

Nutritionist Nan Kathryn Fuchs, Ph.D., editor/writer of *Women's Health Letter* and author of *The Health Detective's 456 Most Powerful Healing Secrets*, finds it appalling that companies are duping consumers into thinking that evaporated cane juice is better than other sweeteners.

"I'm really very angry with the health food industry for putting 'organic cane juice' in so many products and calling them 'health foods,'" Dr. Fuchs says. "It causes the same stimulating effect on insulin as refined sugars even if it does contain tiny amounts of trace minerals."

How Can I Squash My Sugar Cravings? and Other Frequently Asked Questions (FAQs)

It seems that everyone who embarks upon a program to kick sweeteners asks many of the same questions. Here, then, are the most common queries that I receive from members of my free, online KickSugar support group, visitors to my website (www.SugarShock.com) or blog (www.SugarShockBlog.com), and my private coaching clients.

CONNIE, WHAT DO YOU MEAN BY "SUGAR"? WHAT OTHER SWEETENERS SHOULD I AVOID OR CURTAIL?

First and foremost, you should know that I don't mean just "sucrose." It's not common knowledge that "sugar has many disguises," cautions Ann Louise Gittleman, Ph.D., author of *Get the Sugar Out: 501 Simple Ways to Cut the Sugar Out of Any Diet.*

When you read a good label, look for more than just the obvious sucrose, dextrose, and maltose, or other words ending with an "ose." In fact, caloric sweeteners have more than 100 names. Here are the most popular sweeteners used in foods today:

High-fructose corn syrup   Crystalline fructose
Sucrose   Molasses
Brown sugar   Maple syrup

Corn syrup

Invert sugar

Dextrose

Fruit juice concentrates
    (concentrated fruit juice)

Raw sugar

Maltodextrin*

Turbinado sugar

Sugar alcohols or polyols*

Honey

Rice syrup

High-maltose corn syrup

Barley-malt syrup

Powdered sugar

Cane juice

Inulin syrup

Chicory syrup

Tapioca syrup

WHAT ARE SOME FOODS THAT I CAN EAT TO COMBAT MY SUGAR CRAVINGS?

One of the best ways to beat cravings is to begin your day with a nourishing breakfast, experts insist. In fact, "eating breakfast can help you make better dietary decisions throughout the day," exercise physiologist and personal trainer Bob Greene observes in his book, *Bob Greene's Total Body Makeover.*

Other nutrition authorities believe that it's helpful to have ample protein, fiber, and fat at every meal and in most snacks.

"This helps keep blood sugar levels stable by controlling the release of hormones such as insulin and glucagon," says nutritionist and exercise physiologist Jill Vollmuth, C.N.C., who teaches physicians how to implement nutrition in their practice.

Registered dietitian Keri Gans, M.S., R.D., C.D.N., also advises never letting yourself get too hungry. "When you're famished, you're more likely to give in to cravings."

And Mark Hyman, M.D., author of *UltraMetabolism* and former co-medical director of Canyon Ranch health resort in Lenox, Massachusetts, believes that people cutting out sugar should get essential fatty acids by taking pure fish oil and eating low-mercury fish. Dr. Hyman also advises taking two tablespoons of ground flaxseed a day to help balance blood sugar.

In addition, nutrition expert Elizabeth Somer, M.A., R.D., author of *Food & Mood*, believes that drinking plenty of water can be an effective way

---

*Please note that both maltodextrin and sugar alcohols or polyols are not technically sugars. The former is derived from the corn wet-refining process and metabolized rapidly in the body. See sugar alcohols question below for more information.

to halt sugar cravings. "Often, a desire for sweets in the evening is actually a signal that you need fluids," she says.

If water isn't satisfying enough, nutritionist Shari Lieberman, Ph.D., C.N.S., F.A.C.N., suggests making your own fruit water. "Just cut up some strawberries, blueberries, an orange, or a piece of kiwi fruit and then let them sit in the water for a while so you get some of the flavor. And in the winter, you can drink vegetable and chicken broth," says Dr. Lieberman, author of *Dare to Lose*.

"But don't drink extremely sweet beverages such as diet sodas. They will promote sugar and carb cravings," adds Dr. Lieberman, who also considers no-sugar-added protein shakes and unsweetened fiber supplements effective cravings busters.

Others who've helped people kick sweets believe that it's also vital to cut out salt and stop eating corn until you've given up sugar for two months.

In addition, all experts advise keeping nourishing quality carbs on hand at all times—specifically raw, low-sugar vegetables and fruits so that you always have something to eat in a pinch. Broccoli, celery, carrots, cauliflower, Jerusalem artichokes, parsnips, sweet potatoes, jicama, cucumber, red peppers, apples, and strawberries are ideal.

When craving sweet "comfort foods," start picking healthy alternatives. This is a tactic that has worked well for fitness guru and author Kathy Smith. "A favorite of mine is to have a baked apple at night. Or I'll put blueberries in a crystal wine glass, top it with some plain yogurt, toss in some nuts, then add a layer of strawberries, and top it all again with yogurt," says Smith, who believes in turning your snacking time into an "event" by using, for example, crystal or a good piece of china. She also suggests making a cup of herbal tea when you crave sweets.

Nutritionist Dr. Jonny Bowden offers one final, albeit unusual, tip for times when thoughts of sugar overwhelm you. "Try eating something that's *not* sweet. I've found that when your taste buds crave sugar, if you fake them out and give them a sour pickle or a hot pepper or something that tastes completely different, it tricks the brain in some way, and you lose your cravings."

WILL EXERCISE HELP CURB MY CRAVINGS?
Absolutely. Perhaps the tip most often offered by experts is to exercise often— at least several days a week, but more often, if you can. "Physical activity

combats cravings, makes you less prone to bingeing, gives you a pleasurable endorphin rush, and reduces stress," suggests "nutritionist to the stars" Oz Garcia, Ph.D., author of *Look and Feel Fabulous Forever*.

"Exercising also shuts down the appestat—the mechanism in the brain that controls appetite," adds Dr. Nancy Appleton, author of *Lick the Sugar Habit*.

Integrative physician Dr. Fred Pescatore notes that "exercise helps reduce your sugar habit. When you cut out sweets, you'll use up your body's glycogen stores, which will help maintain healthy blood sugar balance. When your body's blood sugar is better maintained, you'll have fewer sugar cravings, which, of course, makes it easier for you to kick sugar. You only need 10 minutes of getting your heart rate up to get this body mechanism to work."

Fitness expert Kathy Smith reassures people that "even as little as 15 minutes a day improves your body's ability to uptake glucose and use it for fuel. The body's not secreting as much insulin when you're exercising."

And as you exercise, Smith notes, not only will your cravings diminish, but you'll also find you have more stamina and endurance for your workouts by reducing refined carbs. In fact, she cites one study that illustrates the benefits low-glycemic food had on bicyclists. "Cyclists pedaled almost 60 percent longer after the low-glycemic, preexercise meal versus the high-GI meal, and they maintained higher blood sugar levels," she notes. "The bottom line: unrefined carbs keep your body's blood sugar level maintained, which, in turn, allows for a steady reservoir of energy that you need to perform well."

Of course, warding off sugar cravings and stabilizing blood sugar levels aren't the only benefits. Exercising regularly also can lower your risk of developing coronary heart disease, high blood pressure, diabetes, stroke, colon and breast cancer, and osteoporosis. It can help you lose weight or maintain it; develop and sustain healthy bones, muscles, and joints; relieve arthritis pain; lessen symptoms of depression and anxiety; boost moods; promote psychological well-being; and make it easier to perform daily tasks.

WHAT OTHER NONFOOD ACTIVITIES DO EXPERTS RECOMMEND TO COMBAT MY CRAVINGS?

Those who've advised sugar addicts recommend that you team up with a buddy who is also curtailing sugar intake, get enough sleep, and reduce stress. And make sure, the experts insist, to take yourself away from tempting situations such as the bakery or ice-cream shop.

"If you can't resist it, don't buy it," urges nutritionist Somer. In other words, get those dessert and quickie-carb snack foods out of the house, out of the office, out of the car. Bear in mind that expression, "Out of sight, out of mind."

Fitness expert Smith also suggests that when the mood for sweet foods strikes, you can do meditation or deep breathing, even if just for a couple of minutes. "Inhale and then exhale to the count of six, then lengthen your breath, and get it up to the count of eight," she recommends.

J. J. Virgin, C.N.S., C.H.F.I., nutritionist for Dr. Phil's "Ultimate Weight Loss Challenge," offers another helpful hint. "Keep yourself busy and occupied, and do what Dr. Phil suggests—replace a bad habit with an 'incompatible one.' So, if you're taking a bath or a shower, you can't be eating a piece of cake," Virgin says. "If you're mowing the lawn, you can't be pigging out on crackers."

Here are some other innovative ideas:

- Do imaginary "urge surfing" to allow your cravings to quickly fade away, suggests relapse prevention expert G. Alan Marlatt, Ph.D., a psychology professor at the University of Washington and director of its Addictive Behaviors Research Center. "Visualize your sugar craving as a wave and simply watch it rise and fall as an observer and don't be 'wiped out' by it. Then, ride the craving like a wave as if you're on a surf board, because it will eventually build, crest, break, and then subside *if* you don't act on it." This imagery, Dr. Marlatt says, helps you to detach from your urges and cravings and reinforces the fact that they're temporary.

- "To combat cravings, visualize the color pink, which is associated with love, or wear rose quartz. It's a way of consciously doing something healing and loving for yourself," suggests herbalist Brigitte Mars, A.H.G., author of *Addiction-Free Naturally*. "Sugar is used at times as a love substitute. The color rose is associated with sweetness, safety, and friendliness."

- "Use fruit-flavored lip gloss or brush your teeth," Dr. Appleton suggests. "The sugar in the toothpaste is not enough to do you any harm, but it's just enough to possibly satisfy your craving."

WHICH NUTRITIONAL SUPPLEMENTS OR VITAMINS CAN HELP CURB MY SUGAR CRAVINGS?

Of course, results can't be guaranteed, and you should consult first with your physician, but specialists suggest a number of supplements that they believe can help ward off intense sugar desires. Make sure to pick supplements that contain no sweeteners, because some companies add sugars as fillers. And bear in mind that supplements haven't been evaluated by the Food and Drug Administration (FDA), and they're not intended to diagnose, treat, cure, or prevent any disease.

Of all supplements, L-glutamine is one of those most often linked to cutting cravings. "Cravings will go away in about 10 minutes if you take 1,000 milligrams of L-glutamine," predicts nutritionally trained Dr. Pescatore.

Chromium is another oft-cited supplement. "Taking 200 micrograms before each meal could really help to keep blood sugar stable so it won't spike and crash," says Dr. Lieberman. "About 80 percent of the population is deficient in chromium, which is essential for production of insulin and the uptake of glucose into the cells. It also could have a beneficial effect on blood lipids."

Nutrition expert Julia Ross, author of *The Mood Cure* and *The Diet Cure*, also suggests taking "biotin, another blood-sugar supporter; tyrosine, a natural stimulant that turns off chocolate and caffeine cravings; 5-HTP, an antidepressant and sleep promoter; and DLPA, which helps eliminate the need for comfort foods."

Now, here's a list of supplements from nutritionist Jill Vollmuth that she believes could help with sugar cravings. (Just bear in mind that this isn't health advice.)

Basic Supplementation:
- A high-quality, professional-grade multivitamin and mineral without iron (unless recommended by your doctor).

To Aid in Alleviating Sugar Cravings:
- Chromium (in amino acid chelate form)—200 micrograms with breakfast, lunch, and dinner.

- High-quality, clean, professional-grade fish oil (from anchovy, sardine, mackerel, or cod)—one gram or one teaspoon per meal at breakfast, lunch, and dinner.

- L-glutamine powder—1 teaspoon (about two to three grams) morning, midday, and evening, mixed in a small amount of water. (You may use more to help cravings, as needed.)

For Additional Help with Cravings:

- 5HTP—50 milligrams per meal (don't take if you're on an SSRI antidepressant or MAOI drug)—with all three main meals.

- Vanadium—100 micrograms at breakfast, lunch, and dinner. (Take at the same time you take chromium. See above.)

- B complex—Take one at breakfast and one at lunch. (Don't take at dinner, because it can energize you.)

WHICH HERBS AND SPICES COULD HELP WARD OFF MY URGES TO SPLURGE ON SWEETS?

Experts say a variety of spices may help defeat those nagging sugar cravings either because they add sweetness to food or because they help regulate blood sugar levels. "For instance," nutritionist Ann Louise Gittleman, Ph.D., says, "cinnamon, cloves, and nutmeg increase your ability to metabolize sugar and remove it from the blood. In particular, cinnamon has a sweet, satisfying, familiar flavor that many associate with holidays. In addition, bay leaf, cayenne, cloves, coriander, dry mustard, and ginger can help regulate your blood sugar levels."

Nutritionist Somer also recommends using anise, cardamom, mace (the fibrous covering on the nutmeg seed, which is available ground), mint, nutmeg, pumpkin pie spice, and others to enhance, season, or flavor sauces and stews, as well as to spice up such foods as winter squash, soups, poultry, fish, salads, broccoli, cucumbers, and grains.

When cravings strike, herbalist Mars recommends sucking on cinnamon sticks, drinking tea made from anise, fennel, or licorice root, or inhaling deeply of aromatic essential oils of anise, cardamom, cinnamon, clove, fennel, nutmeg, rose, and vanilla.

Other experts, including Mars, praise the herb gymnema sylvestre as helpful to normalize blood sugar. "It's known as 'the sugar destroyer,' because it tends to block the body's ability to taste sweets," she says. "Since the molecular arrangement of gymnema is similar to that of glucose, it adheres to the sensors in the taste buds where sugar would be tasted."

Nutritionist Earl Mindell, Ph.D., R.Ph., author of *The Diet Bible* and *The Vitamin Bible*, is also a fan of the herb banaba, which he hails as "the biggest sleeper around. It helps regulate blood sugar and is used extensively by diabetics in the Philippines."

DO YOU HAVE IDEAS TO BEAT SUGAR CRAVINGS WHEN PREGNANT, PMS-ING, OR MENOPAUSAL?

Whether you're going through menstrual, menopausal, or pregnancy hormone shifts, all the cravings advice above will help. In addition, experts say that it can be useful, especially for women with premenstrual symptoms, to keep a cravings diary in which you chart and pinpoint specific situations, emotions, triggers, and times of day when those dessert foods are calling out to you.

If you have PMS, it's helpful to know in advance when you're likely to indulge so you can head off cravings, says Louise Dye, Ph.D., a senior lecturer in biopsychology at the University of Leeds in England and an expert on female-related cravings. That way, as mentioned earlier, you can plan what Dr. Dye calls "environmental intervention" by planning fun activities that take you away from food. In any case, research shows that both PMS and menopausal symptoms are reduced by physical activity.

Specialists also say that right before your period, it's useful to avoid alcohol, because it not only can worsen PMS-related depression, headaches, and fatigue, but also can trigger food cravings.

IF I'M DRINKING COFFEE OR TEA, WILL IT MAKE IT HARDER FOR ME TO QUIT SUGAR?

Good question. Experts do, in fact, recommend cutting back on caffeine while quitting sugar for a number of reasons. "Caffeine is a stimulant, which can actually increase the amount of sugar in the bloodstream," explains Dr. Nancy Appleton in her book *Lick the Sugar Habit*. "When ingested, caffeine stimulates the adrenal glands, which release adrenaline-like substances called catecholamines."

In turn, these "catecholamines cause the heart to pump harder than normal and the liver to release stored sugar, which raises the blood sugar level.

Then, the pancreas secretes insulin to bring the level down to normal. This process," Dr. Appleton notes, "can result in the eventual exhaustion of the pancreas."

The problem is that the "lift" that we get from caffeine is short lived and it "throws the body chemistry out of balance," she continues. "The rush of insulin from the pancreas frequently goes so far beyond restoring normality that the sugar level falls below normal, causing extreme fatigue and other hypoglycemic symptoms. It may be hours before the body's chemistry returns to normal, and if another cup of coffee or tea has been ingested, the cycle of imbalance will continue."

DO WOMEN TEND TO HAVE MORE PROBLEMS THAN MEN WITH SUGAR?

Some scientists do believe that women are harder hit then men. "Women are more vulnerable to sugar addiction and to the effects of sugar, because they have naturally lower levels of beta-endorphins," says Kathleen DesMaisons, Ph.D., author of *Potatoes, Not Prozac*; *Little Sugar Addicts*; and *The Sugar Addict's Total Recovery Program*. "In addition, the monthly fluctuation of hormones exacerbates the beta-endorphin fluctuations and makes sugar cravings worse."

IF MY KIDS ARE GOING TO QUIT DRINKING SOFT DRINKS, IS FRUIT JUICE A BETTER CHOICE?

Actually, a number of health experts say that whole fresh fruits, preferably those low in natural sugars such as apples, strawberries, and blueberries, are always preferable to juice, because they contain nutrients, antioxidants, and fiber, the last of which slows the rate at which your blood sugar is raised. In fact, as cited previously, a growing body of scientific evidence is showing that sweet drinks of any kind—be they soda, sports drinks, or juices (especially those containing high-fructose corn syrup)—can play a role in the development of obesity and other health problems, especially in children.

"Juice is only minimally better than soda," says David Ludwig, M.D., Ph.D., a pediatric obesity specialist at Children's Hospital Boston. "All these beverages are largely the same. They are 100 percent sugar. With the possible exception of milk, children do not need any calorie-containing beverages," adds Dr. Ludwig, noting that some fruit-juice beverages advertised as *healthier* alternatives to soda contain *even more* sugar than the soda itself.

Ultimately, the best thing you can do is to get your kids used to drinking filtered, unflavored water, water with a slice or two of orange tossed in, and later decaffeinated herbal tea.

HOW MUCH SUGAR IS IN A 20-OUNCE BOTTLE OF COCA-COLA?
A 20-ounce bottle of Coca-Cola contains about *16.87 teaspoons of sugar*. You get this figure by multiplying 27 (the number of grams of sugar in a serving) by 2.5 (the number of servings in a bottle), which comes to 67.5 grams of sugar per bottle. Since 1 teaspoon equals approximately 4 grams, you divide the grams (67.5) by 4.

WHAT ARE SOME FOODS THAT CONTAIN "HIDDEN" SUGARS?
You'll find hidden sugars and sweeteners, from sucrose to malted barley, in most processed foods, including many breads and crackers, most salad dressings, most ketchups, many tomato sauces, some mustards, most or many sauces in Chinese and other restaurants, cocktail sauce, sushi rice, soy milk, mayonnaise, and most cough syrups and cough drops. To get more names of foods with hidden sweeteners, sign up for my free e-zine at www.SugarShockBlog.com.

IF I'M GOING TO CUT OUT SUGAR, CAN I AT LEAST HAVE ARTIFICIALLY SWEETENED FOODS?
That's certainly your decision, but bear in mind that, although manufacturers insist their artificially sweetened products are safe and extensively tested, health concerns have been raised about most nonnutritive sweeteners on the market today, including sucralose (Splenda), aspartame (Equal, NutraSweet), saccharin (Sweet'n Low, Sugar Twin, Sucaryl, Weight Watchers), and acesulfame potassium (Sunette, Sweet One). Actually, all independent health authorities I interviewed insist that it's safer to stay away from all *unnatural*, chemically produced, nonnutritive sugar substitutes and choose foods that are *naturally* sweet instead.

"Artificial sweeteners can be just as harmful as sugar," contends Dr. Appleton. Toxicologist and nutritionist Janet Starr Hull, Ph.D., C.N., agrees. "Artificial sweeteners are simply *not* the answer to dieting. Nor are they effective ways to deal with hypoglycemia, diabetes, or insulin resistance.

"Fake sweeteners like sucralose and aspartame are made of unhealthy chemicals with toxic by-products. For example, sucralose (Splenda) contains man-made, chemically produced chlorine, which is carcinogenic, and aspartame (Equal or NutraSweet) converts to formaldehyde, an embalming fluid used to preserve the dead," explains Dr. Hull, author of *Sweet Poison*, which chronicles her near-death experience from a hyperthyroid condition she believes was brought on by "aspartame poisoning." And Dr. Walter Willett also believes that the best choice for sweetening foods is "none of the above. People are not suffering from aspartame or Splenda deficiency. They're suffering from too much sugar."

BUT WON'T ARTIFICIALLY SWEETENED DIET FOODS AND DRINKS HELP ME LOSE WEIGHT?

Actually, some medical experts and nutrition authorities theorize that the opposite can occur. Famous integrative medicine physician Andrew Weil, M.D., notes that "there's not a shred of evidence that the availability or use of artificial sweeteners has helped anyone to lose weight."

Neurosurgeon Russell L. Blaylock, M.D., agrees. "A significant number of people *gain* rather than lose weight, as advertised," says the author of *Excitotoxins: The Taste That Kills*.

That was the case with Cori Brackett of Tucson, Arizona. But when she stopped drinking diet soda, "70 pounds fell right off," recalls Brackett, who produced a documentary about aspartame, entitled *Sweet Misery: A Poisoned World*.

Ralph G. Walton, M.D., professor and chairman of the psychiatry department at Northeastern Ohio University's College of Medicine, tracked this "paradoxical increase in appetite in numerous medical studies. One research study, he says, found that artificial sweetener users took in *more* calories the next day than those eating sucrose. Another of nearly 80,000 women conducted for the American Cancer Society found that artificial sweetener users gained more than nonusers. And still more researchers reported in the *International Journal of Obesity* that rats fed saccharin-sweetened drinks ate three times more calories than rodents given sugar. Scientists speculate that sugar substitutes could play tricks on our brains and bodies, interfere with our automatic process for regulating calorie intake, and play a role in our obesity epidemic.

Nutrition specialist David L. Katz, M.D., M.P.H., an associate professor at the Yale University School of Medicine, also cites studies revealing that artificial sweeteners do nothing to curb sugar cravings and might even *cause* overeating. "The real toxicity of artificial sweeteners is the notion that they are a weight-loss panacea. They are not," Dr. Katz says. "The better way to restrict sugar intake is to learn to prefer less sugar. For that, you must take superfluous sugar and superfluous sweet out of your diet.

"Sugar is addictive, and like all addictive substances, tolerance develops," Dr. Katz continues. "The more you eat, the more you need to get satisfaction. From what we know to date, artificial sweeteners raise this threshold as much as sugar does, so the best way to tame your sweet tooth, and lower your threshold for satisfaction with sweets is to shift to more wholesome, less-processed foods."

CAN ARTIFICIALLY SWEETENED FOODS AND DRINKS TRIGGER CARB CRAVINGS?

Some experts do suspect that artificially sweetened foods and drinks could cause carb cravings. Nutritionist Dr. Gittleman contends that artificial sweeteners are "counterproductive to your weight-loss goals because they suppress or deplete production of serotonin, the neurotransmitter that helps control food cravings. When your serotonin levels plummet, your sugar cravings skyrocket, and this increases the likelihood of bingeing and added pounds. The mere taste of a concentrated sweetener appears to set an instinctual insulin mechanism into place even though it contains zero calories."

As far back as 1983, aspartame's effects on the brain led MIT neuroscientist Richard Wurtman, Ph.D., to point out in *The New England Journal of Medicine* that, in high doses, the sweetener may instill a craving for calorie-laden carbohydrates.

IS THE ARTIFICAL SWEETENER SPLENDA MADE FROM SUGAR AS ITS ADS POINT OUT?

Well, sucralose (brand name Splenda) does start off using sucrose. But, as toxicologist Dr. Hull explains, "It is manufactured in the lab by a very complex chemical process that involves changing the structure of sugar molecules.

"Basically, an alarming chemical soup is created where they actually force chlorine into an unnatural bond with a sugar molecule, substituting three sucrose atoms with three chlorine atoms. So, while sucralose may have begun as sugar, it's really a synthetic chemical."

Furthermore, the consumer children's advocate group Generation Green says, in a complaint to the U.S. Federal Trade Commission about Splenda's misleading advertising, that "following chlorination [of sugar] a further chemical process is applied using phosgene." The Centers for Disease Control website describes phosgene as "a major industrial chemical used to make plastics and pesticides," which at room temperature is a "poisonous gas." The little yellow packets also contain dextrose, a simple form of sugar, and maltodextrin, a digestible carbohydrate derived from chemically modified cornstarch.

IS SUCRALOSE (SPLENDA) SAFE FOR ME TO USE?

Some medical experts are quite skeptical of the no-calorie sweetener's safety despite the fact that it took 20 years and more than 100 studies to get FDA approval before it went on the market in the United States in 1998.

One of the biggest concerns is that Splenda contains the man-made, chemically created chlorine. Before you sniff and say, "Well, that's no big deal," you should know that people tend to mix up *chlorine* with *chloride*, which is naturally occurring in salt as sodium chloride, in minerals as magnesium and potassium chloride, and in deep leafy greens as lithium chloride or calcium chloride. Chloride in its natural form is safe, but Splenda uses an unnatural form of *chlorine*. "That's why we use chlorine filters on tap water—to protect ourselves against its carcinogenic effects," toxicologist and artificial sweetener expert Dr. Janet Starr Hull explained in a phone interview with Connie.

"Industrial-grade chlorine is a carcinogen—any way you slice it," adds Dr. Hull, whose website, www.SplendaExposed.com, posts current independent research and concerns about the sweetener's safety. "Research shows that chlorine in its manufactured form is a carcinogen and toxin.

"Any animal that eats chlorine—especially on a regular basis—is at risk of cancer. Both *The Merck Manual* and *OSHA SARA 120 Hazardous Waste Handbook* even state that emergency procedures should be taken when exposed via swallowing, inhaling, or through the skin. So it's questionable how safe it is for the long term. I'd also caution pregnant women, the elderly, and children to exercise caution with sucralose," Dr. Hull adds. "And it appears that sucralose might raise problems for diabetics—something that was hinted at in an FDA report."

Another problem with sucralose is that when you mix the man-made chlorine with carbon in sucrose, you get a chlorocarbon. "These are pollutants that are toxic to your health," Dr. Hull explains. "So people are ingesting a manufactured grade of chlorine that compounds into a chlorocarbon.

That is not a natural food source, and the body will digest it, contrary to Splenda's marketing claims. And that can be proven."

Thus, Dr. Hull explains, "Splenda/sucralose is simply a chlorinated sugar that's made by taking a molecule of sugar and chemically manipulating it to surrender three hydroxyl groups (hydrogen + oxygen) and replace them with three chlorine atoms. When it's turned into Splenda it becomes a chlorocarbon. In fact, it's in the family of the toxic pesticides Chlordane, Lindane, and DDT."

Nutritionist Dr. Ann Louise Gittleman also worries about Splenda, which is found in more than 4,000 packaged foods and beverages, and which grabs more than 50 percent of the $1 billion U.S. artificial-sweetener market.

"Sucralose is a 'Frankenfood' to me," Dr. Gittleman continues. "I highly suspect that, later in life, users may suffer from the by-products of chlorine, which can act as an estrogen mimic." (In other words, too much estrogen could fuel cancer.)

In addition, Joseph Mercola, D.O., author of *Sweet Deception* (about Splenda) and *The No-Grain Diet*, cautions that research supporting sucralose approval by the FDA is highly questionable. One of the central elements of potential long-term problems is absorption, and they only studied this on eight healthy males.

Dr. Mercola's website, www.mercola.com—the number-one ranked natural health website—posts stories of bad reactions to sucralose, including one by Gypsie M., R.N., 56, a school nurse in Houston, Texas. Gypsie revealed in a phone interview with me that after ingesting products with Splenda, she "developed bad headaches, stomach cramps, flulike aches, joint pains in my feet, joints, and bones, diarrhea, and a feeling of impending doom."

Ultimately, of course, we won't know if Splenda is safe for humans to consume until long-term human studies are conducted. But interestingly, Whole Foods Market is also skeptical of the safety of Splenda and removed all products containing it from their shelves because it didn't fit into the company's goal to promote "real food."

IS IT SAFE TO CONSUME PRODUCTS WITH ASPARTAME?
Well, the FDA insists that aspartame—better known by the brand names NutraSweet and Equal—is "one of the most thoroughly tested and studied food additives the agency has ever approved." What's more, manufacturers using

the no-calorie sugar substitute also insist that their products are completely safe.

But, according to toxicologist Dr. Hull, consumers, through their medical doctors, flooded the FDA with more than 10,000 complaints between 1986 and 1991, reporting 92 different symptoms from aspartame. For example, documented adverse reactions include headaches, dizziness, memory loss, mood swings, nausea, seizures, convulsions, weight gain, sleep problems, reduced libido, loss of blood sugar control, changes in heart rate, breathing difficulties, aggravated PMS symptoms, skin rashes, water retention, vision problems, ear buzzing, diarrhea, stomach cramping, nausea, muscle aches, fatigue, muscular sclerosis–like symptoms, and other neurological problems.

The FDA does acknowledge that "a tiny segment of the population is sensitive to one of the sweetener's by-products [from phenylalanine]," which can aggravate phenylketonuria (PKU), a hereditary, metabolic disease present at birth that affects about 1 in 10,000 people. "People with PKU cannot properly process the isolated amino acid phenylalanine, and they have to follow severely restricted diets. If they ingest a lot of products with phenylalanine, such as aspartame-sweetened drinks and foods, they could develop brain damage, become retarded or even die," Dr. Hull explains.

HOW IS ASPARTAME (NUTRASWEET OR EQUAL) MADE?

It's comprised of 50 percent L-phenylalanine (an amino acid), 40 percent L-aspartic acid (another amino acid), and 10 percent methanol. "Methanol is a wood alcohol that breaks down chemically into formic acid and formaldehyde," Dr. Hull explains. And neurosurgeon Russell L. Blaylock, M.D., who has spent a decade studying the effects of both aspartame and MSG, says that the formaldehyde makes aspartame "a dangerous neurotoxin which can damage the nervous system, and it is a significant carcinogen for many organs."

WHY DO I GET CRAMPS OR THE RUNS AFTER EATING LOW-CALORIE CANDIES, SYRUPS, CHEWING GUM, CAKES, OR BREATH MINTS?

You could be inadvertently consuming sugar alcohols or polyols such as sorbitol, mannitol, maltitol, lactitol, xylitol, and glycerol/glycerin, as well as D-tagatose, isomalt, polydextrose, erythritol, and hydrogenated starch hydrolysate (another name for maltitol). Indeed, a number of sugar-free products, from cookies to medicines to chicken broth, could cause bloating, diarrhea, and stomach cramps.

While sugar alcohols make foods tasty—they're roughly half the sweetness of sugar, low in calories, and raise blood sugar more slowly than sugar—they can cause stomach cramps, bloating, diarrhea, and anal leakage, because, experts say, they're poorly absorbed by our bodies.

"Even small amounts of sorbitol can cause gastrointestinal symptoms," says Jeffrey S. Hyams, M.D., director of Connecticut Children's Medical Center's Department of Digestive Diseases and Nutrition. "People have undergone extensive medical testing for abdominal pain and diarrhea when the problem was simply that they were ingesting excessive amounts of sorbitol."

Interestingly, sugar alcohols aren't considered sugars or artificial sweeteners: Their name comes from the fact that their structure resembles sugar, and they're chemically similar to alcohol. They're typically genetically modified from corn or wheat. Although you can get the runs from the stuff, the FDA classifies sorbitol and xylitol (but not the other polyols) as GRAS (generally recognized as safe) and requires a warning notice only on products containing 15 grams or more, although some companies voluntarily list sugar alcohols if their products have fewer grams.

"Even as little as two grams of any polyol is more than enough to trigger severe intestinal distress in pregnant women, nursing mothers, infants, children, diabetics, hypoglycemics, cardiovascular patients, those on various prescription drugs, seniors, and other health-compromised categories, which is approximately two-thirds of the U.S. population," says Russ Bianchi, a food and beverage formulator.

Back in 1999, the Center for Science in the Public Interest (CSPI) called upon the FDA to require better label warnings on products containing one or more grams per serving of sorbitol or other sugar alcohols. It urged a notice cautioning consumers that the product "may cause diarrhea, bloating, and abdominal pain" and that it's not suitable for children. "Now that so many foods contain sugar alcohols, it's all the more important for the FDA to take action," urges CSPI executive director Dr. Michael Jacobson.

IF I DON'T USE ARTIFICIAL SWEETENERS OR SUGAR ALCOHOLS, HOW CAN I SWEETEN MY FOODS?

There are many ways you can naturally sweeten your foods. Try adding a little juice from oranges, grapes, plums, pears, peaches or other fruits. Toss on some grated or shredded raw or dried apple, raisin, date, or coconut. Add a little coconut juice. Use mashed sweet potatoes or yams. (In fact, Dr. Nancy Appleton even offers a yam-based carob mousse dessert in *Lick the Sugar Habit*.) Try sprinkling your foods with spices such as cinnamon, cloves, nutmeg, ginger, fennel, or pumpkin spice.

You may also wish to learn about the sweet herbal supplement stevia, which millions of people throughout South America and Asia have used as a sweetener for years. Worst-case scenario, add small amounts of maple syrup or raw, washed, organic cane sugar in crystalline form, but please do so *only* if you do *not* have medical reasons such as hypoglycemia to avoid them. And please note that many people are just too sensitive to consume any sweeteners at all.

Finally, before you add sugar or a sugar substitute, ask yourself, "Why do I 'need' this?" You may find that your "need for something sweet has very little to do with a real need," a point raised by Donna F., 41, of Medina, New York, a member of my online KickSugar group. Indeed, maybe your desire for sugar really means that you're looking for emotional food or spiritual sustenance. As I suggest earlier, we recommend learning to relish the natural sweet flavor of fruits and vegetables and change your mind-set from one of deprivation to one of fulfillment.

CAN YOU TELL ME ABOUT STEVIA?

Stevia rebaudiana bertoni is the leaf from a shrub in the chrysanthemum family that's grown and cultivated in parts of South America and Asia, where it's sold as a tabletop sweetener and flavor enhancer. Proponents maintain that "stevioside"—the extract of stevia leaves that becomes a granulated white powder or pale yellow liquid—is about 150 to 300 times sweeter than sugar, has zero calories, and doesn't raise blood sugar levels.

But, in the United States, although "it can impart a sweet taste to foods, it cannot be sold as a sweetener because the FDA considers it an unapproved food additive." The governmental agency, which contends that "toxicological information on stevia is inadequate to demonstrate its safety," has therefore banned its use in foods, beverages, cosmetics, flavors, and pharmaceutical products. But, under the Dietary Supplement Health and Education Act of 1994 (DSHEA), stevia can be sold as a "dietary supplement"; it's illegal, however, to promote it as a sweetener. (Such claims make a company's shipments subject to seizure, fines, or criminal prosecution.) Moreover, an FDA consumer safety officer told me that "the safety of stevia has been questioned by published studies. And no one has ever provided the FDA with adequate evidence that the substance is safe."

On the other hand, stevia's many supporters, which include the American Herbal Products Association, Herb Research Foundation, and the American Botanical Council, as well as integrative physicians and nutritionists, are quick to point out that stevia has been consumed safely by humans for centuries in South Korea, Thailand, Peru, Bolivia, Paraguay, Argentina, Brazil, New Zealand, and Japan, with no known complaints.

Over the years, those who've spoken out in favor of stevia include Julian Whitaker, M.D., Dr. Andrew Weil, the late Dr. Atkins, Dr. Ann-Louise Gittleman, Dr. Joseph Mercola, Dr. Nancy Appleton, and Dr. Earl Mindell.

Proponents also point out that stevia has been used legally in Japan since the 1970s as a sweetener for carbonated drinks, yogurt, candy bars, frozen foods, and chewing gum, and as a tabletop sweetener. Advocates say that stevia is inexpensive to grow, harvest, and produce; is heat sensitive; and is an effective flavor enhancer and preservative.

It should be noted that to become a white powder or clear liquid, stevia undergoes a multistep process not unlike that which sugar undergoes, but you can purchase the whole or ground-up stevia leaf, something I enjoy.

CAN YOU TELL ME ABOUT AGAVE? IS THIS A SAFE, ALTERNATIVE SWEETENER?

Although agave is widely touted on the Internet and in health food stores as safe, natural and low glycemic, it is "a non-GRAS (not generally recognized as safe) label for highly refined fructose, which is metabolized in your body like high fructose corn syrup (HFCS)," according to Russ Bianchi, CEO of Adept Solutions, a global food formulation firm.

Interestingly, agave—which is allegedly derived from the blue agave plant in Mexico—has "*twice* the intensity and sweetness of high-fructose corn syrup," Bianchi says, noting that several countries have all either passed laws banning it or are reviewing its safety. "Even in the United States, after the FDA sent out a warning letter in 2000, a number of health foods companies nervously stopped adding agave nectar to their products."

Experts such as Bianchi also question how agave nectar could be derived from the Mexican plant since, "for some dozen years, there's been a worldwide shortage of blue agave and hardly enough to meet the demand for mescal or tequila alcohol beverages, which also come from agave.

"The bottom line is this: I advise against using agave. I'm really suspicious and concerned about its safety and constitution," Bianchi charges. "I have the same reservations about inulin and chicory, because both are non-compliant with labeling laws and hide the fact that they're highly refined man-made fructose."

I STILL HAVE MORE QUESTIONS. WHAT CAN I DO?

It's great that you want to learn more. For more information, just visit my website or blog at www.SugarShock.com and www.SugarShockBlog.com, where I answer all kinds of questions. And while you're at either site, please sign up for my free e-zine, too. And if you still can't find the answers you're seeking, submit a question to www.SugarShockBlog.com to be considered for a future "Stump the Savvy Sugar Sleuths" column.

Connie's Top 21 Sweet
Sugar-Free Success Secrets
and Strategies

Congratulations. You're about to embark on a way of life that could nurture instead of torture you. Right now pulling the plug on your unhealthy carb habit may seem like a daunting proposition, but I'm convinced that you'll soon feel more energized, centered, focused, and cheerful. Now, because I know how you're feeling, I'll share with you my 21 favorite tips, tactics, secrets, and strategies so you, too, can be successful.

1. SEE YOURSELF FREE.
You now need to convince your mind, heart, and soul to get in the sugar-kicking mood to bring about your desired outcome. Picture yourself completely free of your craving for sweets and relishing life's sweetness instead. Glory in your newfound liberation. Run this image over and over again in your mind. See yourself living the life you want. Know that you've accomplished it.

Visualizing is a powerful tool used by many inspirational leaders, accomplished athletes, prominent statesmen, and influential business owners. "First we visualize what we want, and then we achieve it; because what we visualize, we realize," explains author and motivational speaker Mark Victor Hansen, who used this technique to make *Chicken Soup for the Soul* a big hit. "We see it in our mind's eye, and then it happens," adds Hansen, whose vision paid off handsomely, because although 100-plus publishers initially rejected his and cocreator Jack Canfield's project, the book went on to spawn 100-plus other titles and the series has sold more than 100 million copies.

So see yourself free and success will be yours!

2. CREATE A POWERFUL MANTRA.

Words work well in tandem with visualization. When cookie cravings strike, inwardly repeat a meaningful mantra to squash temptation. Try "I'm in control of what I eat." Or "I only eat healthy foods." Or say, "I am slim and sensual." Perhaps "I'm now a size '8'" works for you. Or "I'm now in perfect health." Just pick a positively worded saying that resonates with you and repeat it often enough until you convince yourself that it's true.

3. VIEW THIS CHALLENGE AS A BLESSING.

Abandon the idea that quitting sweets is a tough, unsavory task. Rather, approach your adventure as an unparalleled opportunity to begin anew. Visionary and self-help guru Bernie S. Siegel, M.D., a tireless advocate of the healing potential in all of us, beautifully captures the sentiment for which you should strive.

"View your sugar addiction as a blessing, not a curse," recommends the author of the number one *New York Times* bestseller *Love, Medicine, and Miracles*. "When you have a major challenge such as kicking a sugar addiction, ask yourself, 'What can I learn from this?' In the end, we thank scary illnesses or situations because they make us better people, and they enable us to fulfill our true possibilities."

4. GET INSPIRED DAILY.

When you're beset by doubt, rely on motivational self-help books, encouraging thoughts, and, if you wish, religious verses. This tactic is simply transformational. Whenever I felt discouraged, down, or frustrated, I pulled out one of my favorites and got enthusiastically recharged right away. These books might lift you up, as they did me:

- *As a Man Thinketh* by James Allen

- *The Language of Letting Go* by Melody Beattie

- *100 Ways to Keep Your Soul Alive* by Frederic and Mary Ann Brussat

- *Chicken Soup for the Soul* and other books by Jack Canfield and Mark Victor Hansen

- *Don't Sweat the Small Stuff . . . and It's All Small Stuff* by Richard Carlson, Ph.D.

- *How to Stop Worrying and Start Living* by Dale Carnegie

- *The Seven Spiritual Laws of Success* by Deepak Chopra

- *Prayer Is Good Medicine* by Larry Dossey, M.D.

- *There's a Spiritual Solution to Every Problem* by Dr. Wayne W. Dyer

- *Creative Visualization* by Shakti Gawain

- *You Can Heal Your Life* by Louise L. Hay

- *The Power of Your Subconscious Mind* by Dr. Joseph Murphy

- *You Can if You Think You Can* by Norman Vincent Peale

To find a number of inspirational thoughts and quotes, just visit my website at www.SugarShock.com, where you can get motivated any time, day or night.

5. PUT SWEETS AND QUICKIE CARBS IN THEIR PROPER PLACE.

To avoid temptation, don't bring harmful foods into your home, car, or workplace. You can't binge on a quart of ice cream if it's not in your freezer. So don't taunt yourself by keeping junk food anywhere near you. And ask for your family's support in this.

As you keep these nutrient-lacking carbs out of sight, get perspective by reminding yourself that you don't need these so-called goodies to have a sweet life.

6. GET A LIFE WITH ZEST AND SPARKLE!

You know that phrase, "Get a life"? It offers simple, brilliant, effective advice. While you're putting your carb habit in its proper place, you need to get involved, go places, have fun, tackle challenges, get a new hobby, and do things you've been wanting to do for years. Build a life that has zest, sparkle, and pizzazz. Grab it with gusto, relish, and appetite. Find delight, contentment, and appreciation for life.

7. PAMPER YOURSELF.

You now need to learn to pamper and reward yourself with nourishing, nurturing, wholesome *nonfood* treats. Take a leisurely bath, listen to uplifting music, get a manicure, take a spa day, buy yourself a present, and, no, it doesn't have to be expensive.

8. BECOME A SAVVY SUGAR SLEUTH.

Now you need to learn sugar's many names and guises so that you can stay away from it. Identify the 20 most commonly used sweeteners listed in chapter 21. When you shop for foods, be dispassionate and detached, and religiously read labels.

9. IF DESSERTS BECKON, ASK YOURSELF WHAT, WHY, AND HOW.

If sugar "calls out" to you, look within for answers and do Sugary Soul-Searching. Pinpoint what's setting you off. Analyze your motivations and feelings. Pose introspective questions. Before you eat something sweet, ask yourself what, why, and how: "What do I *really* want and what's bugging me? Why is that sweet so tempting and why am I consumed by it? How will eating this harm me?"

10. REMEMBER: IF YOU STRAY, YOU CAN GET STRUNG OUT.

Be realistic. Prepare for challenging days when you may find yourself standing motionless in front of a candy store, bakery, or pizza place—with no support nearby.

Before you succumb, run a movie in your mind of how giving in will affect you. Trust me, this kind of Sugary Soul-Searching will help you to quit salivating lickety-split. By tuning in to your feelings, you'll come to your senses and stop yourself.

Now flip the scenario around and ask yourself, "If I don't succumb to temptation, what will happen? How will I feel about myself?" Dwell on the positive outcome. If you say no to those tempting quickie carbs, you'll feel proud and cheerful, right?

11. EMBRACE THE "SIX Ds": DELAY, DISTANCE, DISTRACT, DECODE, DECIDE, AND DELIGHT.

Your well-meaning coworker keeps asking you if you want a donut, and you're close to caving in. Yes, you want one now! Acknowledge and own up to the feeling. Then let the the "Six Ds" come to the rescue. Before you succumb to temptation . . .

- **Delay!** Drink a glass of water and then delay for 15 minutes. Then delay a half hour. Chances are that the craving will pass.

- **Distance!** Make an escape! Shun your favorite bagel joints, candy stores, pizza parlors, supermarkets, or even drugstores when you're in the throes of a craving.

- **Distract!** Do something else! Take a hike. Clean your house. Read a book. Throw yourself into a project. Time will fly, as will your sugar cravings.

- **Decode!** Now it's time to figure out what the heck is going on. In other words, decode your cravings. Determine why you're so sugar obsessed right now.

- **Decide** to respect yourself. Now ignore your "cravings." Watch them subside, and then give yourself nonfood treats.

- **Delight** that you've said no! Really relish your joy, relief, and pride that you successfully took control over your destructive habit.

Use the powerful, effective "Six Ds" over and over again—all throughout the hour, day, week, and so on. You can even choose a different "D" to focus on every day.

12. H.A.L.T.
While doing the Six Ds, you also can inwardly holler, "H.A.L.T.!" to decide which state of mind applies to you: "Hungry, Angry, Lonely, or Tired." This wonderful tactic, I learned, is recommended in 12-step programs. But I urge you to go one step further. Transform your H.A.L.T. to signify that you're "Happy, Alert, Lovable, and Thoughtful."

13. BE GENTLE IF YOU SLIP. USE THE "FALL" FOR YOUR GREATER GOOD.
If you do lapse, be kind to yourself and try these health-enhancing, resolution-building tactics:

- ■ Accept that you're wonderfully imperfect and human.

- ■ Use your goofs to reaffirm your commitment to staying (mostly) sugar free.

- ■ Take extensive notes and chronicle how bad your slip makes you feel.

- ■ Honor, respect, and treasure your mistakes so you can shed light on them. This way, you'll be more likely to stay on the sugar-free path in the future.

- ■ Review these Sweet Sugar-Free Success Secrets and Strategies.

- ■ Give yourself a pep talk.

- ■ Visit www.SugarShock.com to read inspiring Sugar-Free Success Stories.

- ■ Write down why you want to get back on track and kick sweets.

14. RECOGNIZE THAT MOTHER NATURE KNOWS BEST.
When you cut out sugars and quickie, processed carbs, you'll find that many natural veggies, starches, fruits, and herbal teas have a yummy, delectable, satisfying aroma and flavor. Enjoy Mother Nature's gifts such as red peppers, sweet potatoes, jicama, apples, strawberries, blueberries, cashews, walnuts, and carrots. Experiment with herbs and spices such as cinnamon, cloves, ginger, and nutmeg. In short, be grateful and appreciative that you can choose such delicious, nutritious foods.

15. EXPRESS YOURSELF.
Wow! Kicking sugar can give you incredible mental clarity and acuity. It also can make you more creative. So pen a poem about your sugar relationship. If writing's not your thing, then paint a picture, compose a song, hum a tune, choreograph a dance, knit a sweater, plant some flowers, or doodle. Just find a way that best expresses you. Now let this wonderful, revealing poem from a member of my free, online KickSugar group inspire you to action:

Non-Ode to Sugar
by Dee M. of Jacksonville, North Carolina
You say you're my friend, but I know you will kill me in the end.

My affections for you are so strong, but I know this feeling is wrong.
How can I end this relationship? I pray each day not to fall or trip.
I see your dark side, and it's scary, I must confide.
Still you hang around tormenting me—it's so profound.
"Be gone," I say. "Today is a new day!"
I am done with you. Believe me, it's true!
I hide from you no more. I've pushed you out the door.
Now my life is free. You did not conquer me!

16. DINE WITH DIGNITY. ON THE SIDE, PLEASE! ASK SWEET QUESTIONS.

You can still enjoy eating out even though you've kicked sugar. Just assume that many restaurants sprinkle sugar (often liberally) into sauces and dressings to offer "enhanced" flavor. Use these strategies to make your dining experiences enjoyable:

- Tell your server that you're allergic to sugar, honey, or other sweeteners.

- Assume that all salad dressings and sauces are no-nos. Order your salads or entrees plain, with lemon, olive oil, or vinegar on the side.

- Be careful at Chinese, Japanese, or Thai restaurants, because many use sugar.

- Avoid or limit alcohol intake, because booze quickly turns to sugar in your body.

- Skip French bread, crackers, white rice, mashed potatoes, pasta, or other fast-acting carbs. Instead, request more vegetables, preferably steamed.

- If available, order quality carbs like brown rice or a sweet potato.

- Skip the dessert or ask for a fruit plate.

17. SLIP ON THOSE SNEAKERS. POUND THE PAVEMENT. GET A NATURAL HIGH.

Learn that *nothing* is more invigorating than the natural high you get from exercising. Discover, as I have, that no amount of sweet snacks or carb "treats" can hold a candle to the awesome exhilaration of exercise. It's impossible to exaggerate the mood lift, sense of well-being, and upswing in energy you get from joyfully moving.

18. LAUGH IT UP EVERY DAY.

Starting today, chuckle, laugh, and lighten up often. There's no need to be morose, glum, or sullen just because you're kicking an entrenched habit. Instead, crack jokes, read comedy books, or even poke fun at yourself as I did. (See my fun Connie cartoons at www.SugarShock.com.) Or watch funny movies such as *Tootsie*, *Bananas*, or *A Fish Called Wanda*. (Get more ideas at www.filmsite.org.)

19. ADJUST YOUR MIND-SET: THINK FULFILLMENT, NOT DEPRIVATION.

Dwell on what you *gain*, not on what you *lose* by kicking your habit. Approach your new, healthy way of eating with a positive attitude. It's vital to shift your point of view. You're not missing out on cookies, crackers, or chips. Rather, you're gaining health, happiness, energy, and good times. So focus on fulfillment, not deprivation.

20. READ! REREAD! REVIEW! REMEMBER! REACH OUT! RESIST! ROOT! REVEL!

Your success in freeing yourself from sweets will come from having a plan to rely on when temptations taunt you. To win your battle, try my "Eight Rs."

- Firstly, **read, reread, and review** this book. Then, **read** other informative books, such as *Sugar Blues*, *Lick the Sugar Habit*, and *Get the Sugar Out*.

- **Remember** how bad you felt while on sugar. **Remember** that sugar could harm your health, moods, and relationships. **Remember** to stay positive.

- **Reach out** to a savvy physician who understands sugar issues. **Reach out** to my free, online international KickSugar support group and www.SugarShockBlog.com. **Reach out** to family members, friends, colleagues, members of Overeaters Anonymous or another support group. **Reach out** to your Higher Power, if you believe in one.

- **Resist** your sugar cravings and think how proud you'll be when you pass up those formerly tempting "treats."

- Finally, **root** for yourself and **revel** in your amazing accomplishment! Hey, go ahead, pat yourself on the back right now!

21. CULTIVATE GRATITUDE.

I believe that whenever you make a monumental life change, you need to take a thankful snapshot of your life. "Gratitude wakes you up to what is good in your life," the motivational speaker Dr. Bernie Siegel told me in a phone interview. "It refocuses you on seeing the world in a different way. Instead of seeing all your problems, you begin to see some nice things.

"When you do that, you evolve," he continues. "With time, your prayers will become less 'I want to stop eating sugar' to maybe 'I want world peace' or 'I want the whole world to be healthy.'

"When you do this every day, you look at the world differently; you begin to change."

Afterword: Rays of Hope and Signs of Promise

You've now learned that researchers from around the world have conducted considerable groundbreaking research showing that too many sweets and re-fined, fiber-stripped, nutrient-deficient carbs can trigger a cluster of emo-tional and physical problems, from depression to diabetes.

Many experts have warned you that many chronic, degenerative diseases will continue to skyrocket as long as people keep plunging themselves in and out of SUGAR SHOCK! by continually eating these potentially dangerous quickie carbs.

But there's great news, too. Compelling studies clearly demonstrate that you can reverse many of your health woes by removing or scaling back inferior, culprit carbs and instead appreciating nutrient-dense, quality carbs and other top-notch foods, upping your activity level, and keeping blood sugar in control.

Yes, there's hope for the future, especially for our nation's children. Let's look at some promising, pioneering programs now under way.

Appleton, Wisconsin: Diet Boosts Moods and School Grades

When Greg Bretthauer took a position as dean of Appleton Central Alternative High School for at-risk students in Appleton, Wisconsin, many students there were rebellious, ill mannered, depressed, anxious, and difficult to control. Crime was so common that a full-time police liaison officer served the school.

Then, in 1997, Barbara and Paul Stitt, owners of Natural Ovens Bakery in nearby Manitowoc, Wisconsin, brought in fresh fruits, vegetables, lean protein, healthy fats, water, and whole-grain breads and cereals. They got rid of sugar-laden, chemically processed, artificially flavored beverages and junk foods.

Soon thereafter, the teens became more rational, better behaved, and less moody. "Classrooms became calmer, more learning began taking place, and students started getting better grades," reports the former dean. In addition, they attended school more regularly, had improved concentration, required less disciplining, and felt healthier.

To demonstrate how junk food impacts behavior, health, and ability to learn, kids are allowed to occasionally indulge in "forbidden" foods on designated junk food days.

"Within two hours, teachers lose control of the classroom," says Barbara Stitt, Ph.D., author of *Food & Behavior*. "Kids get headaches and stomachaches; they get depressed, angry, tired, or hyper. Many students actually *beg* not to do the junk food day a second time. They quickly learn that junk food causes them to feel miserable."

The Appleton program has been so successful that it's now being implemented throughout the entire Appleton school district of 15,000 students in 25 schools. In addition, the Stitts and Natural Ovens Bakery helped launch a "Peak Performance" program in another 35 midwestern schools and a "Healthy Lifestyles Initiative" in the Perspectives Charter School in Chicago, Illinois.

Lithonia, Georgia: School Goes Mostly Sugar Free

In 1996, then-obese Yvonne Sanders-Butler, Ed.D., was rushed to the emergency room because she was about to have a massive stroke. The five-foot, four-inch, 187-pound, Mississippi native had dangerously high blood pressure, joint pain, allergies, memory problems, depression, frequent nosebleeds, and a huge sugar addiction. After her near-death experience, she joined an overeaters' support group, quit sweets, began eating nourishing foods, started exercising, lost 55 pounds, and regained her health.

Two years later, when Dr. Butler became principal of Browns Mill Elementary School in Lithonia, Georgia, her new students were unruly, unfocused, tardy, often sick, and "larger than the norm." Convinced that "too many bad carbs were responsible" for these problems, she instituted the nation's first largely sugar-free school—against the advice of fellow school administrators, who couldn't envision kids skipping sweets.

Almost overnight, students slimmed down, got more energy, and concentrated better. Disciplinary problems dropped drastically, attendance and test scores soared, visits to the school nurse plummeted, and kids took their new healthy habits home with them.

Dr. Butler, author of *Healthy Kids, Smart Kids*, began other innovative programs, too. Every morning (6:30 a.m.) and afternoon (4:30 p.m.), the school gym becomes a wellness center, where parents, teachers, and community members can work out, take yoga classes, and get help from a fitness trainer.

What's more, the school doesn't hold bake sales but rather raises needed funds selling water, fresh fruit, student art, and school photos, and holding car washes. Birthdays aren't celebrated with cakes and soda but instead by playing educational games and nibbling on fruit, vegetables, chicken salad, soy dishes, and ethnic, nonsugary meals. Students even learn about nutrition and how to read food labels in various classes.

Dr. Butler is so intent on igniting a "wellness revolution" that on one swelteringly hot summer day, after the county signed a new pouring rights contract with Coca-Cola, she staged a one-hour standoff, refusing to permit sugary soft drinks on school premises. She finally allowed bottled water to be stocked instead.

Now, hundreds of educators, parents, and even federal agencies want to learn Dr. Butler's secrets. Her company Ennovy (www.ennovyinc.com) now offers nutrition and fitness coaching to institutions such as Denver, Colorado, schools; her alma mater, Jackson State University; Meharry Medical College; and Morehouse Medical School.

Berkeley, California: Kids Grow Their Grub in "Edible Schoolyard"

Back in 1995, the schoolyard at the urban Martin Luther King Junior Middle School in Berkeley, California, was covered with blacktop, and the school cafeteria closed because it couldn't accommodate the nearly 900 students. Instead, packaged, microwaved food was sold from a shack on the playground.

By 1997, that arid asphalt area was transformed into a one-acre organic garden and the antiquated cafeteria-kitchen was refurbished as a kitchen-classroom. Students now grow and harvest fresh, seasonal produce and make nutritious dishes using fruits and vegetables from their garden.

"The Edible Schoolyard" (www.EdibleSchoolyard.org) is the brain-child of renowned restaurateur Alice Waters (of Chez Panisse fame) and former school principal Neil Smith, and it is funded by the Chez Panisse Foundation.

The program is such a hit that some 3,000 school vegetable gardens have sprouted up at California schools and similar projects have been launched in "just about every state in the nation," says Edible Schoolyard coordinator Marsha Guerrero.

Meanwhile, at Berkeley's 15 other public schools, 10,000 students now learn about nutrition, food, health, sustainable agriculture, and cooking through another project, the School Lunch Initiative, headed by Waters and "renegade chef" Ann Cooper, known for her success at the Ross School in East Hampton, New York.

"We banned foods with high fructose corn syrup and trans fats, got rid of processed foods, and replaced most vendors," Cooper says. "We cook from scratch, serve fresh fruits and vegetables, and put in salad bars. The kids are getting *real* food."

New York City: Chef Changes Palates with Bold, Fresh Flavors

Miso soup. Salmon. Steamed asparagus. Basmati brown rice. Fresh fruit. Salad bar. That's a typical menu at New York City's private Calhoun School since 2002, thanks to world-class chef Robert Surles ("Chef Bobo").

Using fresh foods (usually seasonal), bold flavors, and no refined sugar, Chef Bobo introduced Calhoun's 650 students to nutritious meals, where desserts are relegated to a minor, once-a-week role and served in 1.5 ounce tasting cups. "We want them to understand that fruit is dessert," says the teacher at New York City's French Culinary Institute, a catering business owner and former chef for Yankees player Derek Jeter.

Chef Bobo began by first tossing out sugar-filled ketchup, which was "the only way many kids knew how to eat foods." Then he stopped serving bagels, which initially angered parents. Next, he taught kids about portion control by using tiny taster cups.

"Children now ask for seconds of brussels sprouts, and they're demanding different foods at home," says the chef, whose recipes for pureed cauliflower soup and rutabaga fries are at www.calhoun.org and in *Chef Bobo's Good Food Cookbook*.

New York City: 860,000 Meals Stress Fruits or Vegetables

Serving 860,000 tasty, visually appealing, and nutritious breakfasts and lunches a day at some 1,500 schools across New York City is the challenge of Jorge Leon Collazo, executive chef of the New York City Department of Education's Office of School Food.

Since 2004, Collazo, a former New England Culinary Institute instructor who goes by the name "Chef Jorge," has trained close to 15,000 food service workers in proper vegetable preparation and salad bar standards, introduced more fruits and vegetables, especially from New York state, added plant-based meals to elementary schools in communities of need, unrolled ethnic cuisine entrees familiar to students, and switched white bread with whole wheat. Now, he wants to eliminate trans fats and high-fructose corn syrup. Bringing in organic produce is also "on the radar screen."

Fortunately, overseeing an estimated $125 million-a-year food budget brings clout. Explains SchoolFood's executive director David Berkowitz: "Manufacturers are anxious to sell to New York City because many school districts throughout the country are following what we're doing, pushing the envelope to improve the nutrition of products in their schools."

Nationwide: From Farm Fields to School Cafeterias

Some 500,000 children in 400 school districts in more than 23 states are eagerly eating a variety of vegetables and fruits served in school cafeterias, courtesy of the popular, innovative National Farm to School Program (www.FarmToSchool.org).

"The kids get excited about harvesting carrots and picking strawberries right out of the soil, they get cooking demonstrations from chefs, and they even visit local farms," explains Anupama Joshi, director of the national program, which is coordinated by the Center for Food and Justice at Occidental College and the Community Food Security Coalition. The USDA and the W. K. Kellogg Foundation also provide funding.

"It's a win-win situation. The Farm to School programs teach kids about good nutrition and give them healthy foods at the same time," Joshi says. "That connection, we've found, helps establish eating habits that kids will take with them for a lifetime."

Renowned Integrative Physician Dr. Andrew Weil Seeks to Educate Doctors

Best-selling author Andrew Weil, M.D., is so appalled by the nutrition education physicians receive that he's promoting nutrition and health conferences to teach cutting-edge nutrition information to members of the medical community.

"My goal is for this conference to be a biannual event, where people learn about amazing current research and information that's not included in physician training," says Dr. Weil, who envisions a 300-hour required nutrition program for all medical residents.

"We have to get a new generation of educated health professionals out there," insists Dr. Weil, who also presents a popular annual public forum.

Both events are jointly sponsored by Dr. Weil's University of Arizona Program in Integrative Medicine and the Richard and Hinda Rosenthal Center for Complementary and Alternative Medicine at Columbia University's College of Physicians and Surgeons.

What's more, Dr. Weil's rapidly growing University of Arizona Program in Integrative Medicine offers physicians from around the world extensive in-person and online training in nutrition and mind-body medicine.

More Promising Programs and Developments

Let's look now at other encouraging, health-conscious developments:

- Whole Foods Market, which began in 1980 with one small store, has become the world's leading natural and organic foods supermarket, with 183 stores in North America and the United Kingdom at press time. Meanwhile, Wild Oats Natural Marketplace, founded in 1987, now has 110 stores in 24 states and British Columbia. The success of these publicly traded chains, that avoid high-fructose corn syrup, hydrogenated oils, and artificial additives, shows, as Dr. Ludwig notes, "clearly, huge profits are to be made by providing healthy foods."

- Since 1994, more than 5,000 people who've shed at least 30 pounds and kept it off for a year or longer have shared weight-loss secrets and strategies with the National Weight Control Registry (www.nwcr.ws). " 'Successful losers hardly ever skip breakfast; they eat better carbs, not processed grains, and they get an hour a day of physical activity," says NWCR cofounder James O. Hill, Ph.D.

- Sen. Tom Harkin (D-IA) has sponsored several bills to protect our nation's young from junk food marketers. One enacted proposal required all U.S. schools to formulate a School Wellness Policy by June 30, 2006. Senator Harkin also spearheaded a program for the government to give out fresh fruits and vegetables at some 400 schools in 14 states, including 25 schools on Indian reservations.

- California Governor Arnold Schwarzenegger, former President Bill Clinton, and Arkansas Governor Mike Huckabee have become advocates for healthy diets, exercise, and banning junk food from schools.

- In 2003, after then-obese Governor Huckabee was diagnosed with type 2 diabetes and warned by his doctor that he didn't have long to live, he kicked sugar and lost more than 100 pounds. Now, he runs marathons and oversees "Healthy Arkansas." The state even allows employees to take a half hour a day to exercise.

- "Healthy America" was adopted by the National Governors Association, which Governor Huckabee and Arizona Governor Janet

Napolitano cochaired. Task force members include Governor Schwarzenegger, Iowa Governor Tom Vilsack, South Carolina Governor Mark Sanford, and Tennesseee Governor Phil Bredesen.

- The Institute for Integrative Nutrition (IIN) educates thousands on the power of wholesome, unprocessed foods to improve our health, moods, and lives. IIN, which trains students to become health counselors, was founded in 1993 by health advocate Joshua Rosenthal, M.Sc.Ed., and it is the only holistic nutrition school in the world to integrate Ayurveda, macrobiotics, Chinese medicine, raw foods, Atkins, blood type, and Zone diets, among other methods.

- Meanwhile, award-winning filmmaker/organic farmer/holistic health counselor Amy Kalafa and community organizer/holistic health counselor/former dentist Susan P. Rubin are recruiting 2 million mothers nationwide. The "Two Angry Moms" (www.AngryMoms.org) traveled the country to produce a documentary that reveals the abysmal, nutrient-lacking foods served in schools today, highlights model programs, and inspires people to take action.

- More parents and a coalition of mission-driven food companies launched the "Eat Smart, Grow Strong" campaign "to promote healthy eating at home." Kids' eating habits influence the choices they "make at school, the mall, and everywhere else they eat for the rest of their lives," says cofounder Susan Lamontagne.

- Finally, *Sesame Street*'s renowned Cookie Monster, one of PBS's Muppets famous for scarfing down platefuls of chocolate-chip cookies, began to control his sugar cravings. The beloved, blue furry creature, who used to sing " 'C' is for cookie, that's good enough for me," learned new healthy habits and realized that his favorite sweets are foods to eat "sometimes," not "anytime."

It's Up to Us to Change Ourselves and Influence Others

Ultimately, educating people is the way to bring more healthy foods and slower-digesting, quality carbs into schools, restaurants, grocery stores, and people's homes.

"The idea for quitting smoking was consumer driven," says internist Richard Ash, M.D. "It came from every person who stood up and said, 'This is not healthy.' The same thing applies here: when people demand it, things change."

Dr. Andrew Weil agrees. "This is going to be a grassroots, consumer-led movement. It's going to take enlightened consumers who demand better-quality foods and who require their physicians to be educated in nutrition. We can put pressure on government and companies to change," he said in an interview.

Marion Nestle, Ph.D., author of *What to Eat* and *Food Politics*, insists that "the statement you make with your pocketbook can be quite powerful. Any time you choose a food, you're voting with your fork."

So henceforth vote in a healthy way. Help us make the world a healthier place. That means don't buy or eat sugary foods.

Of course, you may have a powerful habit, but using my strategies and other experts' tactics, you can kick it. Say NO now to sweets for the sake of your moods, health, and happiness.

Cut out or curtail those quickie carbs, and I'm sure that you'll find, as I have, that Life Is Sweeter Without Refined Sweets.

ACKNOWLEDGMENTS FROM AUTHOR CONNIE BENNETT

SUGAR SHOCK! (my first book) was conceived back in April 1998—almost from the minute I gave up sugar on doctors' orders after years of struggling with an on-again, off-again love/hate affair with sweets. Since August 2001, when I began this book in earnest, I've received wholehearted support and "go-get-'em" encouragement from thousands of gracious, generous, warmhearted, dedicated physicians, researchers, nutritionists, obesity experts, consumer health advocates, concerned parents, school administrators, chefs, sugar addicts or people with or at risk for hypoglycemia and diabetes, friends, fellow authors and journalists, friendly bloggers, marketing consultants, healers, and family members. I've been truly blessed to be surrounded, supported, and inspired by such remarkable people, all of whom helped me to bring *SUGAR SHOCK!* to life.

First and foremost, I extend my heartfelt thanks to thousands of amazing, articulate, sugar- or carb-sensitive folks from around the world. You, my fellow "Sugar Kickers," have been incredibly honest, open, and committed to sharing your most intimate thoughts, worries, frustrations, and questions with me. Thanks for revealing exactly what you, my target audience, need and want to know as you embark upon your adventure to cut out the culprit carbs.

In particular, I appreciate those of you who participated in my Fast-Track, Kick-Sugar Countdown Program, my 21-Day, Kick-Sugar Countdown Diet, or my free, online international Yahoo! KickSugar group, which I founded in November 2002 to offer the kind of ongoing support, compassionate encouragement, loving guidance, and helpful information that I *never* received when kicking quickie carbs on my own in 1998.

In addition, I'm tremendously grateful to the hundreds of forward-looking medical professionals, nutrition whizzes, and social activists who kindly provided perspective,

translated medical theories into lay terms, and shared insightful background information with me. I also must single out a handful of experts who frequently bent over backward to arrange time to speak with me, e-mail me follow-up information, and/or
appear in a teleseminar I presented. You were all way beyond astounding!

Those remarkable mentors to whom I'm especially indebted include antisugar pioneer Nancy Appleton, Ph.D.; integrative physician Fred Pescatore, M.D.; nutritionist and
exercise physiologist Jill Vollmuth, C.N.C.; savvy nutritionist Jonny Bowden, Ph.D.,
C.N.S.; knowledgeable food/beverage formulator Russ Bianchi, of Adept Solutions; helpful Commercial Alert cofounder and executive director Gary Ruskin; famed Harvard
researcher and nutritionist Walter C. Willett, M.D., Dr.P.H.; cutting-edge integrative
physician Andrew Weil, M.D.; renowned nutritionist Ann-Louise Gittleman, Ph.D.,
C.N.S.; and inspiring reproductive endocrinologist Deborah Metzger, M.D., Ph.D.

Moreover, I'm beholden to toxicologist and artificial-sweeteners expert Janet Starr-
Hull, Ph.D.; Center for Science in the Public Interest executive director Michael F. Jacobson, Ph.D.; fitness guru Kathy Smith; antiaging physician Alicia Stanton, M.D.;
"nutritionist to the stars" Oz Garcia, Ph.D.; my KickSugar group's founding nutrition
consultant Keri M. Gans, M.S., R.D., C.D.N.; friend and dedicated integrative physician Jill Baron, M.D.; and again my 1998 "saviors" Roberta Ruggiero of the Hypoglycemia Support Foundation and physician Keith DeOrio, M.D.

Moreover, in fall 2005, I was thrilled and fortunate to find the esteemed, pioneering cardiologist, antiaging specialist, and nutritionist Stephen T. Sinatra, M.D.,
F.A.C.C., C.N.S., who came on board as the SUGAR SHOCK! medical consultant.
Wow! Stephen, joining forces with you has given this book "angel wings," as a friend
puts it. Your support and encouragement has been invaluable. It's also quite gratifying
to know that you're one of a rapidly growing number of doctors who really understand the dangers of sweets and refined carbs.

Furthermore, I owe special thanks to renowned dermatologist and best-selling author Dr. Nicholas Perricone, M.D., for being one of my early supporters and for writing the foreword to this book.

My gratitude also goes to my loyal, perceptive, shrewd literary agent Ellen Levine
for being my tireless advocate since fall 2002. Ellen, thank you so much for firmly believing in my project, having a bold vision for it, backing me wholeheartedly for years,
and ultimately hooking me up with Berkley Books.

I'd also like to cite Ellen's husband, Ivan Strausz, M.D., who, just weeks before I
first approached Ellen, had begun to reverse his prediabetes condition simply by removing desserts and breads, losing weight, and exercising regularly. Coincidentally, he
inadvertently demonstrated to my soon-to-be agent the almost miraculous, rejuvenat-
ing powers of identifying and escaping SUGAR SHOCK!

In addition, I gratefully applaud the truly talented, astute, concise editors Judith
Kern and Sandi Gelles-Cole who, at various stages of my project, helped trim and

tighten my lengthy manuscript, give better shape and flow to my considerable research, and make my points with more clarity and panache.

I'm also delighted to have found my enthusiastic, insightful, delightful Berkley Books editor Christine Zika, who gracefully, cheerfully shepherded my manuscript through the publishing process. Thanks, Christine, for your thoughtful suggestions and helpful guidance on how best to make my book "speak" to millions who need this information.

Moreover, I gratefully applaud and appreciate the many folks at The Berkley Publishing Group for their stupendous efforts to put *SUGAR SHOCK!* on the literary map. Kudos to the creative, forward-thinking, and diligent people in so many different departments—sales, editorial, design, copy editing, publicity, and promotion. In particular, I'd like to thank Leslie Gelbman, President, Publisher, and Editor in Chief of Berkley Books, and Susan Allison, Berkley vice president and editorial director, for their vote of confidence and continued support of this book.

I'm also incredibly indebted to some two dozen incredibly knowledgeable and gracious experts who kindly took time to "vet" or verify the accuracy of particular sections of the book pertinent to their area of expertise. Thank you so much, Nancy, Fred, Jill, Jonny, Russ, Janet, Gary, Roberta, and Dr. Metzger (all cited above). More gratitude goes to Ann E. Kelley, Ph.D.; Dharma Singh Khalsa, M.D.; Larry Christensen, Ph.D.; Peter Havel, Ph.D.; Antonio Convit, M.D.; Loren Cordain, Ph.D.; Christine L. Sardo, M.P.H., R.D., L.D.; and J.J. Virgin, C.N.S, C.H.F.I.

Other experts who were especially helpful include Diana Schwarzbein, M.D.; Mark Hyman, M.D.; Bartley G. Hoebel, Ph.D.; Marion Nestle, Ph.D., M.P.H.; Kelly D. Brownell, Ph.D.; Jack LaLanne; Ralph Nader; Joseph Mercola, D.O.; Michael Persinger, Ph.D.; Kathleen DesMaisons, Ph.D.; James O. Hill, Ph.D; Bernie Siegel, M.D.; David L. Katz, M.D.; David S. Ludwig, M.D., Ph.D.; John Banzhaf III; Richard Daynard; John Coale; Jeffrey Wigand, Ph.D.; Ronald Klatz, M.D., and the American Academy of Anti-Aging Medicine; Leonard Marquart, Ph.D., R.D.; Howard J. Shaffer, Ph.D., C.A.S.; Shari Lieberman, Ph.D.; Kay Sheppard, M.A.; Robert Matthews; George Bray, M.D.; Joan Mathews-Larson, Ph.D.; Earl Mindell, Ph.D., R.Ph.; Jeffrey Schaler, Ph.D.; Barry M. Popkin, Ph.D.; Doris Rapp, M.D.; Ira M. Sacker, M.D.; Carden Johnston, M.D.; Patrick Fratellone, M.D.; Vanessa Sands; Ralph G. Walton, M.D.; Gene-Jack Wang, M.D.; Gary Ruskin, and Yvonne Sanders-Butler, Ed.D.

Many others willingly shared information and insights, including Jeraldine Saunders; Elizabeth Somer, M.A., R.D.; Julia Ross, M.A.; Alan Spreen, M.D.; Barbara Stitt, Ph.D.; Paul Stitt, Ph.D.; Alexander G. Schauss, Ph.D.; Forrest Tennant, M.D., Ph.D.; Lora Ruffner; James Turner; Tara Miller, M.S., R.D.; Mary Jo Viederman; Gil Wishire, M.D.; Cori Brackett; Jack Challem; Russell L. Blaylock, M.D.; Nan Kathryn Fuchs, Ph.D.; Lawrence Shiman; James Chow, M.D.; Cheryl Chow; Barry Sears, Ph.D.; Kenneth Snow, M.D.; Neal Barnard, M.D.; Victor Zammit, Ph.D.; Judith Wurtman, Ph.D.; Richard Ash, M.D.; Kenneth Blum, Ph.D.;

representatives of the CDC, FDA, and ADA; and hundreds of others way too numerous to mention.

At this point, I'd also like to single out and express my profound gratitude to the incredibly amazing, astute, articulate, distinguished experts who graciously took time to read and offer endorsements for this book. These kind folks were: Mehmet Oz, M.D.; Arkansas Governor Mike Huckabee; film producer Harvey Weinstein; Christiane Northrup, M.D.; Barbara DeAngelis, Ph.D.; Marilu Henner; Mark Hyman, M.D.; Oz Garcia, Ph.D.; Keith DeOrio, M.D.; Marilyn E. Carroll, Ph.D.; Jill R. Baron, M.D.; Kathy Smith; Naura Hayden; Fred Pescatore, M.D.; Donald I. Abrams, M.D.; Joshua Rosenthal; Roberta Ruggiero; Nancy Appleton, Ph.D.; Dharma Singh Khalsa, M.D.; J.J. Virgin, C.N.S., C.H.F.I.; Kenneth Blum, Ph.D.; Ronald F. Feinberg, M.D., Ph.D.; Russ Bianchi; Mark Victor Hansen; Liz Lipski, Ph.D., C.C.N.; Julia Havey; Dr. Eric Plasker; Cynthia Rowland; Barbara Reed Stitt, Ph.D.; Jimmy Moore; and Devorah Cutler-Rubenstein.

Meanwhile, I also must heartily applaud and express my esteem for the late Robert C. Atkins, M.D., whom I met twice before he passed away, and the late William Dufty, author of *Sugar Blues*, with whom I exchanged e-mails shortly before his death. Both Dr. Atkins and Dufty deserve considerable credit and public esteem for having the courage, conviction, and compassion to warn the world about the innumerable perils of eating too many sweets and processed carbs.

Many fellow investigative journalists and authors also inspired me, especially Eric Schlosser (*Fast Food Nation*), Greg Critser (*Fatland*), and Morgan Spurlock (*Super Size Me*). Likewise, it pleases me that a number of astute reporters from the *New York Times, Chicago Tribune*, and other media outlets also are covering this important story.

Moreover, my fellow intrepid bloggers and self-appointed weight-loss experts Jimmy Moore, Regina Wilshire, Julia Havey, and Dana Carpender deserve more praise.

I'm also especially grateful to my very dear, perceptive friend Tom Smaldone, a savvy former journalist, who eagerly read and critiqued every chapter as soon as I wrote it. Thanks ever so much, Tom, for your tremendous insights; your warm, nurturing, priceless support; your steady stream of teasing, which kept me in good spirits; our many private jokes; and so much more.

Furthermore, I thankfully acknowledge Myra Pinkham, my dedicated, hardworking KickSugar group assistant moderator; former assistant KickSugar moderators Melissa, Erin, and Ruth; Leila Armush, for inspiring me to form KickSugar; and many special "guinea pigs"—especially Jennifer, Ju, Lisa B., Lee Anne, Linda, Lisa, Lynn, and Suzanne—who offered valuable feedback years ago, when I first created my 21-Day, Kick-Sugar Countdown Diet.

Additionally, I'm incredibly indebted to my many hardworking, detail-oriented, awe-inspiring, part-time researchers, research assistants, and fact-checkers from 2001 to 2006, especially the spectacular, dedicated, and now deceased Mary Kittel (to whom I dedicated this book); as well as the astute, amazing Gale Maleskey, R.D.; Jennifer Moore; Carol Turkington; Maureen P. Sangiorgio; Alicia M. Voorhies, R.N.; and Lisa Goldberg, M.S., R.D., C.D.N.

Still more thanks go to other wonderful, part-time helpers over the years, including Lydia Jordan, Bradley Kreit, Jennifer Phillips, Debora Yost, Ernie Tremblay, Joy Darlington, Bonnie Siegler, Sherry Amatenstein, Erin Chapman, Jynelle Athena Gracia, Kate Pickert, Sarah Trabucchi, Allyson Giard, Brooke Fitzsimmons, Karen Berk, Alex Halperin, Jennifer Mundstock, Claudia Caruana, Kathryn Townsend, Staci Sanders, April Crossman, Estelle Sobel, Lisa Iannucci, Fawn Germer, Jennifer Repo, Heather Weisse, Nancy Belzer, and Lynn Grieger, R.D.

A select group of influential, inspirational marketers/mentors and PR whizzes also deserve heaps of glowing praise for their unwavering support, invaluable guidance, and effervescent encouragement: Rick Frishman, Steve and Bill Harrison, Hillary Rivman, Joel Roberts, Mark Victor Hansen, Alex Mandossian, Joan Stewart, Michelle Anton, Robert G. Allen, Anne Leedom, Jack Canfield, Brian Jud, Matt Bacak, Randy Gilbert, Peggy McColl, Michael and Elly Ruge, Warren Whitlock, Martin Wales, Gregory Godek, Bob Austen, Tami DePalma, Suzanne Falter-Barns, and Clayton Makepeace. More thanks are due to Dave Mitchell, Eric Lingenfelter, John Kremer, Mike Stewart, Greg O'Donahue, Mark Whitauer, Jaylee Zeimetz, and VoiceText.com.

I'd also like to single out designer Peter Weber, as well as Kurt Togrul, Scott Wolfson, and Jason Saeler for building www.SugarShock.com; artist Rose Petruzzi for creating the quirky "Sugar Shrew" Connie cartoon character; and Andy Wibbels for setting up my SUGAR SHOCK! blog.

Certainly, I'd be remiss if I didn't thank my many early, enthusiastic, encouraging supporters and advisors, including Nancy Hancock, Naura Hayden, Mark Steisel, Devorah Cutler-Rubenstein, Greg Tobin, Sam Horn, Sterling Lord, Michael Larsen, Tami Booth, Julia VanTine, Carol Gilmore, Mariska Van Aalst, Hazel Dawkins, Dennis Fairchild, Steven Goldsberry, Cynthia Rowland, Bertie Catchings, Dr. Maria Grace, Lisa Delman, Wendy Dubit, Paula Harris, Gina Allchin, Georgia Malone, Sophie Anson, and, of course, Deborah Voorhees, whose idea it was that I write this book in the first place. Moreover, my gratitude galore is due to the highly helpful Maui Writers Conference, the Authors Guild, and the American Society of Journalists and Authors (ASJA).

Also, I'm more thankful than words can say to my incredibly gifted, dedicated, kind acupuncturist Lohkmin Lee, who—without fail—relieved my excruciatingly painful back, arm, and shoulder (from all the sitting/typing), as well as my prolonged book stress.

Further praise is due to the Institute for Integrative Nutrition (IIN), especially the pioneering founder/director Joshua Rosenthal, M.Sc.E.D., along with fellow students, graduates, and staff members, who made my experience there invaluable and rewarding. Special kudos also are due to Kelley Dobbins, Julia Kalish, Robert Notter, Abina

Benson, Anissa Buckley, Amanda Lerner, Pamela Rich, and members of my Fast-Track business coaching team, as well as Glen Colello, Jay Marshall, Amy Kalafa, and Susan Rubin.

Believe it or not, my ex-boyfriend Mark also deserves credit because, by dumping me, he inadvertently inspired me to find a new doctor, learn the truth about and ramifications of my sugar-and-carb habit, and begin a new, more healthy, happy sugar-free way of life.

I'm also obliged to Dr. Gary Ostrow, Mark Angelo, Dave Barrus, Jerry Spiegel, Ken Browning, Craig Nobbs, my family (especially my mom, dad, sister, brother-in-law, and cousins Debbie and Vonnie), Carolyn Mazzenga, Jane Sheahan, Gregg Giannillo, and Douglas Milroy.

This acknowledgment section wouldn't be complete without paying tribute to my Higher Power and Divine Intelligence for giving me strength, persistence, inspiration, and a positive mind-set to pull this off despite numerous challenges.

In addition, I'm thankful to Whole Foods Market, Health Nuts, Evian, Philip Glass, Pavarotti, Yanni, Enya, Basia, Bruce Springsteen, "Jock Jams," Andrea Bocelli, Josh Groban, Celestial Seasonings, and Wisdom Herbs for nourishing and sustaining me as I researched and wrote this book. I also pay homage to the ever-intriguing city of New York, where I love to speedwalk and get charged up and inspired, and my fast Dell computer, which made it possible to rapidly rearrange my thoughts and many facts.

Finally, a million thanks go to you, my dear readers. I treasure you and thank you for reading, absorbing, and getting inspired (I hope) by *SUGAR SHOCK!* I also thank you (optimistically, in advance) for sharing this gift of health with your loved ones.

I truly hope that this book helps your health to blossom, your joy to increase, and your soul to soar.

AFTER-THE-BOOK SUPPORT:

WANT MORE HELP KICKING SWEETS AND QUICKIE CARBS? A SPECIAL INVITATION FROM AUTHOR AND "SUGAR SHREW NO MORE!" CONNIE BENNETT

Dear Readers,

I do hope that *SUGAR SHOCK!* has helped to educate, empower, and inspire you. Because I personally know that the journey from "sugar addiction" to sugar-free delight can be challenging, but ultimately rewarding, I've developed several ways to give you "after-the-book support" so that you can successfully squash your sugar habit. You can:

▪ Visit my blog (www.SugarShockBlog.com) to get gobs of good info such as current SUGAR SHOCK! and other nutrition news; empowering messages; Sugar-Free Success Stories; my free food shopping list; and information about my 21-Day, Kick-Sugar Countdown Diet, which includes tele-coaching (via the phone) and audio e-mails (delivered straight to your in-box).

▪ Learn about my upcoming book signings, seminars, and lectures while you're at my SUGAR SHOCK! blog.

▪ Sign up for my free e-zine and get my list of "Foods With Sly Hidden Sugars" at my website (www.SugarShock.com). Also, make sure to download my free article, "Tips to Find a Sugar-Savvy Doctor." And get lots of other free (sugar-free, of course) goodies there, too.

- Attend one of my free Virtual Book Tours (via phone) with thousands of other would-be Sugar Kickers from around the world. By participating, you'll learn about special bonuses just for you, including replays of informative, entertaining tele-seminars I've conducted with renowned nutritionists, doctors, motivational speakers, and researchers.

- Get warm, nurturing, ongoing, 24/7 support in my free, online, international KickSugar support group on Yahoo! It's really easy to join. Just visit www.Sugar ShockBlog.com and then click on the colorful "Kick Sugar With Us!" link—it's the artwork of people holding hands (because that's what we aim to do, figuratively, of course).

I do hope that you'll join my worldwide community. Don't suffer and struggle alone as I did back in 1998. Indeed, as I've discovered from helping thousands of other folks to kick sugar and quickie carbs, you get much comfort, compassion, and caring just by banding with those of us with similar issues.

So join my thriving kick-sugar family now. Visit www.SugarShock.com and sign up for my mailing list so you won't feel so alone and so that you'll get the information, encouragement, and motivation that you need.

Warmly, and with very high hopes for your life-altering, sugar-free success,

Connie Bennett

Connie Bennett, M.S.J., C.H.H.C.
Author, *SUGAR SHOCK!*
"Sugar Shrew No More!" and
   Kick-Sugar Coach
Founder, The 21-Day,
   Kick-Sugar Countdown Diet
www.SugarShock.com
www.SugarShockBlog.com

INTRODUCTION FROM

CONNIE BENNETT

In spring 1998, I laid the groundwork for *SUGAR SHOCK!* That's because almost immediately after my astute physician "prescribed" that I kick sweeteners and fast-acting carbs to rid me of my 44 baffling, frustrating, excruciating ailments, I plunged into investigative-journalist mode and began to seek out any and all information I could find that would teach me about the far-reaching perils of sweeteners and processed carbohydrates.

My research for this book involved four different components. First off, I personally interviewed (mostly via phone but a few in person) about 300 respected medical experts on the cutting edge—physicians with nutrition training, neuroscientists, medical researchers, obesity experts, food industry analysts and insiders, nutritionists, observers, activists, and public health advocates. You'll find their quotes throughout *SUGAR SHOCK!* In addition, given the massive amount of work this book required over a period of five years, I enlisted the help of several research assistants—astute, experienced, sharp researchers/journalists—to conduct interviews with another 50 or so experts and to provide me with transcripts of their chats.

Secondly, a team of many part-time researchers helped me review dozens, if not hundreds, of medical studies, most of which were recent and all of which were published in respected peer-reviewed medical journals. In the critical, initial stages of my research for *SUGAR SHOCK!*, the industrious, thorough, dedicated Mary Kittel (1969–2004) helped spearhead my research efforts. Mary—a veteran health journalist, who had researched, wrote, and coauthored three books herself—did a stupendous job tracking down, poring over, and clarifying the conclusions in many relevant, top-quality, peer-reviewed studies that linked sugar, high fructose corn syrup, and high-glycemic carbs to a variety of diseases and ailments. Excitedly, we uncovered a huge amount of recent groundbreaking research, most of which received scant or no attention in the press—unless it related to obesity or diabetes. Mary was pivotal in helping me get a clearer picture of how too much sugar and refined carbs could trigger so many different serious ailments.

A third way I conducted research was to connect with my target audience to learn about their needs and interests. In August 2001, when I officially started this book, I chatted online, over the phone, or in person with thousands of self-described current or former "sugar addicts" (mostly hypoglycemics, diabetics, and prediabetics). I also began to offer online support, beginning in other people's support groups. Then on November 16, 2002, I founded my own KickSugar international online support group (on Yahoo!) to encourage, guide, inspire, educate, and network with people having sugar issues. While helping members of KickSugar, they, in turn, provided guidance, impetus, and direction for my research for *SUGAR SHOCK!* because of the kinds of questions, remarks, and articles they posted. Ultimately, my KickSugar group became pivotal in helping me zero in on what specific kinds of information would best help people both understand and conquer their often crippling, mood-destroying, and life-harming sugar or carb addiction. For example, because of members' repeated questions, I added information about how to combat sugar cravings, what supplements could be helpful, whether or not to consume artificial sweeteners, how to positively influence kids to eat right, sugar's societal influence, and much more.

Finally, the fourth way I did research was to read other people's books. In *SUGAR SHOCK!*, I sought to add to the tremendous amounts of research and conclusions made by the talented, insightful Nancy Appleton, Ph.D. (*Lick the Sugar Habit*); William Dufty (*Sugar Blues*); Ann Louise Gittleman, Ph.D. (*Get the Sugar Out*); and John Yudkin, M.D. (*Sweet and Dangerous*). Furthermore, many other experts provided helpful groundwork, including E. M. Abrahamson, M.D., and A. W. Pezet (*Body, Mind & Sugar*); T. L. Cleave (*The Saccharine Disease*); Beatrice Trum Hunter (*The Sugar Trap and How to Avoid It*); Morrison C. Bethea, M.D., Sam S. Andrews, M.D., Luis A. Balart, M.D., and H. Leighton Steward (*SUGAR BUSTERS! Cut Sugar to Trim Fat*); Robert C. Atkins, M.D. (*Dr. Atkins' Diet Revolution* and others); Kathleen DesMaisons, Ph.D. (*Potatoes, Not Prozac*, etc.); Dr. Rachael F. Heller and Dr. Richard F. Heller (*The Carbohydrate Addict's Lifestyle Program* and more); and others.

Of course, *SUGAR SHOCK!* was ultimately made possible because of the many pioneering medical researchers and scientists from around the world who have been—and still are—conducting groundbreaking studies that enable us to reach the conclusions you read here. In addition, physicians and nutritionists are learning and passing on more valuable information.

What follows is a significant selection, though not a complete one (due to space constraints), of medical studies and articles that were helpful when writing this book. Please note that I've included URLs whenever possible, but given the realities of the Internet, where websites get updated often, and the fact that this book was five years in the making, some links cited may no longer be active. Also, in some instances only the URL of an abstract (rather than the full study) is included, because to get the complete article, you need to purchase it online (which I did). If the URL was really lengthy, I simply listed the name of the study, again because of space limitations.

In conclusion, compiling this references section was a massive endeavor involving many research assistants. In particular, I'd like to single out several people who worked long and hard so that I could make my deadlines. Special thanks to the very diligent, hardworking Lydia Jordan and Bradley Kreit, who bent over backward to help me organize these end notes, double-check their accuracy, and see if other references were missing. Additional thanks and gratitude for work on the notes goes to Jennifer Moore, Alicia Voorhees, and other research assistants named in the acknowledgments section.

CHAPTER 1: CONNIE'S STORY: CONFESSIONS OF THE "SUGAR SHREW NO MORE!" AND HOW I CHANCED UPON THE SCARY SUGAR TRUTH

Connie's Note Regarding the Books Mentioned: The books mentioned in this chapter provided me with my initial education about sugar's dangers. In fact, the only way that I was able to realize that I had a whopping 44 hypoglycemic symptoms (which I listed in the sidebar, "Connie, the 'Sugar Shrew' of 1998: My Symptoms") is because after my doctor's diagnosis, I bought some books about hypoglycemia and used a yellow marker pen to highlight all my ailments. Otherwise, I may not have remembered all of these health woes since I no longer suffer from any of them. Below, you'll find books that helped me learn about hypoglycemia and the sugar connection back in 1998. Since my "eureka" sweets-don't-make-me-sweet experience, a few additional books have been published, which you'll find listed elsewhere in the end notes.

Connie's Note Regarding "My Story": While this chapter is sort of like a memoir, I took a little literary license for the sake of clarity and dramatization purposes, as well as the fact that certain incidents are somewhat blurry to me—I was, after all, in a sugar-induced haze back in 1998. For instance, I made some changes to time frame and location. But basically, the story I told in chapter 1—I'm embarrassed to say— is in fact fairly accurate: I was badly hooked on sugar, particularly red licorice, chocolate-covered peanuts, and hard candies; I did suffer from 44 symptoms; my boyfriend did dump me because I became so bitchy after eating a lot of sweets; I did find a wonderful doctor, Dr. Keith DeOrio, who told me to kick sweets; and I did kick the sugar back in 1998. FYI, like millions of Americans, I had heard that sugar wasn't good for you but didn't take action until my life hit rock bottom. In fact, I had even tried to quit several times before, but like most Americans, I just didn't get it together until it became absolutely imperative. As for Mark's and my final break-up incident, the facts are fuzzy, so I created the scene described. Actually, we did go to a wonderful Malibu restaurant, but I don't think that was the night we broke up and he took me home early. Actually, I think we did have a fight that night but still patched it up. In other words, at times, I may have embellished the scenario to make a scene more riveting and readable.

Airola, Paavo O. *Hypoglycemia: A Better Approach*. Phoenix, AZ: Health Plus Publishers, 1977.

Appleton, Nancy. *Lick the Sugar Habit*. Garden City Park, NY: Avery, 1988. (One of my favorite books back in 1998. Nancy Appleton is one of my mentors and heroes.)

Crook, William G. *The Yeast Connection: A Medical Breakthrough*. New York: Vintage Books, 1986.

Donsbach, Kurt W. *Hypoglycemia*. Huntington Beach, CA: International Institute of Natural Health Sciences, 1983.

Dufty, William. *Sugar Blues*. New York: Warner Books, 1975. (One of my favorite books in 1998 when I was kicking sugar.)

Fredericks, Carlton. *New Low Blood Sugar and You*. New York: Pedigree Books, 1985. (Another book that intrigued me.)

Gittleman, Ann Louise. *Get the Sugar Out*. New York: Three Rivers Press, 1996. (One of my favorite books at the time.)

Krimmel, Edward, and Patricia Krimmel. *The Low Blood Sugar Handbook*. Bryn Mawr, PA: Franklin Publishers, 1992.

Light, Marilyn. *Hypoglycemia: One of the Most Widespread and Misdiagnosed Diseases*. New Canaan, CT: Keats Publishing, 1983.

Murray, Michael T. *Diabetes and Hypoglycemia: How You Can Benefit from Diet, Vitamins, Minerals, Herbs, Exercise and Other Natural Methods*. Rocklin, CA: Prima Publishing, 1994.

Ross, Harvey M. *Fighting Depression*. New Canaan, CT: Keats Publishing, 1975. (Sections of this book were fascinating.)

Ruggiero, Roberta. *The Do's and Don'ts of Hypoglycemia: An Everyday Guide to Low Blood Sugar Too Often Misunderstood and Misdiagnosed!* Hollywood, FL: Frederick Fell, 2003.

Saunders, Jeraldine, and Harvey M. Ross. *Hypoglycemia: The Disease Your Doctor Won't Treat*. New York: Kensington Publishing, 1980. (Rereleased in 2002 as *Hypoglycemia: The Classic Healthcare Handbook*.)

Tenney, Louise. *Hypoglycemia: A Nutritional Approach*. Pleasant Grove, UT: Woodland Publishing, 1996.

U.S. Census Bureau. U.S. and World Population Clocks—POPClocks, Population Division. http://www.census.gov/main/www/popclock.html.

CHAPTER 2: DR. SINATRA'S STORY: FROM WITNESSING MY MOM'S DANGEROUS, DIABETIC BLOOD SUGAR SWINGS TO UNMASKING THE CHOLESTEROL AND LOW-FAT MYTHS

American Heart Association. "New Stats Show Heart Disease Still America's No. 1 Killer, Stroke No. 3." http://www.americanheart.org/presenter.jhtml?identifier=3018015.

Fredericks, Carlton. *New Low Blood Sugar and You*. New York: Pedigree Books, 1985.

Life Beat Online. "Heart Disease and Diabetes—What's the Connection?" http://www.lifebeatonline.com/fall2004/news.shtml.

Quinette, P., B. Guillery-Girard, J. Dayan, V. de la Sayette, S. Marquis, F. Viader, B. Desgranges, and F. Eustache. "What Does Transient Global Amnesia Really Mean? Review of the Literature and Thorough Study of 142 Cases." *Brain* 129, no. 7 (2006), doi:10.1093/brain/awl105, http://brain.oxfordjournals.org/cgi/content/abstract/129/7/1640.

Sinatra, Stephen T. *All about me: Hercules the heart*. Wethersfield, CT: Creative Publications, 1981.

———. *Optimum Health: A Natural Lifesaving Prescription for Your Body and Mind*. New York: Bantam Books, 1997.

University of California San Diego. "Statin Effects Study, Statin Adverse Effects." http://medicine.ucsd.edu/SES/adverse_effects.htm.

CHAPTER 3: FROM ENTICEMENT TO ENTRAPMENT: HERE'S THE SHOCKING SUGAR NEWS!

Appleton, Nancy. *Lick the Sugar Habit Sugar Counter*. New York: Avery, 2001.

Ben & Jerry's. "Ingredients and Nutritional Info." http://benjerry.com/our_products/nutritional_info_all.cfm and http://www.benjerry.com/our_products/flavor_details.cfm?product_id=27#.

Bianchi, Russ. "Health and Sweetener Consumption." In *Food Trends*, edited by George Wright, November 2004.

———. "Fruit Juice Concentrate Consumption in the Americas and Europe."

Block, Gladys. "Foods Contributing to Energy Intake in the U.S.: Data from NHANES III and NHANES 1999–2000." *Journal of Food Composition and Analysis* 17, no. 3–4 (2004): 439–47.

Brownell, Kelly D. *Food Fight: The Inside Story of the Food Industry, America's Obesity Crisis, and What We Can Do about It*. New York: McGraw-Hill, 2004.

Cooper, Gail. "Refined Tastes: Sugar, Confectionery, and Consumers in Nineteenth-Century America." *Business History Review: Spring 2004*. http://www.hbs.edu/bhr/archives/bookreviews/78/gcooper_spring2004.pdf.

Corn Refiners Association. http://www.corn.org/web/tapping.htm and http://www.corn.org/web/sweeten.htm.

Gittleman, Ann Louise. *Get the Sugar Out: 501 Simple Ways to Cut the Sugar Out of Any Diet*. New York: Three Rivers Press, 1996.

Harrison, K., and A. L. Marske. "Nutritional Content of Foods Advertised during the Television Programs Children Watch Most." *American Journal of Public Health* 95, no. 9 (2005): 1568–74. http://www.ajph.org/cgi/content/abstract/95/9/1568.

Mann, Jim. "Free Sugars and Human Health: Sufficient Evidence for Action?" Departments of Human Nutrition and Medicine and the Edgar National Centre for Diabetes Research, University of Otago, Dunedin, New Zealand. http://64.233.187.104/search?q=cache:4iyuOsyjnEsJ:www.iuns.org/features/free%2520sugar%2520paper.pdf+The+average+level+of+sugar+consumption

+in+the+United+States+is+nearly+double+the+level+recommended+by+the+World+Health+
Organization+&hl=en&ie=UTF-8.

———. "Sugar Revisited—Again." *Bulletin of the World Health Organization* 81, no. 8 (2003). http://
whqlibdoc.who.int/bulletin/2003/Vol81-No8/bulletin_2003_81(8)_552.pdf.

My Slurpee Cup. "Symptoms of Addiction." http://www.myslurpeecup.com/addicted.html.

NPD Group. "Americans May Be Finding Balance in Their Eating Patterns: The NPD Group Releases
Findings from Its 19th Annual Report on Eating Patterns in America. Port Washington, New York,
Oct. 13, 2004. http://www.npdfoodworld.com/foodServlet?nextpage=pr_body.html&content_id=
2026.

One Life. "The Evolution of Man." http://www.onelife.com/evolve/manev.html.

Popkin, Barry M., and Samara Joy Nielsen. "The Sweetening of the World's Diet." *Obesity Research* 11
(2003): 1325–32.

Schlosser, Eric. *Fast Food Nation: The Dark Side of the All-American Meal*, New York: Perennial,
2002.

Severson, Kim. "Sugar and Alcohol Basic Food Groups for Many Adults: High-Calorie Meals Often
Nutritionally Deficient, UC Berkeley Professor Finds." *San Francisco Chronicle*, June 2, 2004.
http://sfgate.com/cgi-bin/article.cgi?f=/c/a/2004/06/02/MNG0U6V4S436.DTL.

Sherman, Robert B. "A Spoonful of Sugar." Lyrics. National Institutes of Health website.
http://www.niehs.nih.gov/kids/lyrics/spoonful.htm.

Spreen, Allan N. *Nutritionally Incorrect: Why the American Diet Is Dangerous and How to Defend
Yourself*. Pleasant Grove, UT: Woodland Publishing, 1999.

Starbucks. "Beverage Details: Strawberries & Crème Frappuccino Blended Crème."
http://www.starbucks.com/retail/nutrition_beverage_detail.asp?selProducts=230&x=13&y=
6&strAction=GETDEFAULT.

The Sugar Association. "Science Says: The Real Scoop on Sugar Consumption." http://www.sugar.
org/science/consumptionscoop.html.

———. "Sugar Facts: Growing and Processing Sugar." http://www.sugar.org/facts/grow.html#3.

TUFTS Nutrition. Friedman School of Nutrition Science and Policy. From "Where's the Sugar": "The
average level of sugar consumption in the United States is nearly double the level recommended by
the World Health Organization (WHO), which advises that consumption of added sugars should
be limited to 10 percent of calories. This comes to 50 grams for people consuming 2,000 calories
a day or about 12 teaspoons—the equivalent of 12 sugar packets per day. But Americans eat
about 20 teaspoons of sugar a day on average. Added sugar lurks in many foods, including foods
that don't taste sweet." http://nutrition.tufts.edu/news/notes/2003-06.html.

University of California at Berkeley, Research at Berkeley. Press release from Sarah Yang, media
relations. "Junk Food in the U.S. Diet." http://research.chance.berkeley.edu/page.cfm?id=11&
aid=31.

USDA. According to the USDA, every American consumes 12.8 teaspoons of beet and cane sugar a
day, PLUS another 12.8 teaspoons a day in HFCS. This means a total of 25.6 tsp a day.

United States Department of Agriculture. "A Century of Change in America's Eating Patterns: Major
Trends in U.S. Food Supply, 1909–99." http://www.ers.usda.gov/publications/foodreview/
jan2000/frjan2000b.pdf.

———. "Sugar and Sweeteners Outlook—Summary," May 20, 2004, ERS-SSS-240. Approved by
the World Agricultural Outlook Board. http://usda.mannlib.cornell.edu/reports/erssor/specialty/
sss-bb/2004/sss240s.txt.

United States Department of Agriculture, Economic Research Service. "Briefing Room—Sugar and
Sweeteners." http://www.ers.usda.gov/Briefing/Sugar/.

————. HFCS consumption 2003 ERS/USDA Briefing Room—Sugar and Sweetener: Data. http://www.ers.usda.gov/Briefing/Sugar/Data/data.htm.

————. "U.S. Consumption of Caloric Sweeteners, Table 49—U.S. Total Estimated Deliveries of Caloric Sweeteners for Domestic Food and Beverage Use, by Calendar Year." http://www.ers.usda.gov/Briefing/Sugar/Data/Table49.xls

————. "U.S. Consumption of Caloric Sweeteners, Table 50—U.S. Per Capita Caloric Sweeteners Estimated Deliveries for Domestic Food and Beverage Use, By Calendar Year." http://www.ers.usda.gov/Briefing/Sugar/Data/Table50.xls.

————. "U.S. Consumption of Caloric Sweeteners, Briefing Room: Sugar and Sweetener: Data Tables. Table 51—Refined Cane and Beet Sugar: Estimated Number of Per Capita Calories Consumed Daily, by Calendar Year." http://www.ers.usda.gov/Briefing/Sugar/Data/Table51.xls.

————. "U.S. Consumption of Caloric Sweeteners, Briefing Room: Sugar and Sweetener: Data Tables. Table 52—High Fructose Corn Syrup: Estimated Number of Per Capita Calories Consumed Daily, by Calendar Year." http://www.ers.usda.gov/Briefing/Sugar/Data/Table52.xls.

————. "Briefing Room—Diet and Health: Food Consumption and Nutrient Intake Tables." http://www.ers.usda.gov/briefing/dietandhealth/data/foods/table5.htm.

————. "Estimating U.S. Food Consumption," Figure 1. http://www.ers.usda.gov/publications/sb965/sb965o.pdf.

World Health Organization. "Populations with High Sugar Consumption Are at Increased Risk of Chronic Disease, South African Researchers Report." Aug. 28, 2003. http://www.who.int/bulletin/releases/2003/PR0803/en/.

Yang, Sarah. "Junk food in the U.S. Diet." Press release from the media relations department at the University of California at Berkeley, Research at Berkeley. http://research.chance.berkeley.edu/page.cfm?id=11&aid=31.

CHAPTER 4: CLEARING THE CARB CONFUSION: THE PITFALLS OF PROCESSED CARBS AND THE BENEFITS OF QUALITY CARBS

ABC News, "*Cutting Through the Diet Hype*." Produced Nov. 24, 2003.

"ACNielsen Quantifies Impact of Low-Carb Diets." *Business Wire*, Feb. 9, 2004.

Agatston, Arthur. *The South Beach Diet*. New York: Rodale, 2003.

Albert Einstein College of Medicine. "CCARBS: The Controlled Carbohydrate Assessment Registry Bank Study." https://epi.aecom.yu.edu/studies/cca/HomePage.asp?studyID=2/.

American Association of Clinical Endocrinologists Conference on the Insulin Resistance Syndrome, Washington, DC, August 25–26, 2002. "Clinical Endocrinologists Establish Strategies to Detect and Manage the Insulin Resistance Syndrome: An Epidemic Medical Condition That Places One in Three Americans at Higher Risk for Diabetes and Coronary Heart Disease." Washington, DC, Aug. 27, 2002. http://www.aace.com/pub/BMI/press.php.

American Diabetes Association. "American Diabetes Association Applauds New National Diabetes Action Plan." http://www.diabetes.org/for-media/2004-press-releases/National-Diabetes-Action-Plan.jsp.

American Dietetic Association. "Telling People What They Want to Believe: Dean Ornish Looks at Atkins and Other Low-Carb Diets in Journal of the American Dietetic Association." Press release. http://www.eatright.org/Public/Media/PublicMedia_19241.cfm.

Atkins. "Dr. Atkins Timeline." http://atkins.com/atkinslegacy/atkinslegacytimeline.html.

Atkins Exposed.org. Website devoted to unmasking "the truth" about the Atkins diet.

Atkins, Robert. *Dr. Atkins' New Diet Revolution*. New York: Avon, 1992.

Atkins, Veronica. "Statement on Atkins' Death." *USA Today*, February 10, 2004.

Austin, Denise. *Fit and Fabulous After 40*. New York: Broadway Books, 2001.

Bernardini, Robert. *The Truth about Children's Health: The Comprehensive Guide to Understanding, Preventing, and Reversing Disease*. Pri Publishing, 2003.

Boden, Guenther, Karin Sargrad, Carol Homko, Maria Mozzoli, and T. Peter Stein. "Effect of a Low-Carbohydrate Diet on Appetite, Blood Glucose Levels, and Insulin Resistance in Obese Patients with Type 2 Diabetes." *Annals of Internal Medicine* 142, no. 6 (2005): 403–11.

Bowden, Jonny. *Living the Low Carb Life*. New York: Sterling, 2005.

Brehm, B. J., R. J. Seeley, S. R. Daniels, and D. A. D'Alessio. "Weight Loss and Cardiovascular Risk Factors in Healthy Women on a Low Carbohydrate Diet or a Low Fat Diet." *Journal of Clinical Endocrinology and Metabolism* 88, no. 4 (2003): 1617–23.

Brody, Jane E. "Schools Teach 3 C's: Candy, Cookies and Chips." *New York Times*, September 24, 2002.

Challem, Jack. *The Inflammation Syndrome*. New York: John Wiley, 2003.

———. *Syndrome X*. New York: John Wiley, 2000.

Children's Hospital Boston. "Hold the Stuffing: Low-Glycemic Diet May Help Keep Weight Off." Nov. 23, 2004. http://web1.tch.harvard.edu/cfapps/CHdeptPagePressDisplay.cfm?Dept=Press%20Room&PageNbr=125&ParentPage=1.

CNN.com. "Good Carb, Bad Carb? Experts Debate Labels. Should People Really Care That They Digest Potatoes Faster than Carrots?" Posted Sept. 5, 2003. http://www.cnn.com/2003/HEALTH/diet.fitness/09/05/carb.confusion.ap/index.html.

Cordain, Loren. *The Paleo Diet*. New York: John Wiley, 2002.

Cordain, Loren, S. Boyd Eaton, Anthony Sebastian, Neil Mann, Staffan Lindeberg, Bruce A. Watkins, James H. O'Keefe, and Janette Brand-Miller. "Commentary: Origins and Evolution of the Western Diet: Health Implications for the 21st Century." *American Journal of Clinical Nutrition* 81, no. 2 (2005): 341–54. http://www.thepaleodiet.com/articles/Origins%20Paper%20Final.pdf.

Dash, Eric. "Next Up: Low-Carb Nachos?" *New York Times*, June 27, 2004.

Department of Health and Human Services. "HHS, ADA Warn Americans of 'Pre-diabetes', Encourage People to Take Healthy Steps to Reduce Risks." March 27, 2002. http://www.hhs.gov/news/press/2002pres/20020327.html.

Drewnowski, Adam. "Fat and Sugar: An Economic Analysis." *American Society for Nutritional Sciences: Sugar and Fat—From Genes to Culture Symposium* 133 (2003): 829S–830S.

———. "Obesity and the Food Environment: Dietary Energy Density and Diet Costs." *American Journal of Preventive Medicine* 27, no. 31001 (2004): 154–62.

Drewnowski, Adam, N. Darmon, and A. Briend. "Replacing Fats and Sweets with Vegetables and Fruits—a Question of Cost." *American Journal of Public Health*. 94, no. 9 (2004): 1555–59.

Eades, Michael, and Mary Dan Eades. *Protein Power*.

Ebbin, Robert. "Multipaycheck Households Spark Sales." *Restaurants USA*, April 1998. http://www.restaurant.org/research/magarticle.cfm?articleID=296.

FatFreeKitchen.com. "Glycemic Index (GI) & Glycemic Load (GL)." http://www.fatfreekitchen.com/glycemic-index.html.

Foster, Gary D., Holly R. Wyatt, James O. Hill, Brian G. McGuckin, Carrie Brill, B. Selma Mohammed, Philippe O. Szapary, Daniel J. Rader, Joel S. Edman, and Samuel Klein. "A Randomized Trial of a Low-Carbohydrate Diet for Obesity." *New England Journal of Medicine* 348, no. 21 (2003): 2082–90.

French, S. "Pricing Effect on Food Choices." *American Society for Nutritional Sciences: Sugar and Fat—from Genes to Culture Symposium* 133 (2003): 829S–830S.

Gogoi, Pallavi. "News Analysis: The Skinny on Food in 2005—Expect a New Food Pyramid, Labeling Changes to Reveal Artery-Clogging Ingredients, and More Fights over What Constitutes a

Healthy Diet." *Business Week Online,* December 29, 2004. http://www.businessweek.com/bwdaily/dnflash/dec2004/nf20041229_0061_db016.htm.

Greene, Bob. *Get with the Program: Getting Real about Your Weight, Health, and Emotional Well-Being.* New York: Simon & Schuster, 2002.

Groom, Nichola. "South Beach Diet Creator Shuns 'Low-Carb' Label." http://story.news.yahoo.com/news?tmpl=story&cid=571&ncid=751&e=3&u=/nm/20041206/hl_nm/food_southbeach diet_dc.

Harvard School of Public Health. "Carbohydrates: Going with the (Whole) Grain." http://www.hsph.harvard.edu/nutritionsource/carbohydrates.html.

Heller, Richard F., and Rachael Heller. *Carbohydrate Addicted Kids: Help Your Child or Teen Break Free of Junk Food and Sugar Cravings—for Life!* New York: HarperCollins, 1998.

Hidalgo, Jason. "Liquid Candy: Teens and Kids Gulp Down Poor Habits." *Reno Gazette-Journal.* http://www.courier-journal.com/features/health/2003/06/hf-back-soda0605-6447.html.

Hirsch, J. M. "Experts Question Reduced-Sugar Cereals." Associated Press article posted on Yahoo! and other sites, March 20, 2005, 18:37 PST. http://news.yahoo.com/news?tmpl=story&u=/ap/20050321/ap_on_he_me/fit_low_sugar_cereals.

Institute of Food Technologists. "What, When, and Where Americans Eat in 2003." Press release. August 22, 2003. http://www.ift.org/cms/?pid=1000496.

Jenkins, David J. A., Cyril W. C. Kendall, Livia S. A. Augustin, Silvia Franceschi, Maryam Hamidi, Augustine Marchie, Alexandra L. Jenkins, and Mette Axelsen. "Glycemic Index: Overview of Implications in Health and Disease." *American Journal of Clinical Nutrition* 76 (2002); 266–73.

Jenkins, D. J., T. M. Wolever, and R. H. Taylor, et al. "Glycemic Index of Foods: A Physiological Basis for Carbohydrate Exchange." *American Journal of Clinical Nutrition* 34 (1981): 362–66.

Jones, David. "Atkins Killed Our Daughter." *The Daily Mail.* http://www.atkinsexposed.org/atkins/65/Atkins_Killed_Our_Daughter.htm.

Karush, Sarah. "Tony Restaurants Offer Low-Carb, Too; No Price Break for Holding the Potatoes." *Associated Press,* February 16, 2004.

Katz, David. *The Flavor Point Diet.* Emmaus, PA: Rodale, 2005.

———. *The Way to Eat.* Naperville: Sourcebooks, 2002.

Kirchheimer, Sid. "Glycemic Index: New Way to Count Carbs: Evidence Mounts for Low-Glycemic Index Diet to Control Diabetes." http://my.webmd.com/content/article/72/81815.htm?lastselectedguid={5FE84E90-BC77-4056-A91C-9531713CA348.

Lieberman, Shari. *Dare to Lose: 4 Simple Steps to a Better Body,* With Nancy Bruning. New York: Avery, 2002.

Ma, Yunsheng, Barbara Olendzki, and David Chiriboga, et al. "Association between Dietary Carbohydrates and Body Weight." *American Journal of Epidemiology* 161 (2005): 359–67.

McCook, Alison. "Carbohydrate Type, Not Amount, Linked to Obesity." http://www.reutershealth.com/archive/2005/02/16/eline/links/20050216elin003.html.

Mendosa, David. "Revised International Table of Glycemic Index (GI) and Glycemic Load (GL) Values—2002." http://diabetes.about.com/library/mendosagi/ngilists.htm.

Mercola.com. "Update on Atkins' Obesity, 2-25-04." http://www.mercola.com/2004/feb/25/atkins_obesity.htm.

Miller, Christine. "Why Did the Numbers Change?" March 26, 2005. http://www.ediets.com/news/article.cfm?cmi=870253&cid=28.

Mintz, Sidney W. *Sweetness and Power: The Place of Sugar in Modern History.* New York: Penguin Books, 1985.

Mondello, Andrea M. "Low-Fat vs. Low-Carb Headlines Misrepresent Study Results." *Low Carb Living Online*, November 13, 2004. http://forums.lclmag.com/cms/content/view/277/47/.

National Diabetes Information Clearinghouse (NDIC). "Insulin Resistance and Pre-Diabetes." http://diabetes.niddk.nih.gov/dm/pubs/insulinresistance/.

NPD Foodworld. "Americans May Be Finding Balance in Their Eating Patterns: The NPD Group Releases Findings from Its 19th Annual Report on Eating Patterns in America." Port Washington, NY, October 13, 2004. http://www.npdfoodworld.com/foodServlet?nextpage=pr_body.html& content_id=2026.

———. "Eating Patterns in America: Want to Understand the Impact of the Low Carb Craze, Spot Trends in America's Eating Habits and Track the Restaurant Industry?" http://www.npd .com/foodpress/epa.html.

National Restaurant Association. "The Restaurant Industry 2000 Year in Review." http://www .restaurant.org/research/year_in_review.cfm.

Novis. "Consumers Baffled by GI Labels." NUTRAingredients.com, November 24, 2004. http:// nutraingredients.com/news/ng.asp?id=56285&n=dh329&c=eepddtxhprfgmgi.

Nutraingredients.com. "Low-Carb Led 2004 Food Launches," January 5, 2005. http://www.nutrain- gredients-usa.com/news/news-ng.asp?n=57089-low-carb-led.

Opinion Dynamics Corporation. *Dieting in the 21st Century: Low-Carb, Low-Fat, and More.*

———. "The Latest on the Low-Carb Revolution" and "Making Research Matter: Updated Low- Carb Results." Updated February 2005. http://www.opiniondynamics.com/lowcarb.html.

Pawlak, Dorota B., Jake A. Kushner, and David S Ludwig. "Effects of Dietary Glycemic Index on Adi- posity, Glucose, Homeostasis, and Plasma Lipids in Animals." *Lancet* 364 (2004): 778–85.

Pereira, Mark A., Janis Swain, Allison B. Goldfine, et al. "Effects of a Low-Glycemic Load Diet on Resting Energy Expenditure and Heart Disease Risk Factors during Weight Loss." *Journal of the American Medical Association* 292(2004): 2482–90.

Pescatore, Fred. *The Hamptons Diet.* Hoboken: John Wiley, 2004.

PR Web Press Release Newswire. "Low-Fat vs. Low-Carb Study Results Mis-Reported: Study Re- vealed the Real Enemy Is Junk Food," November 24, 2004. http://ca.prweb.com/releases /2004/11/prweb181683.php.

Quaid, Libby. "Popular Diets Tout 'Good Carb' Advice." Associated Press, February 25, 2005.

Reinberg, Steven. "Diet with the 'Right Carbs' Seems to Boost Health." *HealthDayNews*, August 26, 2004. Lifeclinic website. http://www.lifeclinic.com/healthnews/article_view.asp?story=520863.

Reuters.com. "Low-Carb Diets Get New Year's Boost—Survey." http://www.reuters.com/newsArti- cle.jhtml?type=healthNews&storyID=7371408.

Schwarzbein, Diana, and Marilyn Brown. *The Schwarzbein Principle II: The Transition.* Deerfield Beach, FL: Health Communications, 2002.

Sears, Barry. *Enter the Zone.* New York: HarperCollins, 1995.

Sharp, David. "Bread Industry Changing Its Recipe for Success." Associated Press, February. 14, 2005.

Smith, Kathy. *Kathy Smith's Lift Weights to Lose Weight.* With Robert Miller. New York: Warner Books, 2001.

Stafford, Margaret. "Experts Say Low-Carb Craze May Be Over." Associated Press, December 20, 2004. ABCNews website. http://abcnews.go.com/Health/wireStory/?id=345339.

Steward, H. Leighton, Morrison C. Bethea, Sam S. Andrews, and Luis A. Balart. *The New Sugar Busters! Cut sugar to Trim Fat.* New York: Ballantine Books, 2003.

Tanner, Lindsey. "Pediatrics Group Seeks to Eliminate Sodas in Schools." Associated Press, January 4, 2004.

———. "U.S. Teens Fatter than Those in Other Industrialized Countries, Study Says." Associated Press, January 5, 2004.

Taubes, Gary. "What If It's All Been a Big Fat Lie?" *New York Times Magazine*, July 7, 2002.

Tenney, Louise, and Rita Elkins. *Hypoglycemia: A Nutritional Approach*. Today's Health Series, no. 9. Woodland Publishing, 1987.

Trager, Stuart L. "Atkins Lifestyle Fits Government Guidelines." *Atkins corporate webpage*. http://atkins.com/Archive/2005/1/19-715511.html?BrCs=291&BrCg=11279463&BrRc=1049216230.

Warner, Melanie. "Low Carbs? Who Cares? Sugar Is Latest Supermarket Demon." *New York Times*, May 15, 2005.

Webb, Densie. "Glycemic Index: Gateway to Good Health or Grand Waste of Time." *Environmental Nutrition*, November 2002, 1.

Wellness Councils of America. "General Mills Goes Whole-Grain: Food Manufacturer Becomes First to Make All of Its 'Big G' breakfast cereals with whole-grain." Welcoa Newsflash, October 1, 2004. http://www.welcoa.org/freeresources/pdf/general_mills_100104.pdf.

Whitney, Eleanor, and Sharon Rolfes. *Understanding Nutrition*. 7th ed. Minneapolis: West Publishing, 1996.

Willett, Walter C. *Eat, Drink, and Be Healthy: The Harvard Medical School Guide to Healthy Eating*. New York: Simon & Schuster Source, 2001, 94–95.

World Health Organization. "Obesity and Overweight." *WHO Global Strategy on Diet, Physical Activity and Health*. http://www.who.int/hpr/NPH/docs/gs-obesity.pdf.

Yankelovich, Inc. "Food for Life: An Attitudinal and Database Perspective on Food, Diet and Preventive Health Care." *Yankelovich MONITOR Perspective*. http://www.yankelovich.com/products/Food%20For%20Life%20Final%20Presentation%2003-27-06.pdf.

CHAPTER 6: NOT-SO-SWEET ANGLES ON OBESITY AND DIABETES

American Association of Pediatrics Policy Statement. "Soft Drinks in Schools: Committee on School Health." *Pediatrics* 113, no. 1 (2004): 152–54. http://aappolicy.aappublications.org/cgi/content/abstract/pediatrics;113/1/152.

American Beverage Association, website. Press releases and statistics from the ABA (formerly named the National Soft Drink Association). http://www.ameribev.org/about/industrybasics.asp; http://www.ameribev.org/pressroom/bod.asp; http://www.ameribev.org/pressroom/about.asp; http://www.ameribev.org/about/pressreleases.asp.

American Diabetes Association. "Evidence-Based Nutrition Principles and Recommendations for the Treatment and Prevention of Diabetes and Related Complications." *Diabetes Care* 25 (2002): 148–98.

American Diabetes Association, North American Association for the Study of Obesity, American Society for Clinical Nutrition. "Weight Management Using Lifestyle Modification in the Prevention and Management of Type 2 Diabetes: Rationale and Strategies." *Clinical Diabetes* 23, no. 3 (2005): 130–36.

American Heart Association. "Alliance for a Healthier Generation and Industry Leaders Set Healthy School Beverage Guidelines for U.S. Schools," May 3, 2006. http://www.americanheart.org/presenter.jhtml?identifier=3039339.

———. "A Guide for Selecting and Preparing Your Food." http://www.americanheart.org/presenter.jhtml?identifier=499.

American Obesity Association. "Obesity in Youth." http://www.obesity.org/subs/fastfacts/obesity_youth.shtml.

American Psychological Association. "Television Advertising Leads to Unhealthy Habits in Children; Says APA Task Force." http://www.apa.org/releases/childrenads.html.

Applegate, Christina. Celebrity quotes: Christina Applegate: Frosted Flakes. http://www.anecdotage.com/index.php?aid=19556.

Association for the Study of Obesity. "Obesity: The Scale of the Problem." http://www.aso.org.uk/portal.asp?oricmid=161&orictype=header&targetcell=3,0&targetwidth=4&functionname=aso_oric.

BBC News. "Call for Tougher Junk Food Ad Ban." http://news.bbc.co.uk/1/hi/health/5081964.stm.

Bennett, Connie. "Sodas Banned or Restricted in Schools, but Health Advocates Brand Industry Move as a Publicity Stunt," August 17, 2005. http://www.sugarshockblog.com/2005/08/post.html.

Bray, George A., Samara Joy Nielsen, and Barry M. Popkin. "Consumption of High-Fructose Corn Syrup in Beverages May Play a Role in the Epidemic of Obesity." *American Journal of Clinical Nutrition* 79, no. 4 (2004): 537–43.

Burros, Marian. "It'd Be Easier If SpongeBob Were Hawking Broccoli." *New York Times*, January 12, 2005. http://query.nytimes.com/gst/fullpage.html?res=9A05EFDD1638F931A25752C0A9639C8B63&sec=health.

———. "The Snapple Deal: How Sweet It Is." *New York Times*, September 17, 2003. http://query.nytimes.com/gst/fullpage.html?sec=health&res=9C07EED9173AF934A2575AC0A9659C8B63.

Burros, Marian, and Melanie Warner. "Bottlers Agree to a School Ban on Sweet Drinks." *New York Times*, May 4, 2006. http://www.nytimes.com/2006/05/04/health/04soda.html?ex=1304395200&en=80149e91b4b733bb&ei=5088&partner=rssnyt&emc=rss.

Calorie Control Council. "Consumer Use of Low-Calorie, Sugar-Free Foods and Beverages." http://www.caloriecontrol.org/lcchart.html.

Campaign for a Commercial-Free Childhood. "CCFC Member Organizations." http://www.commercialexploitation.org/memberorgs.htm.

———. "Junk-Food Pushers on Defensive as Kids' Advocates Push Back." http://www.commercialexploitation.org/news/junkfooddefensive.htm.

———. "Marketers See Babies' Noses as Pathway to Profits." http://www.commercialexploitation.org/news/articles/babiesnoses.htm.

———. "Marketing to Children: An Overview." http://www.commercialexploitation.org/factsheets/ccfc-facts%20overview.pdf.

———. "TV Ads Market Junk Food to Kids, New Study Finds." http://www.commercialexploitation.org/news/tvadsmarketjunkfood.htm.

Caprio, Sonia. "Obesity and the Metabolic Syndrome in Children and Adolescents." *New England Journal of Medicine* 350, no. 23 (June 2004): 2362–74. http://content.nejm.org/cgi/content/abstract/350/23/2362.

Center for Consumer Freedom. "Ten Dumbest Food Cop Ideas." http://www.consumerfreedom.com/news_detail.cfm?headline=2651.

Center for Disease and Prevention. "BMI—Body Mass Index—About BMI for Adults." http://www.cdc.gov/nccdphp/dnpa/bmi/adult_BMI/about_adult_BMI.htm.

———. Most updated National Center for Health Statistics 2003–2004 National Health and Nutrition Examination Study (NHANES). http://www.cdc.gov/nchs/pressroom/06facts/obesity03_04.htm.

———. "Prevalence of Overweight and Obesity Among Adults: United States, 2003–2004." http://www.cdc.gov/nchs/products/pubs/pubd/hestats/obese03_04/overwght_adult_03.htm.

Center for Science in the Public Interest. "CSPI Applauds Agreement to Get High-Calorie Drinks Out of Schools; Drops Planned Litigation." http://www.cspinet.org/new/200605031.html.

———. "Liquid Candy: How Soft Drinks Are Harming America's Health." http://www.cspinet.org/liquidcandy/index.html.

———. "Soft Drinks Undermining Americans' Health: Teens Consuming Twice as Much 'Liquid Candy' as Milk." News release, October 21, 1998. http://www.cspinet.org/new/soda_10_21_98.htm.

———. "Statement of CSPI Nutrition Policy Director Margo Wootan on the Findings of 'From Wallet to Waistline.'" http://www.cspinet.org/new/pdf/margo_w2w_statement.pdf.

Centers for Disease Control and Prevention. "National Agenda for Public Health Action: A National Public Health Initiative on Diabetes and Women's Health." http://www.cdc.gov/DIABETES/pubs/action/facts.htm.

———. National Center for Health Statistics. "Deaths: Final Data for 2003." http://www.cdc.gov/nchs/products/pubs/pubd/hestats/finaldeaths03/finaldeaths03.htm.

———. "Prevalance of Overweight and Obesity in Adults: United States, 1999–2002." http://www.cdc.gov/nchs/products/pubs/pubd/hestats/obese/obse99.htm.

Commercial Alert. "Coalition Wants Schools to Stop Pushing Junk Food on Children." http://www.commercialalert.org/issues/education/junk-food/coalition-wants-schools-to-stop-pushing-junk-food-on-children.

———. "Soda Deal for Schools Is Weak on Marketing and Enforcement Says Commercial Alert." http://www.commercialalert.org/news/news-releases/2006/05/soda-deal-for-schools-is-weak-on-marketing-and-enforcement-says-commercial-alert.

Connoly, Ceci. "Public Policy Targeting Obesity." *Washington Post*, August 10, 2003. http://www.washingtonpost.com/ac2/wp-dyn/A39239-2003Aug9?language=printer.

CorpWatch. "What's on Channel 1?" Center for Commercial Free Public Education. July 8, 1998. http://www.corpwatch.org/article.php?id=888.

Critser, Greg. *Fat Land: How Americans Became the Fattest People in the World.* Boston: Houghton-Mifflin, 2003.

Davis, Carole, and E. Saltos. "Dietary Recommendations and How They Have Changed Over Time." USDA website. http://www.ers.usda.gov/publications/aib750/aib750b.pdf.

Drewnowski, A. "Obesity and the Food Environment: Dietary Energy Density and Diet Costs." *American Journal of Preventive Medicine* 27, no. 3S (2004): 154–62.

European Audio Visual. "Regulation on Advertising Aimed at Children In EU-Member States and Some Neighbouring States. The Legal Framework." http://www.obs.coe.int/online_publication/reports/childadv.pdf.en.

Forbrugerstyrelsen Press. "Joint Standards for Television Advertising Based on the Legislation on Marketing Practices in the Nordic Countries." *TemaNord* 1991, no. 45. http://www.forbrug.dk/english/dco/dcoguides/guidelines-and-guidances/televisionmarketing0/.

Fredrickson, Donald S., John B. Stanbury, and James B. Wyngarden. *The Metabolic Basis of Inherited Disease.* New York: McGraw-Hill, 1983.

Greenspan, Robyn. "Consumers Becoming Marketing-Resistant." *Internet News*, April 23, 2004. http://www.internetnews.com/stats/article.php/3344701.

Gross, Lee S., Li Li, Earl S. Ford, and Simin Liu. "Increased Consumption of Refined Carbohydrates and the Epidemic of Type 2 Diabetes in the United States: An Ecologic Assessment." *American Journal of Clinical Nutrition* 79 (2004): 774–79.

Gutkowski, Shirley. "Ahhhhh . . . Those Bubbles." http://rdh.pennnet.com/Articles/Article_Display.cfm?Sectionfiltered=Archives&Subsectionfiltered=Display&ARTICLE_ID=160511&KEYWORD=bubbles&x=y.

Havel, Peter J. "Update on Adipocyte Hormones: Regulation of Energy Balance and Carbohydrate/Lipid Metabolism." *Diabetes* 53, no. 1S (2004): S143–51.

Havel, Peter J. et al. "Not All Sugars Are Equal, At Least When It Comes to Weight Gain and Health." *Journal of Clinical Endocrinology and Metabolism* 89, no. 6 (2004).

Hellmich, Nanci. "Child Obesity Worse than Thought, Study Suggests." *USA Today.* http://www .usatoday.com/news/health/2004–06–04-child-obesity_x.htm.

Imperatore, Giuseppina et al. "Prevalence of Impaired Fasting Glucose and Its Relationship with Cardiovascular Disease Risk Factors in U.S. Adolescents." 1999–2000 *Pediatrics* 116, no. 5 (2005): 1122–26. http://pediatrics.aappublications.org/cgi/content/abstract/116/5/1122.

International Diabetes Federation. "Did You Know?" http://www.idf.org/home/index.cfm?node=37.

Jacobson, Michael. "CSPI Applauds Agreement to Get High-Calorie Drinks Out of Schools; Drops Planned Litigation." http://cspinet.org/new/200605031.html.

Johnson, Rachel K., and Carol Frary. "Choose Beverages and Foods to Moderate Your Intake of Sugars: The 2000 Dietary Guidelines for Americans—What's All the Fuss About?" http://jn.nutrition .org/cgi/content/full/131/10/2766S.

Johnson, Richard J., et al. "A Causal Role for Uric Acid in Fructose-Induced Metabolic Syndrome." *American Journal of Physiology—Renal Physiology.* 290(3) (2006): F625–31. http://www .ajprenal.physiology.org/cgi/content/abstract/290/3/F625.

Kahn, C. Ronald. "As Obesity Skyrockets, Joslin Urges Action to Stem the Corresponding Tide of Type 2 Diabetes." http://www.joslin.org/1083_2046.asp.

Kaiser Family Foundation. "The Role of Media in Childhood Obesity," February 2004. http://www.kff.org/entmedia/upload/The-Role-Of-Media-in-Childhood-Obesity.pdf.

Linn, Susan. *Consuming Kids: The Hostile Takeover of Childhood.* New York: New Press, 2004.

Ludwig, David. "Effects of Decreasing Sugar-Sweetened Beverage Consumption on Body Weight in Adolescents: A Randomized, Controlled Pilot Study." *Pediatrics* 117, no. 3 (2006): 673–80.

Mokdad, Ali, et al. "Actual Causes of Death in the United States, 2000." *JAMA* 291 (2004): 1238–45.

———, et al. "The Continuing Epidemics of Obesity and Diabetes in the United States." *JAMA* 286, no. 10 (2001): 1195–1200.

Nader, Ralph. "Big Snapple? Selling the City, Drink by Drink." *Common Dreams,* September 15, 2003. http://www.commondreams.org/views03/0915–10.htm.

The National Academies. "Food Marketing Aimed at Kids Influences Poor Nutritional Choices, IOM Study Finds; Broad Effort Needed to Promote Healthier Products and Diets." http:// www4.nationalacademies.org/news.nsf/isbn/0309097134?OpenDocument.

Nestle, Marion. *Food Politics: How the Food Industry Influences Nutrition and Health.* University of California Press, 2002.

———. *Safe Food: Bacteria, Biotechnology, and Bioterrorism.* University of California Press, 2003.

———. *What to Eat: An Aisle-by-Aisle Guide to Savvy Food Choices and Good Eating.* North Point Press, 2006.

Neville, Kerry. "Portion Distortion." Daily Press. http://www.dailypress.com/features/health/ dp-39328sy0jan14,1,1570536.story?coll=dp-features-healthylife-mix.

New Rules Project. "Curbing the Commercialization of Public Space." http://www.ilsr.org/ newrules/info/publicspace.html.

Nielsen, Samara J., and B. M. Popkin. "Patterns and trends in portion sizes, 1977–1998." *Journal of the American Medical Association* 289(4) (2003): 450–453. http://jama.ama-assn.org/cgi/ content/abstract/289/4/450.

North Carolina School Nutrition Action Committee. "Soft Drink and School Age Children: Trends, Effects, Solutions." http://www.asu.edu/educ/epsl/CERU/Articles/CERU-0203-41-OWI.pdf.

Nutritional Summary for beverage: Coca-Cola Classic. http://www.nutritiondata.com/facts-B00001-01c21da.html.

Ogden, C. L., et. al., "Prevalence of Overweight and Obesity in the United States, 1999–2004." *Journal of American Medicine* 295(13) (2006): 1549–55. http://jama.ama-assn.org/cgi/content/short/295/13/1549.

Olshansky, S. Jay. "A Potential Decline in Life Expectancy in the United States in the 21st Century." *New England Journal of Medicine* 352, no. 11 (2005): 1138–45.

Popkin, Barry M. "U.S. Soft Drink Consumption Grew 135% Since 1977, Boosting Obesity." http://www.unc.edu/news/archives/sept04/popkin091604.html by DAVID WILLIAMSON at UNC News Services.

Preston, Samuel H. "Deadweight? The Influence of Obesity on Longevity." Editorial. *New England Journal of Medicine* 352, no. 11 (2005): 1135–37.

Produce for Better Health Foundation. "Why 5 A Day the Color Way." http://www.5aday.org/html/colorway/colorway_home.php.

Robbins, John. *The Food Revolution: How Your Diet Can Help Save Your Life and Our World*. Berkeley: Conari Press, 2001.

Rozin, P., et al. "The Ecology of Eating: Smaller Portion Sizes in France than in the United States Helps Explain the French Paradox." *Psychological Science* 14, no. 5 (2003).

Ruskin, Gary. "Commercial Alert Criticizes National PTA over Coke Sponsorship." Wednesday, June 4, 2003. http://www.commercialalert.org/index.php/category_id/5/subcategory_id/72/article_id/187.

———. "The Fast Food Trap: How Commercialism Creates Overweight Children." October 31, 2003. http://www.commercialalert.org/issues/education/junk-food/the-fast-food-trap-how-commercialism-creates-overweight-children.

Ruskin, Gary, and Juliet Schor. "Every Nook and Cranny: The Dangerous Spread of Commercialized Culture." http://www.multinationalmonitor.org/mm2005/012005/ruskin.html.

Schlosser, Eric. *Fast Food Nation*. New York: Perennial, 2002.

Schoonover, Heather, and Mark Muller. "Food without Policy: How U.S. Farm Policy Contributes to Obesity." Institute for Agriculture and Trade Policy. http://www.iatp.org/iatp/publications.cfm?accountID=421&refID=80627.

Shape Up America staff. "Diabesity." http://www.shapeup.org/prof/diabesity.php.

Super Size Me. Directed by Morgan Spurlock. Hart Sharp Video, 2004.

Tschöp, Matthias H., et al. "Consuming Fructose-Sweetened Beverages Increases Body Adiposity in Mice." *Obesity Research* 13 (2005): 1146–56.

Teff, K. L., S. S. Elliott, M. Tschöp, T. J. Kieffer, D. Rader, M. Heiman, R. R. Townsend, N. L. Keim, D. D'Alessio, P. J. Havel. "Dietary Fructose Reduces Circulating Insulin and Leptin, Attenuates Postprandial Suppression of Ghrelin and Increases Triglycerides in Women." *J. Clin. Endocrinol. Metab.* 89 (2004): 2963–72. http://www.medicalnewstoday.com/medicalnews.php?newsid=9120.

United States Department of Health and Human Services. "Obesity Still on the Rise, New Data Show." http://www.dhhs.gov/news/press/2002pres/20021008b.html.

USA Today, "Beverage Group: Pull Soda from Primary Schools," August 16, 2005. http://www.usatoday.com/news/health/2005-08-16-soda-schools_x.htm.

Willett, Walter C. *Eat, Drink, and Be Healthy: The Harvard Medical School Guide to Healthy Eating*. New York: Simon & Schuster Source, 2001, 94–95.

Yankelovich Inc. "Yankelovich Study Uncovers Nutritional Naiveté." http://www.yankelovich.com/media/Food%20for%20Life%201%203.17.06.pdf.

Young, Lisa R. and Marion Nestle. "Expanding Portion Sizes in the U.S. Marketplace: Implications for Nutrition Counseling." *Journal of the American Dietetic Association* 103, no. 2 (2003): 231–34.

CHAPTER 7: IS "BIG SUGAR" THE NEXT "BIG TOBACCO"?

"American Morning: Cereal Lawsuit," aired on CNN on March 30, 2005, 07:30 ET. http://transcripts.cnn.com/TRANSCRIPTS/0503/30/ltm.03.html.

Applebee's Restaurant. "Applebee's Launches New Weight Watchers Menu in 1,600 Restaurants." Press release, May 17, 2004. http://www.applebees.com/MediaPressRelease.aspx?id=6.

Arizona Daily Star. "Smucker's Misleads Its Spread, Suit Claims." http://www.dailystar.com/dailystar/relatedarticles/31286.php.

BanTransFats.com. "Plaintiffs' Press Release on Settlement of McDonald's Trans Fat Litigation." http://www.bantransfats.com/mcdonalds.html.

———. "The Oreo Case: Here We Respond to the Most Frequently Asked Questions About the Lawsuit That We Filed Against Kraft Foods in May 2003." http://www.bantransfats.com/theoreocase.html.

BBC News. "Why Some Just Cannot Resist Food," May 16, 2006. http://news.bbc.co.uk/1/hi/health/4986262.stm.

Beaver, John D., Andrew D. Lawrence, Jenneke van Ditzhuijzen, Matt H. Davis, Andrew Woods, and Andrew J. Calder. "Individual Differences in Reward Drive Predict Neural Responses to Images of Food." *Journal of Neuroscience* 26 (2006): 5160–66.

Bennett, Connie. "Appetizing Food Ads Are Linked to Obesity and Eating Disorders, British Study Finds." http://www.sugarshockblog.com/2006/06/appetizing_food.html.

Brownell, Kelly. *Food Fight: The Inside Story of the Food Industry, America's Obesity Crisis, and What We Can Do About It.* New York: McGraw-Hill, 2003.

Center for Science in the Public Interest. "Parents and Advocates Will Sue Viacom and Kellogg." *CSPI Newsroom,* January 18, 2006. http://www.cspinet.org/new/200601181.html and http://cspinet.org/new/pdf/viacom___kellogg.pdf.

———. "Smucker's Spreading Deception, Says CSPI," May 13, 2003. http://www.cspinet.org/new/200305131.html.

Horvitz, Bruce. "Kraft Plans to Start Putting Its Food on a Diet." *USA Today,* July 1, 2003. http://www.usatoday.com/money/industries/food/2003-07-01-kraft_x.htm.

Kraft Foods. "Boys & Girls Clubs of America, the Coca-Cola Company and Kraft Foods Launch $12 Million Youth Health and Wellness Initiative: Triple Play Offers a Game Plan for the Mind, Body and Soul," April 28, 2004. http://www.kraft.com/newsroom/04282004.html.

McDonald's. "McDonald's Launches Balanced Lifestyles Commitment for Children and Celebrates Results of 'McDonald's Go Active! American Challenge' with Bob Greene." Press release, May 25, 2004. http://www.mcdonalds.com/usa/news/2004/conpr_05252004.html#.

Medical Research Council. "New Study Shows Some People Just Can't Resist Food." Press release, May 17, 2006. http://www.mrc.ac.uk/public-press_17_may_2006.

Morgante, Michelle. "San Diego Mother Sues Cereal Makers for Sugar Claims." *Associated Press,* March 28, 2005.

MSN News Staff. "McDonald's Says Goodbye to Super Size." MSN Money, March 3, 2004.

Onion Staff. "Hershey's Ordered to Pay Obese Americans $135 Million." *The Onion,* August 2, 2000. http://www.theonion.com/content/node/28407.

PepsiCo. "Community Information—Pepsi-Cola North America School Policy." http://www.pepsiworld.com/help/faqs/faq.php?category=community_info&page=school_partnership.

Smucker's website. Simply Fruit nutritional information. http://www.smuckers.com/fg/pds/default.asp?groupid=1&catid=16.

TARNIVAL. "What's in Cigarettes?" http://www.tarnival.org/cigarette/ingredients/sugar.html.

World Health Organization Technical Report Series 916. "Diet, Nutrition, and the Prevention of

Chronic Diseases: Report of a Joint WHO/FAO Expert Consultation. Geneva, Switzerland: World Health Organization," April 2003. http://www.fao.org/docrep/005/ac911e/ac911e00.htm.

Zernike, Kate. "Lawyers Shift Focus from Big Tobacco to Big Food." *New York Times,* April 9, 2004. http://query.nytimes.com/gst/fullpage.html?sec=health&res= 9805E6DF1238F93AA35757C0A9629C8B63.

CHAPTER 8: STRANGE BEDFELLOWS: SUGAR, SEX, AND POLITICS

Adams, Mike. "The Food Industry Denies Links Between Foods, Nutrition, and Health: Bad Science Meets Aggressive Marketing." August 7, 2004. http://newstarget.com/001693.html.

Altria Group. "About Altria: Overview." Altria Group is the parent company of Kraft Foods, Philip Morris International, Philip Morris USA, and Philip Morris Capital Corporation. Altria Group is also the largest shareholder in the world's second-largest brewer, SABMiller, with a 36 percent economic interest. http://altria.com/about_altria/1_0_aboutaltriaover.asp.

American Council for Fitness and Nutrition. "American Council for Fitness and Nutrition General Membership List." http://www.acfn.org/about-members/.

American Dietetic Association. "Use of Nutritive and Nonnutritive Sweeteners." http://eatright .org/public/governmentaffairs/92_adap0598.cfm.

Boseley, Sarah. "WHO 'Buried' Report to Please Food Industry." *Guardian,* November 3, 2004. http://www.guardian.co.uk/uk_news/story/0,1341914,00.html.

Brisco, Andrew C. III. "Sugar and Obesity." Editorial from the president and chief executive of the Sugar Association. *New York Times,* February 4, 2004.

Brownell, Kelly. *Food Fight: The Inside Story of the Food Industry, America's Obesity Crisis, and What We Can Do About It.* New York: McGraw-Hill, 2003.

Brownell, Kelly, and Marion Nestle. "The Sweet and Lowdown on Sugar." Editorial. *New York Times,* January 23, 2004.

Bush Greenwatch. "National Dietary Guidelines Rewritten to Favor Industry," October 29, 2004. http://www.bushgreenwatch.org/mt_archives/000217.php.

Burros, Marian. "U.S. Diet Guide Puts Emphasis on Weight Loss." *New York Times,* January 13, 2005.

Case Western Reserve University. "School of Graduate Studies Alumna Named Chair of American Council for Fitness and Nutrition." April 3, 2003. http://cerebrum.cwru.edu/newsrelease/ Nutritionalumna.htm.

Center for Science in the Public Interest. "Big Sugar's 'Thuggish' Tactics Come Under Fire." *CSPI Newsroom,* April 21, 2003. http://cspinet.org/new/200304211.html.

Cordain, Loren, S. Boyd Eaton, Anthony Sebastian, Neil Mann, Staffan Lindeberg, Bruce A. Watkins, James H. O'Keefe, and Janette Brand-Miller. "Commentary: Origins and Evolution of the Western Diet: Health Implications for the 21st Century." *American Journal of Clinical Nutrition* 81 (2005): 341–54.

Fleck, Fiona. "WHO Challenges Food Industry in Report on Diet and Health." *British Medical Journal* 326 (March 2003): 515.

General Mills. "Our Brands: Cocoa Puffs." http://www.generalmills.com/corporate/brands/brand .aspx?catID=50.

Heil, Emily. "Hill Brings Dietary Guidelines to Boil." *Congress Daily,* October 1, 2003.

Iglesias, Gerardo. "Bitter Sugar with Bruno Ribeiro de Paiva." Agricultura Brazil, April 27, 2004. http://www.rel-uita.org/agricultura/azucar-amarga-eng.htm.

Institute for Agriculture and Trade Policy. http://www.iatp.org/.

———"Food without Thought: How U.S. Farm Policy Contributes to Obesity." http://www.iatp .org/iatp/publications.cfm?accountID=421&refID=80627.

Katz, David L. "What the Dietary Guidelines Don't Tell You." *Preventive Medicine*. Column for the *New Haven Register*, January 21, 2005.

Kellogg's website. http://www.frootloops.com.

McConnaughey, Janet. "1 in 3 Children Will Become Diabetic Unless Habits Change, CDC Says." Associated Press, June 15, 2003.

Morgan, Dan. "Sugar Beet Area Not Sweet on Pact." *Washington Post*, September 20, 2004.

Muller, Mark. "A Healthier, Smarter Food System." http://www.iatp.org/iatp/library/admin/uploadedfiles/Healthier_Smarter_Food_System_A.pdf.

Muller, Mark, and H. Schoonover. "Food Without Thought: How U.S. Farm Policy Contributes to Obesity." Institute for Agriculture and Trade Policy. http://www.iatp.org/.

Munoz, Sara Schaefer. "Rebuilding the Pyramid—The USDA's Famous Graphic Is Still in the Mixing Stage; Fighting over the Foundation." *Wall Street Journal*, January 27, 2005.

Nestle, Marion. *Food Politics: How the Food Industry Influences Nutrition and Health*. Berkeley and Los Angeles: University of California Press, 2002: 109–10.

Potrikus, Alaina Sue. "Cafeterias Better but Vending Machines a Problem, Group Says." *Belleville News Democrat*, September 15, 2003.

Quaker Oats website. http://www.capncrunch.com.

Revill, Jo. "Sugar's Secret Sweetener Offer to Health Chiefs: Industry Hopes Cash Will Influence Anti-obesity Drive." *Observer*, October 3, 2004. http://observer.guardian.co.uk/uk_news/story/0,6903,1318564,00.html.

RSSL Food E-news. "WHO Accused of Suppressing a Junk Food Report." November 3–11, 2004. http://www.rssl.com/OurServices/FoodENews/NewsLetter.aspx?ENewsletterID=71#1.

Stanford University General Clinical Research Center. "Insulin Resistance." *Syndrome X, Insulin Resistance and Type 2 Diabetes*. http://syndromex.stanford.edu/InsulinResistance.htm#4.

U.S. Bureau of the Census. *Annual Estimates of the Population by Sex and Selected Age Groups for the United States: April 1, 2000 to July 1, 2003*. http://www.census.gov/popest/national/asrh/NC-EST2003-as.html.

U.S. Department of Agriculture. "Dietary Guidelines for Americans 2005." http://www.healthierus.gov/dietaryguidelines/.

U.S. Department of Agriculture and the U.S. Department of Health and Human Services. "Dietary Guidelines for Americans 2005: Executive Summary." Updated January 12, 2005. http://www.health.gov/dietaryguidelines/dga2005/document/html/executivesummary.htm.

U.S. Department of Health and Human Services. Letter from William R. Steiger, Special Assistant to the Secretary of Health and Human Services, to WHO Director-General J. W. Lee. January 5, 2004. http://www.commercialalert.org/bushadmincomment.pdf.

"What's Really Killing You (And Can You Prevent It?)" A writers briefing, convened by the Writers Guild of America, West, April 15, 2004, and the USC Annenberg Norman Lear Center's Hollywood, Health & Society project, with a panel of health experts "to discuss real threats to the health of Americans, steps to take to prevent them and the role of the entertainment industry." Includes the controversial quote from Susan Finn, Ph.D., R.D., which was picked up by Knight-Ridder. She said at the event: "I would also add that you could take all the vending machines out of schools, and I'm not sure you'd touch the obesity issue at all. You look at the state of West Virginia. They've had the most restrictive vending machine policies in the state of West Virginia for 20 years, and they have the heaviest kids. Now, I'm not throwing a cause-and-effect there. I'm just saying you can take them out, but you have to do a whole lot more than that." http://72.14.209.104/search?q=cache:cLQOrfCTpGsJ:www.learcenter.org/pdf/WhatsKillingYou.pdf+You+can+take+every+vending+machine+out+of+schools,+and+I+

don%27t+believe+you%27d+ touch+the+obesity+issue+in+children&hl=en&gl=us&ct=
clnk&cd=3.

World Health Organization. "Report of the Joint WHO/FAO Expert Consultation on Diet, Nutrition
and the Prevention of Chronic Diseases."

CHAPTER 9: PROOF POURS IN: NEW STUDIES SHOW THAT YOU CAN BECOME DEPENDENT ON SWEETS

American Institute of Unani Medicine website. http://www.unani.com/avicenna%20story%204.htm.

American Society of Addiction Medicine website. http://www.asam.org/info/Whatwedo.htm.

Appleton, Nancy. *Lick the Sugar Habit*. Garden City Park, New York: Avery, 1996. (Originally published as *Lick the Sugar Habit, Not the Candy Bar*. Santa Monica, CA: N. Appleton, 1985.)

Arnold, Tom. Interview by Ellen DeGeneres. *The Ellen DeGeneres Show*, October 13, 2003.

Atkins, Robert C. *Dr. Atkins' New Diet Revolution*. New York: Avon, 2001.

Avena, Nicole M., and B. G. Hoebel. "A Diet Promoting Sugar Dependency Causes Behaviorial Cross-Sensitization to a Low Dose of Amphetamine." *Neuroscience* 122, no. 1 (2003): 17–20.

———. "Amphetamine-Sensitized Rats Show Sugar-Induced Hyperactivity (Cross-Sensitization) and Sugar Hyperphagia." *Pharmacology, Biochemistry and Behavior* 74, no. 3 (2003): 635–39.

Barnard, Neal. *Breaking the Food Seduction*. New York: St. Martin's Press, 2003.

BBC. "Fast Food 'as Addictive as Heroin.' " BBC website.

Blum, Kenneth, E. P. Noble, P. J. Sheridan, A. Montgomery, T. Ritchie, P. Jagadeeswaran, H. Nogami, A. H. Briggs, and J. B. Cohn. "Allelic Association of Human Dopamine D2 Receptor Gene in Alcoholism." *Journal of the American Medical Association* 263, no. 15 (1990): 2055–60.

Blum, Kenneth, J. G. Cull, E. R. Braverman, and D. E. Comings. "Reward Deficiency Syndrome." *The American Scientist* 84 (1996): 132–45. http://www.recoveryemporium.com/AmSci.htm.

Brink, P. J. "Addiction to Sugar." *Western Journal of Nursing Research* 15, no. 3 (1993): 280–81.

Brookhaven National Laboratory. "More Clues About Obesity Revealed by Brain-Imaging Study, June 20, 2002. http://www.bnl.gov/bnlweb/pubaf/pr/2002/bnlpr062002.htm.

———. "New Food-Addiction Link Found, Mere Sight/Smell of Food Spikes Levels of Brain 'pleasure' chemical," May 20, 2002. http://www.bnl.gov/bnlweb/pubaf/pr/2002/bnlpr052002.htm.

———. "Scientists Find Link Between Dopamine and Obesity, February 1, 2001. http://www.bnl.gov/bnlweb/pubaf/pr/2001/bnlpr020101.htm.

Bruinsma, Kristen, and Douglas L. Taren. "Chocolate: Food or Drug?" *Journal of the American Dietetic Association* 99, no. 10 (1999): 1249–56.

Campbell, Una C., and Marilyn E. Carroll. "Reduction of Drug Self-Administration by an Alternative Non-drug Reinforcer in Rhesus Monkeys: Magnitute and Temporal Effects." *Psychopharmacology* 147, no. 4 (2000): 418–25.

Carroll, Marilyn E., A. D. Morgan, W. J. Lynch, U. C. Campbell, and N. K. Dess. "Intravenous Cocaine and Heroin Self-Administration in Rats Selectively Bred for Differential Saccharin Intake: Phenotype and Sex Differences." *Psychopharmacology* 161, no. 3 (2002): 304–13.

Chocolate Manufacturers Association website. http://www.chocolateusa.org/resources/statistical-information.asp.

Colantuoni, Carlo, Pedro Rada, Joseph McCarthy, Caroline Patten, Nicole M. Avena, Andrew Chadeayne, and Bartley G. Hoebel. "Evidence That Intermittent, Excessive Sugar Intake Causes Endogenous Opioid Dependence." *Obesity Research* 10, no. 6 (2002): 478–88.

Colantuoni, Carlo, J. Schwenker, J. McCarthy, P. Rada, B. Ladenheim, J. L. Cadet, G. J. Schwartz,

T. H. Moran, and B.G. Hoebel. "Excessive Sugar Intake Alters Binding to Dopamine and Mu-Opioid Receptors in the Brain." *NeuroReport* 12, no. 16 (2001): 3549–52.

Days of Wine and Roses. Directed by Blake Edwards, 1962.

DesMaisons, Kathleen. *Potatoes, Not Prozac*. New York: Fireside, 1999.

Diagnostic and Statistical Manual of Mental Disorders. 4th ed. Washington, D.C.: American Psychiatric Association, 2000, 191–209.

Drewnowski, Adam. "Taste and Food Preferences in Human Obesity." In *Taste, Experience, and Feeding*, edited by Elizabeth D. Capaldi with Terry L. Powley. Washington, DC: American Psychological Association, 1990.

Dufty, William. *Sugar Blues*. New York: Warner Books, 1975.

Galic, M. A., and M. A. Persinger. "Voluminous Sucrose Consumption in Female Rats: Increased 'Nippiness' During Periods of Sucrose Removal and Possible Oestrus Periodicity." *Psychological Reports* 90, no. 1 (2002): 58–60.

Gosnell, B. "Sucrose Intake Predicts Rate of Acquisition of Cocaine Self-Administration." *Psychopharmacology* 149, no. 3 (2000): 286–92.

Heller, Rachael F., and Richard F. Heller. *The Carbohydrate Addict's Diet*. New York: Signet, 1993.

Hetherington, Marion M., and Jennifer I. MacDiarmid. "Chocolate Addiction: A Preliminary Study of Its Description and Its Relationship to Problem Eating." *Appetite* 21, no. 3 (1993): 233–46.

———. "Pleasure and Excess: Liking for and Overconsumption of Chocolate." *Physiology and Behavior* 57, no. 1 (1995): 27–35.

Horovitz, Bruce. "Jumpin' Jelly! Doughnuts Dominate Dining Growth." *USA Today*, May 27, 2003.

Kampov-Polevoy, Alexey B., James C. Garbutt, and David S. Janowsky. "Association Between Preference for Sweets and Excessive Alcohol Intake: A Review of Animal and Human Studies." *Alcohol and Alcoholism* 34, no. 3 (1999): 386–95.

Kampov-Polevoy, Alexey B., M. V. Tsoi, E. E. Zvartau, N. G. Neznanov, and E. Khalitov. "Sweet Liking and Family History of Alcoholism in Hospitalized Alcoholic and Non-alcoholic Patients." *Alcohol and Alcoholism* 36, no. 2 (2001): 165–70.

Kelley, Anne, M. J. Will, T. L. Steininger, M. Zhang, and S. N. Haber. "Restricted Daily Consumption of a Highly Palatable Food (Chocolate Ensure) Alters Striatal Enkephalin Gene Expression." *European Journal of Neuroscience* 18, no. 9 (2003): 2592–98.

Lam, Michael. *An Insider's Guide to Natural Medicine*. http://www.drlam.com.

Le Magnen, J. "A Role for Opiates in Food Reward and Food Addiction." In *Taste, Experience, and Feeding*, edited by Elizabeth D. Capaldi with Terry L. Powley. Washington, DC: American Psychological Association, 1990.

———. "Palatability: Concept, Terminology, and Mechanisms." *Eating Habits: Food, Physiology and Learned Behaviour*, edited by Robert A. Boakes, David A. Popplewell, and Michael J. Burton. New York, NY: John Wiley & Sons, 1987.

Leon, M. J., N. Volkow, et al. "Cortisol Reduces Hippocampal Glucose Metabolism in Normal Elderly but Not in Alzheimer's Disease." *Journal of Clinical Endocrinology and Metabolism* 82, no. 10 (1997): 3251–59.

Levine, A. S., C. M. Kotz, and B. A. Gosnell. "Sugars and Fats: The Neurobiology of Preference." *Journal of Nutrition* 133, no. 3 (2003): 831–34.

Macinnis, Peter. *Bittersweet: The Story of Sugar*. Australia: Allen & Unwin, 2003.

The Man with the Golden Arm. Directed by Otto Preminger, 1954.

McCloy, James, and R. F. McCloy. "Enkephalins, Hunger and Obesity." *Lancet* 2, no. 8134 (1979): 156.

Mercola, Joseph. *The No-Grain Diet*. New York: Penguin Group, 2003.

Mesley, Wendy. "Can We Be Addicted to Junk Food?" CBC Marketplace, broadcast October 29, 2002. http://www.cbc.ca/consumers/market/files/food/junkfood_addiction/index.html.

Mundell, E. J. "Rat Studies Show Evidence of 'Sugar Dependence.'" *Reuters Health*, June 18, 2001.

National Center for Chronic Disease Prevention, Centers for Disease Control and Prevention. http://www.cdc.gov/nccdphp.

National Institute on Drug Abuse. "Director's Page." http://www.drugabuse.gov/about/welcome/Volkowpage.html.

Nordlie, Tom. "UF College of Medicine Researchers Report Link Between Overeating, Obesity and Addiction." Press release. University of Florida Health Science Center, July 8, 2004. http://www.napa.ufl.edu/2004news/foodaddiction.htm.

O'Doherty, J., E. T. Rolls, S. Francis, R. Bowtell, and F. McGlone. "Representation of Pleasant and Aversive Taste in the Human Brain." *Journal of Neurophysiology* 85, no. 3 (2001): 1315–21.

Pescatore, Fred. *The Hamptons Diet*. Hoboken, NJ: John Wiley & Sons, 2004.

Reuters. "Is junk food immoral. Socially responsible investment funds are weighing the issue of fast food and fat." July 11, 2003.

Ross, Julia. *The Mood Cure: The 4-Step Program to Rebalance Your Emotional Chemistry and Rediscover Your Natural Sense of Well-Being*. New York: Viking, 2002.

Rudin, Ronald, A. *The Craving Brain: The Biobalance Approach to Controlling Addicitons*. New York: HarperCollins, 1997.

Schroeder, B. E., J. M. Binzak, and A. E. Kelley. "A Common Profile of Prefrontal Cortical Activation Following Exposure to Nicotine- or Chocolate-Associated Contextual Cues." *Neuroscience* 105, no. 3 (2001): 535–45.

Shaffer, Howard J. "What Is Addiction: A Perspective." Harvard Medical School, Division on Addictions. http://www.divisiononaddictions.org/html/whatisaddiction.htm.

The Simpsons: "Sweets and Sour Marge." 1308 DABF03. Original airdate: January 20, 2002. http://www.thesimpsons.com/episode_guide/index.htm.

The Simpsons: "The Heartbroke Kid." 1617 F71342 SI-1611. Original airdate: May 1, 2005. http://www.thesimpsons.com/episode_guide/index.htm.

Society for the Study of Ingestive Behavior. http://www.ssib.org/sponsors.html.

Tuomisto, T., M. M. Hetherington, M. F. Morris, M. T. Tuomisto, V. Turjanmaa, and R. Lappalainen. "Psychological and Physiological Characteristics of Sweet Food 'addiction.'" *International Journal of Eating Disorders* 25, no. 2 (1999): 169–75.

Volkow, N. D., G. J. Wang, et al. "Effects of Alcohol Detoxification on Dopamine D2 Receptors in Alcoholics: A Preliminary Study." *Psychiatry Research: Neuroimaging* 116, no. 3 (2002): 163–72.

Volkow, Nora D., Joanna S. Fowler, and Gene-Jack Wang. "The Addicted Human Brain: Insights from Imaging Studies." *Journal of Clinical Investigation* 11 (2003): 1444–51.

Wang, Gene-Jack, and Nora D. Volkow, et al. "Brain Dopamine and Obesity." *Lancet* 357, no. 9253 (1999): 354–57.

———. "The Role of Dopamine in Motivation for Food in Humans: Implications for Obesity." *Expert Opinion: Therapeutic Targets* 6, no. 5 (2002): 601–9.

Yanovski, Susan. "Sugar and Fat: Cravings and Aversions." *Journal of Nutrition* 133, no. 3 (2003): 829S–830S; 835S–837S.

CHAPTER 10: SUGARY SNACKS CAN MINIMIZE YOUR MEMORY

Aljada, A., H. Ghanim, P. Mohanty, T. Syed, A. Bandyopadhyay, and P. Dandona. "Glucose Intake Induces an Increase in Activator Protein 1 and Early Growth Response 1 Binding Activities, in the

Expression of Tissue Factor and Matrix Metalloproteinase in Mononuclear Cells, and in Plasma Tissue Factor and Matrix Metalloproteinase Concentrations." *American Journal of Clinical Nutrition* 80, no. 1 (2004): 51–57.

Aljada, A., P. Mohanty, H. Ghanim, T. Abdo, D. Tripathy, A. Chaudhuri, and P. Dandona. "Increase in Intranuclear Nuclear Factor KappaB and Decrease in Inhibitor KappaB in Mononuclear Cells After a Mixed Meal: Evidence for a Proinflammatory Effect." *American Journal of Clinical Nutrition* 79 (April 2004): 682–90.

Alzheimer's Disease Education and Referral Center. "Alzheimer's Disease: Unraveling the Mystery." http://www.alzheimers.org/unraveling/09.htm.

Alzheimer's Prevention Foundation International. http://www.alzheimersprevention.org.

Benton, David, and S. Nabb. "Carbohydrate, Memory, and Mood." *Nutrition Reviews* 61, no. 5 (2003): S61–S67.

Benton, D., and M. P. Ruffin, et al. "The Delivery Rate of Dietary Carbohydrates Affects Cognitive Performance in Both Rats and Humans." *Psychopharmacology* 166 (February 2003): 86–90.

Benton, D., and J. Sargent. "Breakfast, Blood, Glucose and Memory." *Biology of Psychology* 33 (1992): 207–210.

Chowka, Peter Barry. "William B. Grant: A Dietary Approach to Alzheimer's." Dialogue with the Experts. http://members.aol.com/pbchowka/grant.html.

Convit, Antonio, Oliver T. Wolf, Chaim Tarshish, and Mony J. de Leon. "Reduced Glucose Tolerance Is Associated with Poor Memory Performance and Hippocampal Atrophy Among Normal Elderly." *Proceedings of the National Academy of Sciences* 100, no. 4 (2003): 2019–22.

Hyman, Mark. *UltraMetabolism: The Simple Plan for Automatic Weight Loss.* New York: Simon & Schuster, 2006.

Khalsa, Dharma Singh. *Brain Longevity.* New York: Warner Books, 1997.

Messier, C., et al. "Effect of Age and Glucoregulation on Cognitive Performance." *Neurobiology of Aging* 24, no. 7 (2003): 985–1003.

Mohanty, P., W. Hamouda, R. Garg, A. Aljada, H. Ghanim, and P. Dandona. "Glucose Challenge Stimulates Reactive Oxygen Species (ROS) Generation by Leucocytes." *Journal of Clinical Endocrinology and Metabolism* 85, no. 8 (2000): 2970–73.

National Institute of Health. "Brain Basics: Know Your Brain." www.ninds.nih.gov/health.

Neergaard, Lauran. "Blood Sugar Linked to Old Age Memory Loss." *Associated Press*, February 3, 2003.

Novartis Starlix. "What Is Impaired Glucose Tolerance?" http://www.starlix.info/media_center/content/pages/impaired_gluc.

Rodgers, Anne Brown. "Alzheimer's Disease: Unraveling the Mystery." Alzheimer's Disease Education and Referral Center website. www.alzheimers.org.

Schubert, Markus, Jens C. Bruning, and C. Ronald Kahn, et al. "Role for Neuronal Insulin Resistance in Neurodegenerative Diseases." *Proceedings of the National Academy of Science* 101, no. 9 (2004): 3100–5.

Science Blog. "High Sugar Blood Levels Linked to Poor Memory." www.scienceblog.com/community/modules.php?name=News&file=article&sid=903.

U.S. Census Bureau 2000 figures. www.census.gov/main.

Vaisman, N., et al. "Effect of Breakfast Timing on the Cognitive Functions of Elementary School Students." *Archives of Pediatric and Adolescent Medicine* 150 (1996): 1089–92.

CHAPTER 11: SWEETS CAN SOUR YOUR MOODS

Agatson, Arthur. *The South Beach Diet.* Emmaus, PA: Rodale Press, 2003.

American Heart Association. Omega-3 Fatty Acid Recommendations. http://www.americanheart.org/presenter.jhtml?identifier=4632.

Amsterdam, Jay, and Greg Maislin. "Hormonal Responses During Insulin-Induced Hypoglycemia in Manic-Depressed, Unipolar Depressed, and Healthy Control Subjects." *Journal of Clinical Endocrinology and Metabolism* 73, no. 3 (1990): 541–48.

Anderson, Richard A. "Elevated Intakes of Supplemental Chromium Improve Glucose and Insulin Variables in Individuals with Type 2 Diabetes." *Diabetes* 46 (Nov. 1997): 1786–91

Appleton, Nancy. *Lick the Sugar Habit.* Garden City Park, NY: Avery 1988.

Benton, David. "Carbohydrate Ingestion, Blood Glucose, and Mood." *Neuroscience and Biobehavioral Reviews* 26, no. 3 (2002): 293–308.

Bilici, Mustafa, Hasan, Efe, M. Arif Koroglu, et al. "Antioxidative Enzyme Activities and Lipid Peroxidation in Major Depression: Alterations by Antidepressant Treatments." *Journal of Affective Disorders* 64 (2001): 43–51.

Christensen, Larry, and C. Redig. "Effect of Meal Composition on Mood." *Behavioral Neuroscience* 107, no. 2 (1993): 346–53.

Christensen, Larry, and L. Pettijohn. "Mood and Carbohydrate Cravings." *Appetite* 36, no. 22 (2001): 137–45.

Davidson, Jonathan, Kurian Abraham, Kathryn Connor, and Malcolm McLeod. "Effectiveness of Chromium in Atypical Depression: A Placebo-Controlled Trial." *Society of Biological Psychiatry* 53 (2003): 261–64.

DesMaisons, Kathleen. *Potatoes, Not Prozac.* New York: Simon and Schuster, 1999.

Donohoe, R. T. and D. Benton. "Blood Glucose Control and Aggressiveness in Females." *Personality and Individual Differences* 26, no. 5 (1999): 905–11.

Drevets, Wayne C. "Neuroimaging Studies of Mood Disorders." *Society of Biological Psychiatry* 48 (2000): 813–29.

Drevets, Wayne C., Joseph L. Price, Mark E. Bardgett, et al. "Glucose Metabolism in the Amygdala in Depression: Relationship to Diagnostic Subtype and Plasma Cortisol Levels." *Pharmacology, Biochemistry and Behavior* 71 (2002): 431–47.

Food and Behavior Research (FAB). http://www.fabresearch.org.

Geary, Amanda. *The Food and Mood Handbook: Find Relief at Last from Depression, Anxiety, PMS, Cravings and Mood Swings.* London: Thorsons, 2001.

Giugliano, Dario, Antonio Ceriello, and Giuseppe Paolisso. "Oxidative Stress and Diabetic Vascular Complications." *Diabetes Care* 19, no. 3 (1996): 257–63.

Gold, A. E., K. M. MacLeod, B. M. Frier, and I. J. Deary. "Changes in Mood During Acute Hypoglycemia in Healthy Participants." *Journal of Personality and Social Psychology* 68, no. 3 (1995): 498–504.

Kinsbourne, Marcel. "Sugar and the Hyperactive Child." *New England Journal of Medicine* 330 (February 3, 2004): 355–56.

Leonard, Brian E., and Cai Song. "Stress and the Immune System in the Etiology of Anxiety and Depression." *Pharmacology, Biochemistry and Behavior* 54, no. 1 (1996): 299–303.

———. "Stress, Depression, and the Role of Cytokines." *Advances in Experimental Medicine and Biology* 461 (1999): 251–65.

Liu, Jianghong, Adrian Raine, Peter H. Venables, and Sarnoff A. Mednick. "Malnutrition at Age 3 Years and Externalizing Behavior Problems at Ages 8, 11, and 17 Years." *American Journal of Psychiatry* 161 (November 2004): 2005–13.

Lustman, Patrick, Ryan Anderson, Kenneth B. Freedland, et al. "Depression and Poor Glycemic Control: A Meta-analysis of the Literature." *Diabetes Care* 23, no. 7 (2000): 934–37.

Matthews, Keith, Alasdair Rooney, and Richard Day. "Depression, Appetite and Eating." *Food Cravings and Addictions*, September 2001.

McLeod, Malcolm. Dr. Malcolm McLeod's Chromium Connection Blog. *"Studies Prove Chromium Reduces Carb Cravings."* http://chromiumconnection.com/blog/2005/12/studies-proves-chromium-reduces-carb.html.

McLeod, Malcolm, Bradley N. Gaynes, and Robert N. Golden. "Chromium Potentiation of Antidepressant Pharmacotherapy for Dysthymic Disorder in 5 Patients." *Journal of Clinical Psychiatry* 60 (April 1999): 237–40.

McLeod, Malcolm, and Robert Golden. "Chromium Treatment of Depression." *International Journal of Neuropsychopharmacology* 3 (2000): 311–14.

Mental Health Foundation. "Changing Diets, Changing Minds: How Food Affects Mental Health and Behaviour." www.mentalhealth.org.uk/html/content/changing_minds.pdf.

———. "Feeding Minds: The Impact of Food on Mental Health." http://www.mentalhealth.org.uk/html/content/feedingminds_exec_summary.pdf.

———. "Food and Mental Health." http://www.sustainweb.org/mhealth_index.asp.

———. "Food and Mental Health Campaign." http://www.mentalhealth.org.uk/page.cfm?pagecode=PRFM#reports.

Mercer, Michele, and Mark Holder. "Food Cravings, Endogenous Opiod Peptides, and Food Intake." *Appetite* 39 (1997): 325–52.

Musante, Linda, Frank Treiber, Harry Davis, et al. "Hostility: Relationship to Lifestyle Behaviors and Physical Risk Factors." *Behavioral Medicine* 18, no. 1 (Spring 1992).

National Institute of Mental Health. National Institutes of Health. "An Overview That Summarizes Research into the Causes, Diagnosis, Prevention, and Treatment of Depression." 1999. http://www.nimh.nih.gov/publicat/depresfact.cfm?textSize=L.

———. National Institutes of Health. "Depression in Children and Adolescents." http://www.nimh.nih.gov/HealthInformation/depchildmenu.cfm.

———. "Mental Health and the Family: Mental Health Statistics." http://www.nmha.org/infoctr/factsheets/15.cfm.

———. "Summary of Statistics Describing the Prevalence of Mental Disorders in America 2001." http://www.nimh.nih.gov/publicat/numbers.cfm.

National Mental Health Association. "Children's Mental Health Statistics." http://www.nmha.org/children/prevent/stats.cfm.

Omega-3 Information Service. http://www.omega-3info.com/research.htm.

Pelchat, Marcia. "Of Human Bondage: Food Craving, Obsession, Compulsion, and Addiction." *Physiology and Behavior* 76 (2002): 347–52.

Rados, Carol. "FDA, EPA Revise Guidelines on Mercury in Fish." *FDA*, May–June 2004. http://www.fda.gov/fdac/features/2004/304_fish.html.

Ronzio, Robert. *The Encyclopedia of Nutrition and Good Health.* New York: Facts on File, 2003.

Ross, Julia. *The Mood Cure.* New York: Viking, 2002.

Schauss, Alex. *Diet, Crime and Delinquency.* Rev. ed. Berkeley: Parker House, 1981.

———. "Nutrition and Behavior." *Journal of Applied Nutrition* 35, no. 1 (1983): 30–43.

———. *Nutrition and Behavior.* New Caanan, CT: Keats, 1985.

———. "Nutrition and Behavior: Complex Interdisciplinary Research." *Nutrition and Health* 3 (1984): 9–37.

Sears, Barry. *Enter the Zone.* New York: HarperCollins, 1995.

Somer, Elizabeth. *Food and Mood.* 2nd ed. New York: Henry Holt & Co., 1999.

Stitt, Barbara R. *Food and Behavior.* Manitowoc, WI: Natural Press, 1997.

Stoll, Andrew L., W. Emanuel Severus, Marlene P. Freeman, et al. "Omega-3 Fatty Acids in Bipolar Disorder." *Archives of General Psychiatry* 56, no. 5 (1999): 407–12.

Surwit, R. S., R. B. Williams, I. C. Siegler, et al. "Hostility, Race, and Glucose Metabolism in Nondiabetic Individuals." *Diabetes Care* 25, no. 5 (2002): 835–39.

Timonen, Markku, et al. "Insulin Resistance and Depression: Cross Sectional Study." *BMJ* 330 (January 2005): 17–18. http://bmj.bmjjournals.com/cgi/content/full/330/7481/17.

Tintera, John. "*What You Should Know about Your Glands.*" Weston A. Price Foundation. http://www.westonaprice.org/archive/archive_tintera.html.

Turkington, C., and Joseph Harris. *The Encyclopedia of the Brain and Brain Disorders.* 2nd ed. New York: Facts on File, 2002.

Turkington, C., and E. F. Kaplan. *Making the Antidepressant Decision: How to Choose the Right Treatment Option for You or Your Loved One.* New York: Contemporary Books, 2001.

Weber, B., U. Schweiger, M. Deuschle, and I. Heuser. "Major Depression and Impaired Glucose Tolerance." *Exp Clinic Endocrinolo Diabetes* 198 (2000): 187–90.

Westover, Arthur N., and Lauren B. Marangell. "A Cross-National Relationship Between Sugar Consumption and Major Depression." *Depression and Anxiety* 16 (2002): 118–120.

Willner, Paul, David Benton, and Emma Brown, et al. "Depression Increases Craving for Sweet Rewards in Animal and Human Models of Depression and Craving." *Psychopharmacology* 136 (1998): 272–83.

Wurtman, Judith. *Managing Your Mind and Mood Through Food.* New York: Rawson Assoc., 1986.

———. *The Serotonin Solution.* New York: Ballantine Books, 1996.

Yamamoto, Takashi. "Brain Mechanisms of Sweetness and Palatability of Sugars." *Nutrition Review* 61, supp. 1 (May 2003): 5–9.

CHAPTER 12: A SWEET TOOTH COULD TRASH YOUR RELATIONSHIPS AND SEX LIFE

About.com. "Can't Get No Satisfaction: Women's Sexual Health and Diabetes." http://diabetes.about.com/cs/sexuality/a/aafemalesexdysf.htm.

Airola, Paavo. *Hypoglycemia: A Better Approach.* Phoenix, AZ: Health Plus Publishers, 1977.

American Diabetes Association. *Diabetes A to Z: What You Need to Know about Diabetes—Simply Put.* 4th ed. Alexandria, VA: American Diabetes Association, 2000.

Appleton, Nancy. *Lick the Sugar Habit.* Garden City Park, NY: Avery, 1988.

Basson, R., et al. "Report of the International Consensus Development Conference on Female Sexual Dysfunction: Definition and Classifications." *Journal of Urology* 163 (March 2000): 888–93.

Blackstone, Margaret. *Beat Diabetes! How I Overcame Diabetes and You Can Too!* Avon, MA: Adams Media Corporation, 2000.

Chow, James, and Cheryl Chow. *Hypoglycemia for Dummies.* New York: Wiley, 2003.

Contactmusic.com. "Weinstein Weight Loss," May 28, 2006. http://www.contactmusic.com/new/xml feed.nsf/mndwebpages/weinstein%20weight%20loss_28_05_2006.

Costabile, Raymond. "Optimizing Treatment for Diabetes Mellitus Induced Erectile Dysfunction." *Journal of Urology* 1709 (August 2003): S35–S39.

De Berardis, G., F. Pellegrini, M. Franciosi, M. Belfiglio, B. Di Nardo, S. Greenfield, S. H. Kaplan, M. C. Rossi, M. Sacco, G. Tognoni, M. Valentini, and A. Nicolucci. "Identifying Patients with Type 2 Diabetes with a Higher Likelihood of Erectile Dysfunction: The Role of the Interaction Between Clinical and Psychological Factors. Quality of Care and Outcomes in Type 2 Diabetes Study Group." *Clinical Urology* 169, no. 4 (2003): 1422–28.

DesMaisons, Kathleen. *Potatoes, Not Prozac: A Natural, Seven-Step Dietary Plan to Stabilize the Level of Sugar in Your Blood, Control Your Cravings, and Lose Weight.* New York: Fireside, 1998.

Dubey, Anita. "Complications: Diabetes and Sexual Dysfunction. Canadian Diabetes Association." http://www.diabetes.ca/Section_About/sexualdys.asp.

Feldman, H. A., I. Goldstein, D. G. Hatzichristou, et al. "Impotence and Its Medical and Psychological Correlates: Results of the Massachusetts Male Aging Study." *Journal of Urology* 151, no. 1 (1994): 54–61.

Goldstein, Patrick. "The Big Picture: Playing Dirty to the Max." *Los Angeles Times,* January 20, 2004, sec. E, 1.

Haas, Elson. *The New Detox Diet: The Complete Guide for Lifelong Vitality with Recipes, Menus, and Detox Plans.* With Daniella Chace. Berkeley, CA: Celestial Arts, 2004.

Haberman, Maggie. "Movie Boss Licks M&M Addiction." *New York Daily News,* October 4, 2004.

Hayden, Naura. *How to Satisfy a Woman Every Time . . . and Have Her Beg for More!* New York: Bibli O'Phile Books, 2001.

Hoebel, Bartley G. "Excessive Sugar Intake Alters Binding to Dopamine and Mu-Opiod Receptors in the Brain." *Neuroreport* 12, no. 16 (2001): 3549–52.

The Hypoglycemia Support Foundation website. www.hypoglycemia.org.

Joslin Diabetes Center Sexual Function Clinic. "Sexual Dysfunction and Diabetes." http://www.joslin.harvard.edu/education/library/sexual_dysfunction.shtml.

Kilo, Charles, and Joseph R. Williamson. *Diabetes: The Facts That Let You Regain Control of Your Life.* New York: John Wiley & Sons, 1987.

Lamm, Steven. *The Hardness Factor: How to Achieve Your Best Health and Sexual Fitness at Any Age.* With Gerald Secor Couzens. New York: HarperCollins, 2005.

Lincoln, Thomas A., and John A. Eaddy. *Beating the Sugar Blues: Proven Methods and Wisdom for Controlling Hypoglycemia.* Alexandria, VA: American Diabetes Association, 2001.

Lisle, Douglas J., and Alan Goldhamer. *The Pleasure Trap: Mastering the Hidden Force That Undermines Health and Happiness.* Summertown, TN: Healthy Living Publications, 2003.

LowCarbFreedom.com. "Fits of Anger? You Might Have Type II Diabetes, Like Harvey Weinstein of Miramax Pictures," October 4, 2004. http://www.lowcarbfreedom.com/2004/10/fits_of_anger_y.html.

McCool, Martha Hope, and Sandra Woodruff. *My Doctor Says I Have a Little Diabetes: A Guide to Understanding and Controlling Type 2, Non-insulin-Dependent Diabetes.* New York: Avery, 1999.

McGill, Hannah. "What Harvey Did Next: After Building Up a Multi-Million-Dollar Production Empire, the Future Looks Uncertain for Harvey and Bob Weinstein." *Herald* (Glasgow), November 20, 2004, 10.

Meirelles, Janet. *Diabetes Is Not a Piece of Cake.* Lake Oswego, OR: Lincoln Publishing, 1997.

Mendelsohn, Naomi. "Winning the Uphill Battle: Sexual Dysfunction and Diabetes." *Sexual Health: Love, Lust and Life.* savvyHEALTH.com. http://www.savvyhealth.com/disp.asp?doc_id=27.

Mnookin, Seth. "How Harvey Weinstein Survived His Mid-life Crisis (for Now)." *New York Magazine,* October 11, 2004, 40. http://www.newyorkmetro.com/nymetro/news/people/features/9985/index.html.

Myers, M. G., Jr., et al. "The IRS-1 Signaling System." *TIBS* 19, no. 7 (1994): 289–93.

Rubin, Alan L. *Diabetes for Dummies.* New York: Hungry Minds, 2001.

Sarkadi, Anna, and Urban Rosenqvist. "Intimacy and Women with Type 2 Diabetes: An Exploratory Study Using Focus Group Interviews." *Diabetes Educator* 29, no. 4 (2003): 641–52.

Saunders, Jeraldine, and Harvey M. Ross. *Hypoglycemia: The Classic Healthcare Handbook.* New York: Kensington Publishing, 2002.

Schwarzbein, Diana. *The Schwarzbein Principle: The Truth about Losing Weight, Being Healthy, and Feeling Younger.* Deerfield Beach, FL: Health Communications, 1999.

Shimer, Porter. *New Hope for People with Diabetes.* Roseville, CA: Prima Publishing 2001.

Shiri, R., J. Koskimaki, M. Hakama, J. Hakkinen, T. L. Tammela, H. Huhtala, and A. Auvinen. "Effect of Chronic Diseases on Incidence of Erectile Dysfunction." *Urology* 62, no. 6 (2003): 1097–1102.

Superiorpics.com Entertainment News, May 28, 2006. http://news.superiorpics.com/2006/05/28/.

Thrash, Agatha M., and Calvin L. Thrash. *Diabetes and the Hypoglycemic Syndrome.* Seale, AL: New Lifestyle Books, 1993.

Whitaker, Julian. *Reversing Diabetes: Reduce or Even Eliminate Your Dependence on Insulin or Oral Drugs.* New York: Warner Books, 2001.

White, M. F., et al. "The Insulin Signaling System." *Journal of Biological Chemistry* 1994, no. 269: 1–5.

Widdicombe, Ben. "Gossip: Gatecrasher: Is Harvey Weinstein Back on the M&M's?" *New York Daily News*, March 6, 2005.

———. "Gossip: Gatecrasher." *New York Daily News*, November 7, 2004.

Yale Diabetes Center. *Diabetes Facts and Guidelines 2003–2004.* 57.

CHAPTER 13: IT MIGHT *NOT* BE "ALL IN YOUR HEAD": WHAT YOUR DOCTOR DOESN'T KNOW OR BELIEVE ABOUT HYPOGLYCEMIA

ADAM Health Illustrated Encyclopedia s. v. "Hypoglycemia." http://www.nlm.nih.gov/medlineplus/ency/article/000386.htm#Definition.

Airola, Paavo. *Hypoglycemia: A Better Approach.* Scottsdale, AZ: Health Plus Publications, 1977.

American Diabetes Association, the Endocrine Society, and the American Medical Association. "Statement on Hypoglycemia." Editorial. *Journal of the American Medical Association* 223 (1973): 682.

Appleton, Nancy. *Lick the Sugar Habit.* New York: Avery, 1996.

Atkins corporate website. http://www.atkins.com.

Atkins, Robert. *Dr. Atkins Vita-Nutrient Solution.* New York: Simon & Schuster, 1999.

Benton, David. "Carboyhydrate Ingestion, Glucose and Mood." *Neuroscience and Biobehavioral Reviews* 26, no. 3 (2002): 293–308.

Centers for Disease Control. "A–Z Index of Topics in Alphabetical Order." http://www.cdc.gov/az.do.

Chow, Cheryl, and James Chow. *Hypoglycemia for Dummies.* New York: Wiley, 2003.

Claymon, Charles, ed. *The American Medical Association Family Medical Guide.* New York: Random House, 1994.

CNN.com. "Diseases and Conditions: Hypoglycemia." From MayoClinic.com. http://www.cnn.com/HEALTH/library/DS/00198.html.

Coleman, Lee. "In Diseases: A Look at the Current Crop of Chic Complaints." *Cosmopolitan*, July 1980.

Dufty, William. *Sugar Blues.* New York: Warner, 1975.

Fairview Clinical Laboratories. "Glucose Testing and Diagnosis of Diabetes: Revised ADA Criteria." *Scope: Lab Focus,* September 2003. http://64.233.179.104/search?q=cache:XEC2itd9wG4J:labguide.fairview.org/newsletters/LF0903.pdf+michael+steffes+and+%22hypoglycemic+disorders%22&hl=en.

Flagg, Marianne. "Hypoglycemia (Low Blood Sugar)." http://www.yalenewhavenhealth.org/hv-iframe.asp?hvurl=/Library/HealthGuide/IllnessConditions.

Flegg, Anita. "How Do Doctors Test for Hypoglycemia?" http://www.anitaflegg.com/Oct112002.

———. *Hypoglycemia: The Other Sugar Disease.* Ottawa, Ontario, Canada: Book Coach Press, 2003.

Fredericks, Carlton. *New Low Blood Sugar and You.* New York: Perigree, 1985.

Fried, Susan K., and Salome P. Rao. "Sugars, Hypertriglyceridemia, and Cardiovascular Disease." *American Journal of Clinical Nutrition* 78, no. 4 (2003): 873S–880S.

Garg, K. N., and S. Sharan. "Alcoholic Hypoglycemia: Its Relation to Blood Ethanol Concentration." *Indian Journal of Pharmacology* 9, no. 2 (1977): 167–69.

Gittleman, Ann Louise. *Get the Sugar Out: 501 Simple Ways to Cut the Sugar Out of Any Diet.* New York: Three Rivers Press, 1996.

Gyland, S. Letter to the editor. *Journal of the American Medical Association* 152, no. 18 (1953).

Harris, S. "Hyperinsulinism and Dysinsulinism." *Journal of the American Medical Association* 83 (September 1924): 729.

The History of Health. Health, Wealth and Happiness! website. http://www.relfe.com/history_1.html.

Hoffman, Ronald. "Hypoglycemia." *Conscious Choice*, July 1999. http://www.consciouschoice.com /1999/cc1207/hmd1207.html.

———. "Sugar Disease." http://www.drhoffman.com/page.cfm/131.

Hunter, Rachel. "The New Food Medicine: Living Proof . . . It Really Does Work!" *First for Women*, August 1994, 42–43.

Hypoglycemia Association Inc. "Symptoms of Hypoglycemia and Hypoadrenocorticism." Bulletin #44. http://www.fred.net/slowup/habul44.html.

Hypoglycemia Homepage, Holland. "Glucose Tolerance Test." http://hypoglykemie.nl/gtt.htm.

The Hypoglycemia Support Foundation website. http://www.hypoglycemia.org.

Idema, Lars. Hypoglycemia Homepage, Holland (personal website). http://hypoglykemie.nl.

Joslin Diabetes Center. "Is Low Blood Glucose (Hypoglycemia) Dangerous?" http://www.joslin. org/Beginners_guide_654.asp.

Krapp, Kristine, and Jacqueline Long, eds. *Gale Encyclopedia of Alternative Medicine.* Belmont, CA: Thomson Gale, 2001.

Krimmel, Edward, and Patricia Krimmel. *The Low Blood Sugar Handbook: You Don't Have to Suffer.* Bryn Mawr, PA: Franklin, 1992.

Larson, Joan Mathews. "Hypoglycemia and Alcoholism." In *Seven Weeks to Sobriety.* http://www .healthrecovery.com/alcoholism_hypoglycemia.html.

Lewellen, Ted. "Comment: The Hypoglycemia-Aggression Hypothesis." *Current Anthropology* 25 (February 1985): 31–32.

Lewis, Laura. "The Low Down on Low Blood Sugar!" December 1999. http://www.lauralewis .com/archives/article12–99b.html.

MedicineNet.com. "Diabetes Overview: Glucose." http://www.medterms.com/script/main/art.asp? ArticleKey=3608.

MedlinePlus Medical Encyclopedia. http://www.medlineplus.org.

Morris, Bob. "At Lunch with Fran Lebowitz: Words Are Easy, Books Are Not." *New York Times,* August 10, 1994.

National Diabetes Information Clearinghouse of the National Institute of Diabetes and Digestive and Kidney Diseases. "Hypoglycemia." http://www.nlm.nih.gov/medlineplus/hypoglycemia/ html.

National Institute of Diabetes and Digestive and Kidney Diseases, National Institute of Health, National Diabetes Information Clearinghouse. Information regarding "Hypoglycemia." http://diabetes.niddk .nih.gov/dm/pubs/hypoglycemia/index.htm.

Nutrimed Labs. "The Sugar Paradox." http://www.nutrimed.com/SUGAR.HTM.

Perkins, Cynthia. "Holistic Help with Cynthia: Do You Have Undiagnosed Hypoglycemia?" http://www.holistichelp.net/hypoglycemia.html.

Plesman, Jurriaan. "What Is Hypoglycemia?" The Hypoglycemic Health Association of Australia. http://www.hypoglycemia.asn.au/.

Ruggiero, Roberta. *The Do's and Don'ts of Low Blood Sugar.* Hollywood, FL: Lifetime, 1983.

Ross, Harvey. *Fighting Depression: How to Lift the Cloud That Darkens Millions of Lives*. New Canaan, CT: Keats, 1992.

Sachs, G. S., D. J. Printz, D. A. Kahn, et al. *The Expert Consensus Guideline Series: Medication Treatment of Bipolar Disorder 2000*. A Postgraduate Medicine Special Report, April 2000. The McGraw-Hill Companies, Inc. http://www.psychguides.com/gl-treatment_of_bp2000.html.

Saunders, Jeraldine, and Harvey Ross. *Hypoglycemia: The Classic Healthcare Handbook*. New York: Kensington, 2002.

Schindehette, Susan, Karen Grigsby Bates, Michelle Caruso, Laura Schiff, Joanna Blonska, Ellen Tumposky, Olivia Abel, and Jennifer Longley. "Going to Extremes." *People*, October 18, 1999.

Snow, Kenneth J. "Hypoglycemia." http://www.emedicine.com/med/topic1123.htm.

Spataro, Sue. "Living with Hypoglycemia." Pinksunrise.com Family Health Center. http://www.families-first.com/whc/hypoglycemia1.htm.

Starlanyl, Devin. "Reactive Hypoglycemia (RHG): FM/MPS Perpetuating Factor." http://www.tidalweb.com/fms/rhg.shtml.

Steffes, Michael W. "Hypoglycemic Disorders." *New England Journal of Medicine* 332 (1995): 1144–52.

Swisher, Natalie. "Healthy Woman: Hungry or Hypoglycemic?" *M&F Hers*. March 2003, 120–21.

Tintera, John. "What You Should Know about Your Glands." Weston A. Price Foundation. http://www.westonaprice.org/archive/archive_tintera.html.

Turner, B., et al. "The Effect of Evening Alcohol Consumption on Next-Morning Glucose Control in Type 1 Diabetes." *Diabetes Care* 24, no. 11 (2001): 1888–93.

UCSF Children's Hospital at UCSF Media Center. "Intensive Care Nursery House Staff Manual: Neo-Natal Hypoglycemia." http://www.ucsfhealth.org/childrens/health_professionals/manuals/52_Hypoglycemia.pdf.

United States National Institutes of Health. "Diagnosing and Treating Low Blood Sugar Levels." http://clinicaltrials.gov/ct/gui/show/NCT00001276;jsessionid=DF576B960DFD9AB94D62B5A2D9F8CDD4?order=1.

Walsh, John. "Tales of the City: The Ups and Downs of Roy and Pam." *Independent*, February 19, 2004.

Weight Loss Control. "How Dieting Influences Your Metabolism." http://www.weightlosscontrol.com/metabolism.htm.

Wesson, Kenneth. "Brain Basics for the Teaching Professional." Sciencemaster. http://www.sciencemaster.com/columns/wesson/wesson_part_05.php.

Wolever, Thomas, et al. "Long-Term Effect of Varying the Source or Amount of Dietary Carbohydrate on Postprandial Plasma Glucose, Insulin, Triacylglycerol, and Free Fatty Acid Concentrations in Subjects with Impaired Glucose Tolerance." *American Journal of Clinical Nutrition* 77, no. 3 (2003): 612–21.

CHAPTER 14: SUGAR'S ROLE IN "THE CHRONIC BIG KILLERS": DIABETES, CANCER, HEART DISEASE, AND OBESITY

Abbassi, F., T. McLaughlin, C. Lamendola, H. S. Kim, A. Tanaka, T. Wang, K. Nakajima, and G. M. Reaven. "High Carbohydrate Diets, Triglycerides-Rich Lipoproteins, and Coronary Heart Disease Risk." *American Journal of Cardiology* 85 (2000): 45–48.

ABC Seven News. "Army of Navajo Families Fights Diabetes," June 17, 2004. http://www.wjla.com/news/stories/0604/153760.html.

American Diabetes Association. "Complications Associated to Type 2 Diabetes." http://www.diabetes.org/type-2-diabetes/complications.jsp.

———. "Diabetes Statistics." http://www.diabetes.org/diabetes-statistics.jsp.

———. "Direct and Indirect Costs of Diabetes in the United States." http://www.diabetes.org/diabetes-statistics/cost-of-diabetes-in-us.jsp.

———. "Identifying Symptoms for Diabetes." http://www.diabetes.org/diabetes-symptoms.jsp.

———. "The Scoop on Sugar." http://www.diabetes.org/youthzone/the-scoop-on-sugar.jsp.

———. "Standards of Medical Care in Diabetes—2006." http://care.diabetesjournals.org/cgi/content/full/29/suppl_1/s4.

———. "Statement Regarding Sugar." http://www.diabetes.org/nutrition-and-recipes/nutrition/sweeteners.jsp.

———. "Sugar and Sugar Substitutes." http://www.diabetes.org/for-parents-and-kids/diabetes-care/sugar.jsp.

American Heart Association. "AHA Scientific Statement, AHA Dietary Guidelines, Revision 2000: A Statement for Healthcare Professionals from the Nutrition Committee of the American Heart Association." http://circ.ahajournals.org/cgi/content/full/102/18/2284.

———. "Dietary Guidelines." http://www.americanheart.org/presenter.jhtml?identifier=1330.

———. "Heart Disease Still No. 1 Killer, 2006 Statistics Update Reports." http://www.americanheart.org/presenter.jhtml?identifier=3038611.

———. "Metabolic Syndrome." http://www.americanheart.org/presenter.jhtml?identifier=4756.

———. "Metabolic Syndrome May Be an Important Link to Stroke," February 6, 2004. http://www.americanheart.org/presenter.jhtml?identifier=3018936.

———. "Profiling High Blood Pressure as a "Silent Killer." http://www.americanheart.org/presenter.jhtml?identifier=2114.

Apovian, Caroline M. "Sugar-Sweetened Soft Drinks, Obesity, and Type 2 Diabetes." Editorial. *JAMA* 292 (2004), 978–79.

Archer, S. L., K. Liu, A. R. Dyer, K. J. Ruth, D. R. Jacobs, Jr., L. Van Horn, J. E. Hilner, and P. J. Savage. "Relationship Between Changes in Dietary Sucrose and High Density Lipoprotein Cholesterol: The CARDIA Study. Coronary Artery Risk Development in Young Adults." *Annals of Epidemiology* 8, no. 7 (1998): 433–38 http://www.ncbi.nlm.nih.gov/entrez/query.fcgi?cmd=retrieve&db=pubmed&list_ uids=9738689&dopt=Abstract.

Augustin, L. S., L. Dal Maso, C. La Vecchia, M. Parpinel, E. Negri, S. Vaccarella, C. W. Kendall, D. J. Jenkins, and S. Francesch. "Dietary Glycemic Index and Glycemic Load, and Breast Cancer Risk: A Case-Control Study." *Annals of Oncology* 12, no. 11 (2001): 1533–38.

Augustin, L. S., S. Gallus, C. Bosetti, F. Levi, E. Negri, S. Franceschi, L. Dal Maso, D. J. Jenkins, C. W. Kendall, and C. La Vecchia. "Glycemic Index and Glycemic Load in Endometrial Cancer." *International Journal of Cancer* 105, no. 3 (2003): 404–7.

Beresford, S. A., et al. "Low-Fat Dietary Pattern and Risk of Colorectal Cancer: The Women's Health Initiative Randomized Controlled Dietary Modification Trial." *Journal of the American Medical Association.* 295, no. 6 (2006): 643–54.

Bernstein, Richard. *Diabetes Solution: The Complete Guide to Achieving Normal Blood Sugars.* Boston: Little Brown and Company, 2003.

Borugian, M. J., S. B. Sheps, A. S. Whittemore, A. H. Wu, J. D. Potter, and R. P. Gallagher. "Carbohydrates and Colorectal Cancer Risk among Chinese in North America." *Cancer Epidemiology, Biomarkers and Prevention* 11, no. 2 (2002): 187–93.

Brehm, B. J., R. J. Seeley, S. R. Daniels, and D. A. D'Alessio. "Weight Loss and Cardiovascular Risk Factors in Healthy Women on a Low Carbohydrate Diet or a Low Fat Diet." *Journal of Clinical Endocrinology and Metabolism* 88, no. 4 (2003): 1617–23.

Brillat-Savarin, Jean Anthelme. *The Physiology of Taste.* France: Author, 1825.

CACRC. "An Interview with Gerald Reaven: Syndrome X: The Risks of Insulin Resistance," September 2000. http://www.cacr.ca/news/2000/0009reaven.htm (accessed March 27, 2005).

Carbohydrate Awareness Council website. http://www.carbaware.org/about/team.htm.

CBS News Online. "60 Minutes: Why Is America So Fat?" July 14, 2004. http://www.cbsnews.com/stories/2004/07/12/60II/main628877.shtml.

Centers for Disease Control and Prevention. National Center for Chronic Disease Prevention and Health Promotion. "National Diabetes Fact Sheet." http://www.cdc.gov/diabetes/pubs/general05.htm#impaired.

———."Profiling the Leading Causes of Death in the United States." http://www.cdc.gov/nccdphp/publications/factsheets/ChronicDisease/pdfs/00_ChronicDieaseAllStates.pdf.

———. National Center for Health Statistics. FastStats A to Z. "Deaths/Mortality." http://www.cdc.gov/nchs/fastats/deaths.htm.

———. FastStats A to Z. "Deaths: Preliminary Data for 2004." http://www.cdc.gov/nchs/products/pubs/pubd/hestats/prelimdeaths04/preliminarydeaths04.htm.

Center for Science in the Public Interest. "America: Drowning in Sugar, Experts Call for Food Labels to Disclose Added Sugars." Press release, August 3, 1999. http://www.cspinet.org/new/sugar.html.

———. "Sugar Consumption 'Off The Charts' Say Health Experts: HHS/USDA Urged to Commission Review of Sugar's Health Impact." Press release, December 30, 1998. http://www.cspinet.org/new/sugar.htm.

Chen, I. H. "Results of the Second National Health and Nutrition Examination Survey (NHANES II)." *Spine* 19, no. 10 (1994): 1193–94.

Children's Hospital Boston. "Hold the Stuffing: Low-Glycemic Diet May Help Keep Weight Off: Dieters Have Higher Metabolism, Feel Less Hungry," Press release, November 23, 2004. http://www.childrenshospital.org/cfapps/CHdeptPagePressDisplay.cfm?Dept=Press%20Room&PageNbr=125&ParentPage=1.

CNN. "Janklow Takes the Stand in His Defense: Says He Remembers Nothing about Fatal Crash," December 6, 2003. http://www.cnn.com/2003/LAW/12/06/janklow.trial.ap/index.html.

———. "Law Center: Janklow to Quit After Manslaughter Verdict: South Dakota Congressman Facing Jail Term," December 10, 2003. http://www.cnn.com/2003/LAW/12/08/janklow.trial.ap/.

Cordain, Loren, Michael R. Eades, and Mary D. Eades. "Hyperinsulinemic Diseases of Civilization: More Than Just Syndrome X." *Comparative Biochemistry and Physiology* Part A 136 (2003): 95–112.

Cordain, Loren, S. Boyd Eaton, Anthony Sebastian, Neil Mann, Staffan Lindeberg, Bruce A. Watkins, James H. O'Keefe, and Janette Brand-Miller. "Commentary: Origins and Evolution of the Western Diet: Health Implications for the 21st Century." Commentary. *American Journal of Clinical Nutrition* 81, no. 2 (2005): 341–54.

Diabetes in Control. "Low-Carb Diet Controls Diabetes Without Weight Loss or Insulin Use." http://www.diabetesincontrol.com/modules.php?name=News&file=article&sid=3601.

Diabetes Prevention Program (DPP). http://diabetes.niddk.nih.gov/dm/pubs/preventionprogram/.

Dominguez, Alex. "Waistline Good Indicator of Diabetes Risk." *AP News Wire*, March 22, 2005. http://life.channels.netscape.ca/life/article.adp?id=20050322131409990011.

Ebbeling, Cara B., Michael M. Leidig, Kelly B. Sinclair, Linda G. Seger-Shippee, Henry A. Feldman, and David S. Ludwig, "Effects of an Ad Libitum Low-Glycemic Load Diet on Cardiovascular Disease Risk Factors in Obese Young Adults." *American Journal of Clinical Nutrition* 81, no. 5 (2005): 976–82.

Engeland, Anders, Tone Bjørge, Anne Johanne Søgaard, and Aage Tverdal. "Body Mass Index in Adolescence in Relation to Total Mortality: 32-Year Follow-Up of 227,000 Norwegian Boys and Girls." *American Journal of Epidemiology* 157 (2003): 517–23. http://aje.oupjournals.org/cgi/content/full/157/6/517-FNI.

Favero A., M. Parpinel, and M. Montella. "Energy Sources and Risk of Cancer of the Breast and Colon-Rectum in Italy." *Advances in Experimental Medicine and Biology* 472 (1999): 51–55.

Ford, E. S., and S. Liu. "Glycemic Index and Serum High-Density Lipoprotein Cholesterol Concentration among U.S. Adults." *Archives of Internal Medicine* 161, no. 4 (2001): 572–76. http://www.ncbi.nlm.nih.gov/entrez/query.fcgi?cmd=Retrieve&db=pubmed&dopt=Abstract&list_uids=11252117&query_hl=10&itool=pubmed_DocSum.

Foster, Gary D., Holly R. Wyatt, James O. Hill, Brian G. McGuckin, Carrie Brill, B. Selma Mohammed, Philippe O. Szapary, Daniel J. Rader, Joel S. Edman, and Samuel Klein. "A Randomized Trial of a Low-Carbohydrate Diet for Obesity." *New England Journal of Medicine* 348, no. 21 (2003): 2082–90.

Fox News. "Janklow Convicted of All Counts in Traffic Death, December 8, 2003. http://www.foxnews.com/story/0,2933,105154,00.html.

Framingham Heart Study. "The Framingham Heart Study." http://www.framingham.com/heart/index.htm.

Franceschi, S., L. Dal Maso, L. Augustin, E. Negri, M. Parpinel, P. Boyle, D. J. Jenkins and C. La Vecchia. "Dietary Glycemic Load and Colorectal Cancer Risk." *Annals of Oncology* 12, no. 2 (2001): 173–78.

Fried, S. K., and S. P. Rao. "Sugars, Hypertriglyceridemia, and Cardiovascular Disease." *American Journal of Clinical Nutrition* 78, no. 4 (2003): 873S-880S. http://www.ncbi.nlm.nih.gov/entrez/query.fcgi?cmd=Retrieve&db=pubmed&dopt=AbstractPlus&list_uids=14522752&query_hl=4&itool=pubmed_DocSum.

Gannon, Mary C., and Frank Q. Nuttall. "Control of Blood Glucose in Type 2 Diabetes Without Weight Loss by Modification of Diet Composition." *Nutrition and Metabolism* 3 (2006): 16.

———. "Effect of a High-Protein, Low-Carbohydrate Diet on Blood Glucose Control in People with Type 2 Diabetes." *Diabetes* 53, no. 9 (2004): 2375–82.

Gaziano, Michael J., Charles H. Hennekens, Christopher J. O'Donnell, Jan L. Breslow, and Julie E. Buring. "Fasting Triglycerides, High-Density Lipoprotein, and Risk of Myocardial Infarction." *Circulation* 96 (1997): 2520–25.

Goodwin, Pamela J., Marguerite Ennis, Kathleen I. Pritchard, Maureen E. Trudeau, Jarley Koo, Yolanda Madarnas, Warren Hartwick, Barry Hoffman, and Nicky Hood. "Fasting Insulin and Outcome in Early-Stage Breast Cancer: Results of a Prospective Cohort Study." *Journal of Clinical Oncology* 20, no. 1 (2002): 42–51.

Gotto, Antonio M., Jr. "Triglyceride: The Forgotten Risk Factor." *Circulation* 97 (1998): 1027–28.

Gray, Liz. "Does the Food Pyramid Diet Lead to Additional Diseases in Diabetics? Research Says . . . Yes." *Native American Times*, April 22, 2004. http://nativetimes.com/index.asp?action=displayarticle&article_id=4329.

Gross, Lee S., Li Li, Earl S. Ford, and Simin Liu. "Increased Consumption of Refined Carbohydrates and the Epidemic of Type 2 Diabetes in the United States: An Ecologic Assessment." *American Journal of Clinical Nutrition* 79 (2004): 774–79.

Harvard School of Public Health. "Frequent Consumption of Sugar-Sweetened Beverages Linked to Greater Weight Gain and Type 2 Diabetes in Women." Press release, August 24, 2004. http://www.hsph.harvard.edu/press/releases/press08242004.html.

Health Professional Follow-Up Study. http://www.hsph.harvard.edu/hpfs/.

Higginbotham, Susan, Zuo-Feng Zhang, I-Min Lee, Nancy R. Cook, Edward Giovannucci, Julie E. Buring, and Simin Liu. "Dietary Glycemic Load and Risk of Colorectal Cancer in the Women's Health Study." *Journal of the National Cancer Institute* 96 (2004): 229–33.

Hitti, Miranda. "High Carb Diet Linked to Breast Cancer: Associations Seen in Study of Mexican Women." WebMD Health website, August 6, 2004. http://my.webmd.com/content/article/92/101647.htm?lastselectedguid=%7B5FE84E90-BC77-4056-A91C-9531713CA348%7D.

Hochgeschwender U., J. L. Costa, P. Reed, S. Bui, and M. B. Brennan. "Altered Glucose Homeostasis in Proopiomelanocortin-Null Mouse Mutants Lacking Central and Peripheral Melanocortin." *Endocrinology* 114, no. 12 (2003): 5194–5202.

Hodge A. M., D. R. English, K. O'Dea, and G. G. Giles. "Glycemic Index and Fiber as Risk Factors for Type 2 Diabetes in the MCCS." *Diabetes Care* 27, no. 11 (2004): 2701–6.

———. "Increased Diabetes Incidence in Greek and Italian Migrants to Australia: How Much Can Be Explained by Known Risk Factors." *Diabetes Care* 27, no. 10 (2004): 2330–34.

Howard, B. V., et al. "Low-Fat Dietary Pattern and Risk of Cardiovascular Disease: The Women's Health Initiative Randomized Controlled Dietary Modification Trial." *JAMA* 295, no. 6 (2006): 655–66.

———. "Low-Fat Dietary Pattern and Weight Change Over 7 Years: The Women's Health Initiative Dietary Modification Trial." *JAMA* 295, no. 1 (2006): 39–49.

Howard, Barbara V., and Judith Wylie Rosett. "Sugar and Cardiovascular Disease: A Statement for Healthcare Professionals from the Committee on Nutrition of the Council on Nutrition, Physical Activity, and Metabolism of the American Heart Association." *Circulation* 106 (2002): 523–27.

James, Janet, Peter Thomas, David Cavan, and David Kerr. "Preventing Childhood Obesity by Reducing Consumption of Carbonated Drinks: Cluster Randomized Controlled Trial." *British Medical Journal* 328 (2004): 1237–41.

Jeppesen, Jørgen, Hans Ole Hein, Poul Suadicani, and Finn Gyntelberg. "Triglyceride Concentration and Ischemic Heart Disease: An Eight-Year Follow-Up in the Copenhagen Male Study." *Circulation* 97 (1998): 1029–36.

Liu, Simin, et al. "A Prospective Study of Dietary Glycemic Load, Carbohydrate Intake, and Risk of Coronary Heart Disease in U.S. Women." *American Journal of Clinical Nutrition* 71 (2000): 1455–61.

Liu, Simin, JoAnn E. Manson, Julie E. Buring, Meir J. Stampfer, Walter C. Willett, and Paul M. Ridker. "Nutritional Status, Dietary Intake, and Body Composition: Relation Between a Diet with a High Glycemic Load and Plasma Concentrations of High-Sensitivity C-Reactive Protein in Middle-Aged Women." *American Journal of Clinical Nutrition* 75 (March 2002): 492–98.

Liu, Simin, JoAnn E. Manson, Meir J. Stampfer, Michelle D. Holmes, Frank B. Hu, Susan E. Hankinson, and Walter C. Willett. "Carbohydrate Metabolism and Diabetes: Dietary Glycemic Load Assessed by Food-Frequency Questionnaire in Relation to Plasma High-Density-Lipoprotein Cholesterol and Fasting Plasma Triacylglycerols in Postmenopausal Women." *American Journal of Clinical Nutrition* 73 (2001): 560–66.

Liu, Simin, Walter C. Willett, Meir J. Stampfer, Frank B. Hu, Mary Franz, Laura Sampson, Charles H. Hennekens, and JoAnn E. Manson. "Lipids and Cardiovascular Risks: A Prospective Study of Dietary Glycemic Load, Carbohydrate Intake, and Risk of Coronary Heart Disease in U.S. Women." *American Journal of Clinical Nutrition* 71, no. 6 (2000): 1455–61.

Lombardo Y. B., S. Drago, A. Chicco, P. Fainstein-Day, R. Gutman, J. J. Gagliardino, and C. L. Gomez Dumm. "Long-Term Administration of a Sucrose-Rich Diet to Normal Rats: Relationship Between Metabolic and Hormonal Profiles and Morphological Changes in the Endocrine Pancreas." *Metabolism* 45, no. 12 (1996): 1527–32.

McKeown, Nicola M., James B. Meigs, Simin Liu, Edward Saltzman, Peter W. F. Wilson, and Paul F. Jacques. "Metabolic Syndrome/Insulin Resistance Syndrome/Pre-Diabetes: Carbohydrate Nutrition,

Insulin Resistance, and the Prevalence of the Metabolic Syndrome in the Framingham Offspring Cohort." *Diabetes Care* 27 (2004): 538–46.

Medical News Today. "Men with Cardiovascular Disease May Be at Considerably Increased Risk for Death Even When Their Blood Sugar Level Remains in the 'Normal' Range." http://www.medicalnewstoday.com/medicalnews.php?newsid=37730.

Mercola.com. "Sugar and Cancer." http://www.mercola.com/2000/oct/8/sugar_cancer.htm.

———. "High Triglycerides Risk for Heart Attack." http://www.mercola.com/1998/archive/triglycerides_risk_for_heart_attack.htm.

———. "Triglycerides May Predict Heart Risk." http://www.mercola.com/1997/archive/heart_risk.htm.

Meyer, Katie A., Lawrence H. Kushi, David R. Jacobs, Jr., Joanne Slavin, Thomas A. Sellers, and Aaron R. Folsom. "Carbohydrate Metabolism and Diabetes: Carbohydrates, Dietary Fiber, and Incident Type 2 Diabetes in Older Women." *American Journal of Clinical Nutrition* 71 (April 2000): 921–30.

Michaud, Dominique S., Simin Liu, Edward Giovannucci, Walter C. Willett, Graham A. Colditz, and Charles S. Fuchs. "Dietary Sugar, Glycemic Load, and Pancreatic Cancer Risk in a Prospective Study." *Journal of the National Cancer Institute* 94, no. 17 (2002): 1293–1300.

Moerman C. J., H. B. Bueno de Mesquita, and S. Runia. "Dietary Sugar Intake in the Aetiology of Biliary Tract Cancer." *International Journal of Epidemiology* 22, no. 2 (1993): 207–14.

Moss, Ralph. *The Cancer Zone.* http://www.thecancerzone.com/civ.html.

———. "The Pima Indians, Obesity and Diabetes." http://diabetes.niddk.nih.gov/dm/pubs/pima/obesity/obesity.htm.

Nakagawa, T., H. Hu, S. Zharikov, K. R. Tuttle, R. A. Short, O. Glushakova, X. Ouyang, D. I. Feig, E. R. Block, J. Herrera-Acosta, J. M. Patel, and R. J. Johnson. "A Causal Role for Uric Acid in Fructose-Induced Metabolic Syndrome." *American Journal of Physiology—Renal Physiology* (October 18, 2005), doi:10.1152/ajprenal.00140.2005.

National Diabetes Fact Sheet, 2005. http://diabetes.org/uedocuments/NationalDiabetesFactSheetRev.pdf.

National Diabetes Information Clearinghouse. "The Pima Indians, Pathfinders for Health." http://diabetes.niddk.nih.gov/dm/pubs/pima/index.htm.

National Health and Nutrition Examination Survey. "Prevalence and Associated Risk Factor Findings in the U.S. Population from the 3rd National Health and Nutrition Examination Survey, 1998–1994." *Annals of Internal Medicine* 2003, no. 163: 427–36.

Nurses' Health Study I. http://www.channing.harvard.edu/nhs/history/index.shtml#histI.

Nurses' Health Study II. http://www.channing.harvard.edu/nhs/history/index.shtml#histII.

Oglesby, Alan K., et al. "The Association Between Diabetes Related Medical Costs and Glycemic Control: A Retrospective Analysis." *Cost Effectiveness and Resource Allocation* 4 (2006). http://www.pubmedcentral.nih.gov/articlerender.fcgi?artid=1369002.

Park, Y. W., S. Zhu, L. Palaniappan, S. Heshka, M. R. Carnethon, and S. Heymsfield. "The Metabolic Syndrome: Prevalence and Associated Risk Factor Findings in the U.S. Population from the Third National Health and Nutrition Examination Survey, 1988–1994." *Archives of Internal Medicine* 163, no. 4 (2003): 427–36.

Pereira, Mark, Janis Swain, Allison B. Goldfine, Nader Rifai, and David S. Ludwig. "Effects of a Low-Glycemic Load Diet on Resting Energy Expenditure and Heart Disease Risk Factors During Weight Loss." *JAMA* 292 (2004): 2482–90.

Port, Sidney C., Noel G. Boyle, Willa A. Hsueh, Manuel J. Quiñones, Robert I. Jennrich, and Mark O. Goodarzi. "The Predictive Role of Blood Glucose for Mortality in Subjects with Cardiovascular Disease." *American Journal of Epidemiology* 163, no. 4 (2006): 342–51; doi:10.1093/aje/kwj027.

PR Web. "Light Bulbs and Low-Carb Diets." http://www.prweb.com/releases/2005/11/prweb311399.htm.

Prentice, R. L., et al. "Low-Fat Dietary Pattern and Risk of Invasive Breast Cancer: The Women's Health Initiative Randomized Controlled Dietary Modification Trial." *JAMA* 295, no. 6 (2006): 629–42.

Reich, J. "Iatrogenic Causes Blamed for 3rd Leading Cause of Death Deficiencies in U.S. Medical Care." *JAMA* 284, no. 17 (2001): 2184–85.

Reinberg, Steven. "Diet with the 'Right Carbs' Seems to Boost Health: Low-Glycemic-Index Plan Is Better Than Low-Fat or Low-Carb Diets, Study Says." HealthDay, August 26, 2004. http://www.healthday.com/view.cfm?id=520863.

Romieu, Isabelle, Eduardo Lazcano-Ponce, Luisa Maria Sanchez-Zamorano, Walter Willett, and Mauricio Hernandez-Avila. "Carbohydrates and the Risk of Breast Cancer among Mexican Women." *Cancer Epidemiology Biomarkers and Prevention* 13 (2004): 1283–89.

Samaha, Frederick F., Nayyar Iqbal, Prakash Seshadri, Kathryn L. Chicano, Denise A. Daily, Joyce McGrory, Terrence Williams, Monica Williams, Edward J. Gracely, and Linda Stern. "A Low-Carbohydrate as Compared with a Low-Fat Diet in Severe Obesity." *New England Journal of Medicine* 348, no. 21 (2003): 2074–81.

Sanders, T. A. "High- versus Low-Fat Diets in Human Diseases." *Current Opinion in Clinical Nutrition and Metabolic Care* 6, no. 2 (2003): 151–55.

Sanjoaquin, M. A., P. N. Appleby, M. Thorogood, J. I. Mann, and T. J. Key. "Nutrition, Lifestyle and Colorectal Cancer Incidence: A Prospective Investigation of 10,998 Vegetarians and Non-vegetarians in the United Kingdom." *British Journal of Cancer* 90, no. 1 (2004): 118–21.

Saydah, S. H., Catherine M. Loria, Mark S. Eberhardt, and Frederick L. Brancati. "Abnormal Glucose Tolerance and the Risk of Cancer Death in the United States." *American Journal of Epidemiology* 157, no. 12 (2003): 1092–1100.

Schulze, Matthias B., Simin Liu, Eric B. Rimm, JoAnn E. Manson, Walter C. Willett, and Frank B Hu. "Carbohydrate Metabolism and Diabetes: Glycemic Index, Glycemic Load, and Dietary Fiber Intake and Incidence of Type 2 Diabetes in Younger and Middle-Aged Women." *American Journal of Clinical Nutrition* 80 (August 2004): 348–56.

Schulze, Matthias B., JoAnn E. Manson, David S. Ludwig, Graham A. Colditz, Meir J. Stampfer, Walter C. Willett, and Frank B. Hu. "Sugar-Sweetened Beverages, Weight Gain, and Incidence of Type 2 Diabetes in Young and Middle-Aged Women." *JAMA* 292, no. 8 (2004): 927–34.

Second National Health and Nutrition Examination Survey. http://www.cdc.gov/nchs/data/series/sr_01/sr01_038.pdf.

Sheard, N., et al. "Dietary Carbohydrate (Amount and Type) in the Prevention and Management of Diabetes." *Diabetes Care* 27 (2004): 2266–71.

Shim, Hyunsuk, Yoon S. Chun, Brian C. Lewis, and Chi V. Dang. "A Unique Glucose-Dependent Apoptotic Pathway Induced by c-Myc." *Proceedings from the National Academy of Sciences, USA* 95, no. 4 (1998): 1511–16.

Siegler, Bonnie. *Diabetes.* Interview with Halle Berry. Third quarter 2003, 8.

———. "Halle Berry: My Battle with Diabetes." *Daily News,* December 13, 2005. http://www.daily-mail.co.uk/pages/live/articles/health/healthmain.html?in_article_id=371528&in_page_id=1774.

Silink, Martin. Keynote address, Rotary District 9830, Hobart College, March 3, 2006. http://lanecove.rotarnet.com.au/Rotacove%2030%20May%2006.pdf.

Silvera, S. A., M. Jain, G. R. Howe, A. B. Miller, and T. E Rohan. "Dietary Carbohydrates and Breast Cancer Risk: A Prospective Study of the Roles of Overall Glycemic Index and Glycemic Load." *International Journal of Cancer* 114, no. 4 (2005): 653–58.

Slaughter, Adele. "Patti LaBelle Sings Out about Diabetes Danger." *USA Today,* November 28, 2001. http://www.usatoday.com/news/health/spotlight/2001-11-28-labelle-diabetes.htm.

Slyper, Arnold, Jason Jurva, Joan Pleuss, Raymond Hoffmann, and David Gutterman. "Origonal Research Communication: Influence of Glycemic Load on HDL Cholesterol in youth." *American Journal of Clinical Nutrition* 81, no. 2 (2005): 376–79.

Stefansson, Vilhjamur. *Cancer: A Disease of Civilization?* New York: Hill and Wang, 1960.

Tauber, Michelle, Julie Jordan, and David J. Searls. "The 50 Most Beautiful People 2003: Halle Berry." *Time*, May 12, 2003, 72.

Trager, Stuart. "Statement by Stuart Trager, M. D., Chair, Atkins Physicians Council on February 10, 2004, Report on Dr. Atkins Weight at the Time of His Death." Neil Rogers Show website. http://news.neilrogers.com/news/articles/2004021102.html.

U.S. Census Bureau. "U.S. Population Passes 290 Million: Mountain and Coastal States Fastest-Growing." Press release, December 18, 2003. http://www.census.gov/PressRelease/www/releases/archives/population/001624.html.

Warburg, Otto. "On the Origin of Cancer Cells." *Science* 123, no. 3191 (1956): 309–14.

Willett, Walter, JoAnn Manson, and Simin Liu. "Glycemic Index, Glycemic Load, and Risk of Type 2 Diabetes." *American Journal of Clinical Nutrition* 76, no. 1: 274S–280S. July 2002. Presented at a symposium held at Experimental Biology 2001, Orlando, Florida, April 1, 2001.

Wolever, T. M., and D. J. Jenkins. "The Use of the Glycemic Index in Predicting the Blood Glucose Response to Mixed Meals." *American Journal of Clinical Nutrition* 43 (1986): 167–72.

Wolever, T. M., D. J. Jenkins, V. Vuksan, A. L. Jenkins, G. S. Wong, and R. G Josse. "Beneficial Effect of Low-Glycemic Index Diet in Overweight NIDDM Subjects." *Diabetes Care* 15 (1992): 562–64.

World Health Organization website. "Diabetes: The Cost of Diabetes," September 2002. http://www.who.int/mediacentre/factsheets/fs236/en/.

Yang, Eun Ju, Jean M. Kerver, Yi Kyung Park, Jean Kayitsinga, David B. Allison, and Won O. Song. "Carbohydrate Intake and Biomarkers of Glycemic Control among U.S. Adults: The Third National Health and Nutrition Examination Survey (NHANES III)." *American Journal of Clinical Nutrition* 77, no. 6 (2003): 1426–33.

Yudkin, John. *Sweet and Dangerous*. New York: Bantam Books, 1979.

Zack, Jinny, and W. D. Currier. *Sugar Isn't Always Sweet: Living With, Understanding, and Managing Hypoglycemia*. Brea, CA: Uplift Books, 1983.

CHAPTER 15: *FOR WOMEN ONLY*: TOO MUCH SUGAR CAN AFFECT FERTILITY, PMS, AND MENOPAUSE

Appleton, Nancy. *Lick the Sugar Habit Sugar Counter: Discover the Hidden Sugar in Your Food*. New York: Avery/Penguin Putnam, 2001.

Arthritis Foundation. "What's in a Name: Fibro vs. CFS." http://www.arthritis.org/resources/news/news_fibro_cfs.asp.

Augustin, L. S., et al. "Glycemic Index and Glycemic Load in Endometrial Cancer." *International Journal of Cancer* 105, no. 3 (2003): 404–7.

Centers for Disease Control and Prevention. "Candidiasis," December 2003. http://www.cdc.gov/ncidod/dbmd/diseaseinfo/candidiasis_t.htm.

CFIDS Association of America Website. http://cfids.org/profresources/media.asp.

Cordain, L., et al. "Hyperinulemic Diseases of Civilization: More Than Just Syndrome." *Comparative Biochemistry and Physiology*, Part A, June 20, 2003.

Daniells, Stephen. "Low-Carb Diet May Help Women with Ovary Problems." http://www.nutraingredients.com/news/ng.asp?n=67217-pcos-low-carb-diabetes.

Douglas, C. C., B. A. Gower, B. E. Darnell, F. Ovalle, R. A. Oster, and R. Azziz. "Role of Diet in the Treatment of Polycystic Ovary Syndrome." *Fertility and Sterility* 85, no. 3 (2006): 679–88.

Dye, L., and J. E. Blundell. "Menstrual Cycle and Appetite Control: Implications for Weight Regulation." *Human Reproduction* 12, no. 6 (1997): 1142–51.

Dye, L., P. Warner, and J. Bancroft. "Food Craving During the Menstrual Cycle and Its Relationship to Stress, Happiness or Relationship and Depression: A Preliminary Enquiry." *Journal of Affective Disorder* 34 (1995): 157–64.

Endicott, Jean. *Premenstrual Changes, Syndromes, and Disorders.* National Institute of Mental Health (January 1, 1986).

Endometriosis Association. "What Is Endometriosis?" http://www.endometriosisassn.org/endo.html.

Feinberg, Ronald. *Healing Syndrome O: A Strategic Guide to Fertility, Polycystic Ovaries, and Insulin Imbalance.* New York: Penguin, 2004.

Hetherington, Marion. *Food Cravings and Addiction.* Leatherhead, Surrey, England: Leatherhead Food International, 2001.

InterNational Council on Infertility Information Dissemination, Inc., website. http://www.inciid.org/faq.php?cat=infertility101&id=2#68.

Kittel, Mary. *Stay Fertile Longer.* With Deborah Metzger. Emmaus, PA: Rodale Books, 2004, 244.

"Low-Carb Diet May Help Women with Ovary Problems." http://www.nutraingredients.com/news/ng.asp?n=67217-pcos-low-carb-diabetesdup.

Lowcarbezine website. "Low Carb and Fertility Continued," August 3, 2004. http://www.holdthetoast.com/httblog/archives/000009.html.

Mayo Clinic website. http://www.mayoclinic.com.

Mercer, M., and M. Holder. "Food Cravings, Endogenous Opioid Peptides, and Food Intake: A Review." *Appetite* 29, no. 3 (1997): 325–52.

Michener, Q., et al. "The Role of Low Progesterone and Tension as Triggers of Premenstrual Chocolate and Sweets Craving: Some Negative Experimental Evidence." *Physiology and Behavior* 67, no. 3 (1999): 417–20.

National Institute of Allergy and Infectious Diseases. "Chronic Fatigue Syndrome," May 2004. http:\\www.niaid.nih.gov/factsheets/cfs.htm.

National Women's Health Information Center. "Vaginal Yeast Infections," July 2002. http://www.4woman.gov/faq/yeastinfect.htm.

Prevention's Ultimate Guide to Women's Health and Wellness. Emmaus, PA: Rodale Books, 2002.

Shaw, G., et al. "Neural Tube Defects Associated with Maternal Periconceptional Dietary Intake of Simple Sugars and Glycemic Index." *American Journal of Clinical Nutrition* 78, no. 5 (2003): 972–78.

Somer, Elizabeth. *Food and Mood: The Complete Guide to Eating Well and Feeling Your Best.* New York: Henry Holt 1999.

Teitlebaum, J., et al. "Effective Treatment of Chronic Fatigue Syndrome and Fibromyalgia—A Randomized Double-Blind, Placebo-Controlled, Intent to Treat Study." *Journal of Chronic Fatigue Syndrome* 8 (2001).

Wagner, John J., and Charles I. Chavkin. "Neuropharmacology of Endogenous Opioid Peptides." http://www.acnp.org/g4/GN401000050/CH050.html.

Wurtman, J. J. "Depression and Weight Gain: The Serotonin Connection." *Journal of Affective Disorders* 29 (1993): 183–92.

CHAPTER 16: *FOR YOUR BEAUTY*: SUGAR GLUTTING COULD GIVE YOU PIMPLES, WRINKLES, AND MORE

Centers for Disease Control and Prevention. "Disease Information: Candidiasis." www.cdc.gov/ncidod/dbmd/diseaseinfo/candidiasis_g.htm.

Cordain, Loren. "Cereal Grains: Humanity's Double-Edged Sword." *World Reverend Nutritional Diet* 84 (1999): 19–73.

———. "Omega-3 Fatty Acids and Acne—Reply." *Archives of Dermatology* 139 (July 2003): 942–43.

Cordain, Loren, et al. "Hyperinsulinemic Diseases of Civilization: More Than Just Syndrome X." 136, no. 1 (2003): 95–112.

Cordain, Loren, Staffan Lindeberg, Magdalena Hurtado, Kim Hill, S. Boyd Eaton, and Jennie Brand-Miller. "Acne Vulgaris: A Disease of Western Civilization." *Archives of Dermatology* 138 (December 2002): 1584–90.

James, Kat. "Hair Today, Gone Tomorrow: Control Your Hair Loss Naturally." *Better Nutrition*, April 2003.

Melton, Lisa. "Age Breakers: Rupturing the Body's Sugar Protein Bonds Might Turn Back the Clock." *Scientific American*, July 2000.

Mercola, Joseph. "Bread May Be the Culprit Behind Acne." *Archives of Dermatology*, December 2002. http://www.mercola.com/2002/dec/25/bread_acne.htm.

Pearson, Helen. "Chips Means Zits? Study Supports Belief That Diet Is to Blame for Adolescent Acne." *Nature Science Update*, December 2, 2002.

Purba, Martalena, Antigone Kouris-Blazos, Naiyana Wattanapenpaiboon, et al. "Skin Wrinkling: Can Food Make a Difference?" *Journal of the American College of Nutrition* 20, no. 1 (2001): 71–80. http://www.jacn.org/cgi/content/full/20/1/71.

RMIT University. "Big Brother Scenario Set to Tackle Acne Problem." Press release, December 19, 2003. http://www.rmit.edu.au/browse;ID=tce1y9d2448r1;STATUS=A?QRY=big%20brother%20scenario&STYPE=ENTIRE.

———. "Extreme Diets Not the Answer." Press Release, November 3, 2003. http://www.rmit.edu.au/browse;ID=lsilxfoap2on;STATUS=A?QRY=Neil%20Mann&STYPE=ENTIRE.

———. "Researchers to Study Spotty Problem." Press release, December 4, 2002. http://www.rmit.edu.au/browse;ID=povym33ol5691;STATUS=A?QRYNeil%20Mann&STYPE=ENT.

———. "RMIT Study to Ease Teenage Acne Blues." Press release, February 13, 2004. http://www.rmit.edu.au/browse;ID=akojxfmz30vtz;STATUS=A?QRY=Neil%20Mann&STYPE=ENTIRE.

———. "Young Male Volunteers Needed for Pimple Study." Press release, June 2, 2003. http://www.rmit.edu.au/browse;ID=2jrk0spt1xb1;STATUS=A?QRY=Department%20of%20Food%20.

CHAPTER 17: *FOR PARENTS*: HELP YOUR YOUNG SUGAR BRATS END THEIR FITS OF FURY

Appleton, Nancy. *Lick the Sugar Habit*. Garden City Park, New York: Avery, 1996. Originally published as *Lick the Sugar Habit, Not the Candy Bar*. Santa Monica, CA: N. Appleton, 1985. Special thanks to Dr. Appleton for the "Close to Home" cartoon by John McPherson, p. 148. Close to Home © 1993 John McPherson. *Lick the Sugar Habit* reprinted the cartoon with permission of Universal Press Syndicate.

———. *Stopping Inflammation: Relieving the Cause of Degenerative Diseases*. Garden City Park, NY: Square One Publishers, 2005.

Chen, M. Y., and J. C. Liao. "Relationship Between Attendance at Breakfast and School Achievement among Nursing Students." *Journal of Nursing Research* 10, no. 1 (2002): 15–21.

Child Trends. "Guide to Effective Programs for Children and Youth: Child and Adolescent Trial for

Cardiovascular Health (CATCH)," December 31, 2001. http://www.childtrends.org/Lifecourse/programs/ChildandAdolesentTrialforCardiovascularHealth.htm.

DesMaisons, Kathleen. *Little Sugar Addicts: End the Mood Swings, Meltdowns, Tantrums, and Low Self-Esteem in Your Child Today*. New York: Three Rivers Press, 2004.

Donnelly, Shannon. "Let's Heal Ourselves: Actress Brings Anecdotes of Tragedy, Hope to HOW." Interview with Marilu Henner. *Palm Beach Daily News*, January 30, 2005.

Hayman, Laura L., Christine L. Williams, Stephen R. Daniels, Julia Steinberger, Steve Paridon, Barbara A. Dennison, and Brian W. McCrindle. "Cardiovascular Health Promotion in the Schools: A Statement for Health and Education Professionals and Child Health Advocates from the Committee on Atherosclerosis, Hypertension, and Obesity in Youth (AHOY) of the Council on Cardiovascular Disease in the Young, American Heart Association." *Circulation* 110, no. 15 (2004): 2266–75.

Hypoglycemia Support Foundation website. http://www.hypoglyecemia.org.

Luepker, R. V., C. L. Perry, S. M. McKinlay, P. R. Nader, G. S. Parcel, E. J. Stone, L. S. Webber, J. P. Elder, H. A. Feldman, C. C. Johnson, S. H. Kelder, and M. Wu. "Outcomes of a Field Trial to Improve Children's Dietary Patterns and Physical Activity: The Child and Adolescent Trial for Cardiovascular Health (CATCH)." *JAMA* 275, no. 10 (1996): 768–76.

McGinnis, Marianne. "Hold the Sugar: Kids Are Consuming Way More Than Is Healthy." *Prevention*, January 2005.

Nader, P. R., E. J. Stone, L. A. Lytle, C. L. Perry, S. K. Osganian, S. Kelder, L. S. Webber, J. P. Elder, D. Montgomery, H. A. Feldman, M. Wu, C. Johnson, G. S. Parcel, and R. V. Luepker. "Three-Year Maintenance of Improved Diet and Physical Activity: The CATCH Cohort." *Archives of Pediatrics and Adolescent Medicine* 153, no. 7 (1999): 695–704.

Perry, C. L., D. E. Sellers, C. Johnson, S. Pedersen, K. J. Bachman, G. S. Parcel, E. J. Stone, R. V. Luepker, M. Wu, P. R. Nader, and K. Cook. "The Child and Adolescent Trial for Cardiovascular Health (CATCH): Intervention, Implementation, and Feasibility for Elementary Schools in the United States." *Health Education and Behavior* 24, no. 6 (1997): 716–35.

Rapp, Doris. *Allergies and the Hyperactive Child*. New York: Simon and Schuster, 1980.

———. *Is This Your Child? Discovering and Treating Unrecognized Allergies*. New York: William Morrow, 1991.

———. *Our Toxic World: A Wake-Up Call*. Buffalo, New York: Environmental Medical Research Foundation, 2004.

Ruggiero, Roberta. *The Do's and Don'ts of Hypoglycemia: An Everyday Guide to Low Blood Sugar*. Hollywood, FL: Frederick Fell, 2003.

Schwartz, Marlene, Eunice Y. Chen, and Kelly D. Brownell. "Trick, Treat, or Toy: Children Are Just as Likely to Choose Toys as Candy on Halloween." *Journal of Nutrition, Education and Behavior* 35, no. 4 (2003): 207–9.

Smith, Lendon. *Feed Your Kids Right*. New York: Dell, 1981.

CHAPTER 19: WITHOUT SUGAR, WHAT'S LEFT TO EAT? PLENTY!

Environmental Protection Agency. "Management Measures for Agricultural Sources." http://www.epa.gov/nps/MMGI/Chapter2/ch2-1.html.

Environmental Working Group. "Overexposed: Organophosphate Insecticides in Children's Food." http://www.ewg.org/reports_content/ops/download.pdf.

———. "Report Card: Pesticides in Produce." http://www.foodnews.org/reportcard.php.

———. "They Are What They Eat: Kids' Food Consumption and Pesticides." http://www.ewg.org/reports_content/apples/kidseat.pdf.

"Natural and Organic Claims." Letter to producers from Robert C. Post, Director, Labeling and Additives Policy Division, Food Safety and Inspection Service, United States Department of Agriculture, March 8, 1999. http://www.fsis.usda.gov/OPPDE/larc/Claims/Organic_Claims.htm.

Organic Trade Association. "Nutritional Considerations." http://www.ota.com/organic/benefits/nutrition.html.

———. "10 Good Reasons to Go Organic," http://ota.com/organic_and_you/10reasons.html.

Whole Foods Market. "Majority of Americans Are Unaware Most Meat and Poultry Is Raised with Antibiotics, Growth Hormones; Nationwide Survey Shows Americans Want Term 'Natural' Meat to Mean No Antibiotics, Hormones, By-Products." http://www.wholefoodsmarket.com/company/ pr_06-01-04.html.

CHAPTER 20: TOP 10 FOOD-LABEL MISCONCEPTIONS ABOUT SWEETENERS

American Diabetes Association. "Evidence-Based Nutrition Principles and Recommendations for the Treatment and Prevention of Diabetes and Related Complications." Position statement. *Diabetes Care* 25 (2002): 148–98.

Appleton, Nancy. *Lick the Sugar Habit Sugar Counter: Discover the Hidden Sugar in Your Food.* New York: Avery, 1996.

Arizona State University East National Food and Agricultural Policy Project. "Slotting Fees: Symptom of a More Fundamental Problem?" March 2001. http://nfapp.east.asu.edu/policy/2001/04/pb01-04.htm.

Armenian Medical Network. "How to Read Food Labels." www.dental.am/eng/diet/5.html.

Biermann, June, and Barbara Toohey. *The Diabetic's Book.* New York: Perigee Books, 1992.

Brecher, S. J., M. M. Bender, V. L. Wilkening, et al. "Status of Nutrition Labeling, Health Claims, and Nutrient Content Claims for Processed Foods: 1997 Food Label and Package Survey." *Journal of American Dietetic Association* 100 (2000): 1057–62.

Browne, Mona Boyd. *Label Facts for Healthful Eating.* Dayton, OH: The Mazer Corporation, 1993.

Burger King website. www.burgerking.com.

Challem, Jack. "Fructose: Maybe Not So Natural . . . and Not So Safe." *Nutrition Reporter.* http://www.thenutritionreporter.com/fructose_dangers.html.

Center for Science in the Public Interest. "America: Drowning in Sugar—Experts Call for Food Labels to Disclose Added Sugars." Press release, August 3, 1999. http://www.cspinet.org/new/sugar.html.

———. "Consumer Group Petitions FDA to Require 'Diarrhea' Notice on Foods That Contain Sorbitol." Press release, September 27, 1999. http://www.cspinet.org/new/sorbitol_pr.html.

———. "Petition to the FDA to Require Better Sugar Labeling on Foods." http://64.233.161.104/search?q=cache:u3LhCWPOT8IJ:www.cspinet.org/reports/sugar/sugarpet1.pdf+Ronald+Krauss,+head+of+Molecular+Medicine+at+Lawrence+Berkeley+Laboratories+in+California+and+triglycerides+part+of+the+Missing+&hl=en&ie=UTF-8.

———. "Request for Regulatory Action to Prohibit Misleading Claims by the J.M. Smucker Company," May 13, 2003. http://cspinet.org/new/pdf/smuckers_complaint.pdf.

———. "Smucker's Spreading Deception, Says CSI," May 13, 2003. http://www.cspinet.org/new/200305131.html.

Child Health Alert newsletter. Vol. 16, September 1997. www.childhealthalert.com/newsletters/sep97.htm.

CNN.com. "Adding Nutrition Info to Menus Considered," February 21, 2005. http://www.cnn.com/2005/HEALTH/diet.fitness/02/21/nutrition.labels.ap/index.html.

Dannon Company website. http://www.dannon.com/dn/dnstore/cgi-bin/ProdSubEV_Cat_240859_SubCat_261774_NavRoot_200.htm.

DesMaisons, Kathleen. *Potatoes, Not Prozac*. New York: Simon & Schuster, 1999.

Duyff, Roberta Larson. *American Dietetic Association Complete Food and Nutrition Guide*. 2nd ed. Hoboken, NJ: John Wiley & Sons, 2002.

Federal Register. Vol. 65, June 26, 2000. http://www.accessdata.fda.gov/scripts/oc/ohrms/dailylist.cfm?yr=2000&mn=6&dy=26.

Federal Trade Commission. "Slotting Allowances and the Antitrust Laws." Testimony presented by Williard K. Tom, October 29, 1999. http://www.ftc.gov/os/1999/10/slotting991020.htm (accessed January 11, 2005).

Finke, Michael. "Did the Nutrition Labeling and Education Act Affect Food Choices in the United States?" Selected conference paper. *The American Consumer and the Changing Structure of the Food System*. Economic Research Service, USDA, May 4–5, 2000, Arlington, VA.

Finke, Michael S., and D. Weaver. "The Relationship Between the Use of Sugar Content Information on Nutrition Labels and the Consumption of Added Sugars." *Food Policy* 28, no. 3 (2003): 213–19(7).

Fischer, Howard. "Smucker's Mislabels Its Spread, Suit Claims." *Arizona Daily Star*, July 24, 2004. http://www.dailystar.com/dailystar/relatedarticles/31286.php.

Food and Nutrition Board. Dietary Reference Intakes for Energy, Carbohydrate, Fiber, Fat, Fatty Acids, Cholesterol, Protein, and Amino Acids (Macronutrients). Washington, DC: National Academies Press, 2002. http://books.nap.edu/books/0309085373/html/209.html#pagetop (accessed January 19, 2005).

Foodintol.com. "The Trouble with Sugar Free: How Sorbitol Causes Irritable Bowel Syndrome," August 25, 2003. http://www.foodintol.com/food_intolerance/hot_ibs.htm (accessed January 19, 2005).

Forristal, Linda Joyce. "In the Kitchen with Mother Linda: The Murky World of HFCS." *Wise Traditions in Food, Farming and the Healing Arts*, fall 2001. http://www.westonaprice.org/motherlinda/cornsyrup.html#forristal.

Fuchs, Nan Kathryn. *The Nutrition Detective: A Woman's Guide to Treating Your Health Problems through the Foods You Eat*. Los Angeles: Jeremy P. Tarcher, 1985.

Galles, Gary A. "The Market for Space in the Market." *The Freeman* 50, no. 3 (2000). http://www.libertyhaven.com/theoreticalorphilosophicalissues/economics/economicissues/marketspace.shtml (accessed January 10, 2005).

Gittleman, Ann Louise. *Get the Sugar Out: 501 Simple Ways to Cut the Sugar Out of Any Diet*. New York: Three Rivers Press, 1996.

Hyams, Jeffrey S., N. L. Etienne, A. M. Leichtner, et al. "Carbohydrate Malabsorption Following Fruit Juice Ingestion in Young Children." *Pediatrics*, July 1988, 64–68.

International Food Information Council. "Sugar and Low-Calorie Sweeteners." www.ific.org/nutrition/sugars/index.cfm.

International Jelly and Preserve Association. "How Fruitspreads Measure Up." http://www.jelly.org/spreadcalc.html.

KidsHealth. "Figuring Out Food Labels." http://kidshealth.org/kid/stay_healthy/food/labels.html (accessed January 11, 2005).

Kraft Foods website. "Low-Fat Wheat Thins—Nutrition Information." http://www.kraftfoods.com/main.aspx?s=product&m=product/product_display&u3=******4400000013**.

Letter to Joe Levitt, Director of the Center for Food Safety and Applied Nutrition at the Food and Drug Administration. "Re: Request for Regulatory Action to Prohibit Misleading Labeling Claims by the J.M. Smucker Company," May 13, 2003.

Lifeclinic website. http://www.lifeclinic.com/focus/nutrition/food-label.asp. Accessed January 30, 2004.

Loeb, Neal, of Watertown, Wisconsin, individually and on behalf of all other Wisconsin consumers similarly situated, v. J.M. Smucker Co. in Orrville, Ohio. Complaint. Case No. 03CV2641, Case Code 30703.

National Heart, Lung and Blood Institute. "Tipsheet—Reading Food Labels." http://nhlbisupport. com/chd1/Tipsheets/reading-labels-tips.htm.

National Honey Board. "Honey's Nutrition and Health Facts." Press release, July 2001. http:// www.honey.com/pressrm/research/nutri.html.

"Natural Claims." Memo from Robert G. Hibbert, Director, SLD, to Branch Chiefs, SLD, November 22, 1982. www.fsis.usda.gov/OPPDE/larc/Policy%20Memos.pdf (see policy memo #55).

The Semi-Daily Journal of Economist Brad DeLong: Fair and Balanced Almost Every Day. "Only in California." A remark posted about the Odwalla's company's use of "evaporated cane juice," a term that the FDA considers illegal. Posted by DeLong on August 11, 2003. http://www.j-brad-ford-delong.net/movable_type/2003_archives/001942.html (accessed April 2, 2005).

Sheppard, Kay. *From the First Bite: A Complete Guide to Recovery from Food Addiction.* New York: Health Communications, 2000.

Sizer, Frances, and Eleanor Whitney. *Nutrition: Concepts and Controversies.* Belmont, CA: Wadsworth, 1997.

Smucker's Company website. Simply Fruit nutritional information. http://www.smuckers.com/fg/pds/ default.asp?groupid=1&catid=16.

Steward, H. Leighton, Morrison C. Bethea, Sam S. Andrews, and Luis A. Balart. *The New Sugar Busters.* New York: Ballantine Books, 2003.

Stonyfield Farms. Nutrition labels. http://www.stonyfield.com/nutritionlabels/Label.cfm?LabelID=2.

———. Nutrition labels. http://www.stonyfield.com/nutritionlabels/Label.cfm?LabelID=18.

———. Nutrition labels. http://www.stonyfield.com/nutritionlabels/Label.cfm?LabelID=30.

———. All Natural Fat Free Yogurts. http://www.stonyfield.com/OurProducts/AllNaturalYogurts. cfm#javascript:void(0).

———. Organic Whole Milk Yogurt: Strawberries & Cream. http://www.stonyfield.com/OurProducts/ WholeMilkYogurt.cfm#javascript:void(0).

Teff, Karen L., Sharon S. Elliott, Matthias Tschöp, Timothy J. Kieffer, Daniel Rader, Mark Heiman, Raymond R. Townsend, Nancy L. Keim, David D'Alessio, and Peter J. Havel. "Dietary Fructose Reduces Circulating Insulin and Leptin, Attenuates Postprandial Suppression of Ghrelin, and Increases Triglycerides in Women." *Journal of Clinical Endocrinology and Metabolism* 89 (2004): 2963–72.

U.S. Food and Drug Administration. "The Food Label," May 1999. http://www.fda.gov/ opacom/backgrounders/foodlabel/newlabel.html.

U.S. Food and Drug Administration. Center for Food Safety and Applied Nutrition (CFSAN). "Frequently Asked Questions about GRAS," December 2004. http://www.cfsan.fda.gov/~dms/ grasguid.html.

———. "How to Understand and Use the Nutrition Facts Label," November 2004. http://vm .cfsan.fda.gov/~dms/foodlab.html.

Yankee Grocery. "Maple Syrup Nutritional Information." http://www.yankeegrocery.com/ maple_nutrition.html#nutritionaldata.

CHAPTER 21: HOW CAN I SQUASH MY SUGAR CRAVINGS? AND OTHER FREQUENTLY ASKED QUESTIONS (FAQS)

Acesulfame-K Toxicity Information Center. http://www.holisticmed.com/acek/.

Alexander, Kelly. "Sweet Relief? A Sugar Snob Taste-Tests Splenda and Other Sweeteners." *Slate*, September 11, 2002. http://slate.msn.com/id/2070686/.

Allan, Christian B., and Wolfgang Lutz. *Life Without Bread: How a Low-Carbohydrate Diet Can Save Your Life*. New York: Keats 2000.

American Beverage Association website. http://www.ameribev.org/default.asp.

American Cancer Society. "Aspartame." http://www.cancer.org/docroot/PED/content/PED_1_3X_ Aspartame.asp?sitearea=PED (accessed April 2, 2005).

———. "Common Questions about Diet and Cancer." http://www.cancer.org/docroot/PED/content/ PED_3_2X_Common_Questions_About_Diet_and_Cancer.asp.

American Diabetes Association. Picture of check from Equal to the American Diabetes Assocation. http://www.diabetes.org/ada/jg3.jpg.

———. "Sweeteners." http://www.diabetes.org/nutrition-and-recipes/nutrition/sweeteners.jsp.

———. "Type 2 Diabetes." http://www.diabetes.org/type-2-diabetes.jsp.

American Dietetic Association. "ADAF Receives Grant to Support NCND." *ADA Courier* 32, no. 1 (1993).

———. "Organic Foods Versus Conventional Foods." www.eatright.org/cps/rde/xchg/ada/hs.xsl/ home_4143_ENU_HTML.htm.

———. "Straight Answers about Aspartame." http://www.eatright.org/cps/rde/xchg/ada/hs.xsl/ nutrition_1030_ENU_HTML.htm.

———. "Sugar Alcohols: New Drink or Food Additive?" http://www.eatright.org/cps/rde/xchg/ ada/hs.xsl/home_4383_ENU_HTML.htm.

Appleton, Nancy. *Lick the Sugar Habit*. Garden City Park, NY: Avery Publishing, 1988.

Aspartame Consumer Safety Network website. http://www.aspartamesafety.com/.

Aspartame (NutraSweet) Toxicity Info Center. http://www.holisticmed.com/aspartame/.

Austin Business Journal. "Texas Consumer Group Is Sour on Splenda Sweetener," January 31, 2005. http://www.bizjournals.com/austin/stories/2005/01/31/daily6.html.

Bailey, Bill. "What Is *Stevia Rebaudiana* and Is It Safe?" http://www.lowcarbnexus.com/articles/stevia. html.

Barrett, Stephen. "Stevia: Is It safe?" http://www.quackwatch.org/04ConsumerEducation/QA/ stevia.html.

Bastin, Sandra. "Nonnutritive Sweeteners." University of Kentucky Cooperative Extension Service, 2000. http://www.ca.uky.edu/agc/pubs/fcs3/fcs3105/fcs3105.pdf.

Bidwell, Jean, and Beth Regan. "Regulatory History of Saccharin." *Saccharin*. http://enhs.umn .edu/saccharin/reghistory.html.

Blaylock, Russell L. *Excitotoxins: The Taste That Kills*. Santa Fe, NM: Health Press, 1997.

Bonvie, Linda, Bill Bonvie, and Donna Gates. *The Stevia Story*. Atlanta: Body Ecology Diet, 1997.

Bouchez, Colette. "Dietitians Say Splenda Is Not the Same as Sugar." *WebMD Medical News,* February 16, 2005. http://my.webmd.com/content/article/100/105877.htm.

Bowden, Jonny. *Living the Low Carb Life: From Atkins to the Zone, Choosing the Diet That's Right for You*. New York: Sterling Publishing, 2004.

Bowen, James. "Splenda Is Not Splendid." http://www.pacifichealth.info/?m=200501.

Braly, James, and Ron Hoggan. *Dangerous Grains: Why Gluten Cereal Grains May Be Hazardous to Your Health*. New York: Avery, 2002.

Bressler, Jerome. "Establishment Inspection Report—the Bressler Report." U.S. Food and Drug Administration, EIR: G.D. Searle, Searle Laboratories. *Summary of Findings* (FDA), August 1977. http://www.dorway.com/bressler.txt.

Burrington, Kimberlee J. "Prolonging Bakery Product Life." *Food Product Design*, July 1998. http://www.foodproductdesign.com/articles/463/463_0798DE.html.

Butchko, Harriet H. Correspondence regarding "Adverse Reactions to Aspartame: Double-Blind

Challenge in Patients from a Vulnerable Population." *Biological Psychiatry* 36, no. 3 (1994): 206–7.

Cabot, Sandra. "Aspartame Makes You Fatter!" http://www.aspartame.com/aspartam.htm.

Calorie Control Council. "Consumer Use of Low-Calorie, Sugar-Free Foods and Beverages." http://www.caloriecontrol.org/lcchart.html.

———. "Low-Calorie Sweeteners: Acesulfame Potassium." http://www.caloriecontrol.org/acesulf .html.

———. "Low-Calorie Sweeteners: Saccharine." http://www.caloriecontrol.org/sacchar.html.

———. Memorandum from Beth Hubrich to Judy Tidwell. "Misinformation about Aspartame," December 16, 2003. http://allergies.about.com/cs/aspartame/a/bluc_bhubrich.htm.

———. "Most Popular Low-Calorie, Sugar-Free Products." http://www.caloriecontrol.org/popsugfree.html.

———. "The 'Multiple Ingredient Approach'; The Secret to Good Tasting Light Foods and Beverages." http://www.caloriecontrol.org/mia.html.

———. Saccharin website. www.saccharin.org.

Carney, Beth. "It's Not All Sweetness for Splenda; Although the Sugar Substitute's British Maker, Tate & Lyle, Has Seen Its Stock Rise Smartly, Analysts Doubt This High Will Last." *Business Week Online*, January 19, 2005.

Cauchon, Dennis. "FDA Advisers Tied to Industry." *USA Today*, September 25, 2000.

Center for Science in the Public Interest. "CSPI's Guide to Food Additives." http://www.cspinet .org/reports/chemcuisine.htm.

———."Food Products Containing Sorbitol." http://www.cspinet.org/new/ssachart.html.

———. "Food Products Containing Sugar Alcohols Other Than Sorbitol." http://www.cspinet .org/new/sachart.html.

———. Letter to National Toxicology Program Board of Scientific Counselors' Report on Carcinogens Subcommittee, October 24, 1997. http://www.cspinet.org/reports/saccomnt.htm.

Chemistry in Action. "What's in a Sweetener?" 50 (1997). http://www.ul.ie/%7Echildsp/CinA/ Issue50/HomePage.html.

Committee on Toxicity of Chemicals in Food, Consumer Products and the Environment. *Annual Report 2000.* http://www.food.gov.uk/multimedia/pdfs/cotcomcocrep_cot.pdf.

Congressional Record. "Aspartame Safety Act." vol. 131, no. 106 (1985): S10820–S10847.

Constantine, Alex. "Aspartame Corruption Expose." http://www.alkalizeforhealth.net/Lsweetdebate7 .htm.

Cooking with Stevia website. http://www.cookingwithstevia.com/stevia_faq.html.

Cornell Cooperative Extension Food and Nutrition. "Acesulfame Potassium Approved for Beverages," July/August 1998.

Crossen, Cynthia. *Tainted Truth: The Manipulation of Fact in America.* New York: Simon & Schuster, 1994.

Davidson, T. L., and S. E. Swithers. "A Pavlovian Approach to the Problem of Obesity." *International Journal of Obesity* 28, no. 7 (2004): 933–35.

DeAngelis, Catherine D. "Conflicts of Interest and the Public Trust." *Journal of the American Medical Association* 284 (2000): 2237–38.

DesMaisons, Kathleen. *The Sugar Addict's Total Recovery Program.* New York: Ballantine, 2000.

The Diabetes Monitor. "Is Stevia Safe? Depends Who You Ask." http://www.diabetesmonitor.com/ stevia.htm.

Donn, Jeff. "Respected Journal Says Conflicts Compromising Science." *Associated Press*, May 18, 2000.

Dorland's Illustrated Medical Dictionary, s.v. "cyclamate." MerckSource website. http://

www.mercksource.com/pp/us/cns/cns_hl_dorlands.jspzQzpgzEzzSzppdocszSzuszSzcommonzSz dorlandszSzdorlandzSzdmd_a-b_00zPz.htm.

Duffy, Valerie B., and Madeleine Sigman-Grant. "Position of the American Dietetic Association: Use of Nutritive and Nonnutritive Sweeteners." *Journal of the American Dietetic Association* 104, no. 2 (2004): 255–75.

Duprey, Rich. "Splenda's Ads: Sugar-Coated?" *Motley Fool*, February 15, 2005. http://www .fool.com/News/mft/2005/mft05021507.htm.

Duyff, Roberta Larson. *The American Dietetic Association Complete Food and Nutrition Guide.* Hoboken, NJ: John Wiley & Sons, 2002.

Eades, Michael R., and Mary Dan Eades. *Protein Power.* New York: Bantam Books, 1996.

Executive Health's Good Health Report. "Q&A: Is Newly FDA Approved Sweetener Sucralose Good for You?" 35, no. 2 (1998): 6.

Fairburn, Christopher G., and G. Terence Wilson, eds. *Binge Eating: Nature, Assessment, and Treatment.* New York: Guilford Press, 1993.

Franz, Marion, et al. *"Evidence-Based Nutrition Principles and Recommendations for the Treatment and Prevention of Diabetes and Related Complications." Diabetes Care* 25 (2002):148–98. http://care.diabetesjournals.org/cgi/content/full/25/1/148?ijkey=08e8543e42e3749447ee4e12ec85 b7418f63711c&keytype2=tf_ipsecsha.

Fumento, Michael. "Why Is Big Sugar Bitter about Splenda?" *Scripps Howard News Service*, February 3, 2005.

Gallo-Torres, Julia, and Lynn Domblaster. *"How Sweet It Is."* PreparedFoods.com. http://www .preparedfoods.com/CDA/Archives/58dedfd391788010VgnVCM100000f932a8c0.

Garbow, Joel R., John J. Likos, and Stephen A. Schroeder. "Structure, Dynamics, and Stability of Cyclodextrin Inclusion Complexes of Aspartame and Neotame." *Journal of Agricultural and Food Chemistry* 49 (2001): 2053–60.

Generation Green. Letter from Rochelle Davis, Executive Director, and Robert M. Brandon, Project Director, to Division of Advertising Practices, Bureau of Consumer Protection, Federal Trade Commission, January 13, 2005. http://www.generationgreen.org/2005_01-FTC-letter.htm.

———. "Splenda Marketing Campaign Seeks to Mislead, Confuse Consumers: Generation Green Asks the FTC to Investigate," January 13, 2005. http://www.generationgreen.org/2005-01_ lead-story.htm.

Gilbert, Sue. "Splenda: Safe during Pregnancy?" http://parenting.ivillage.com/pregnancy/psafe/0,,8x92,00 .html?arrivalSA=1&cobrandRef=0&arrival_freqCap=1&pba=adid=11036807.

Gittleman, Ann Louise. *The Fat Flush Plan.* New York: McGraw-Hill, 2002.

———. *Get the Sugar Out: 501 Simple Ways to Cut the Sugar Out of Any Diet.* New York: Three Rivers Press, 1996.

Gogoi, Pallavi. "How Far from Sugar Is Splenda?" *Business Week Online*, February 2, 2005. http:// www.businessweek.com/technology/content/feb2005/tc2005022_7832_tc024.htm.

Gold, Mark D. "Aspartame/NutraSweet Toxicity Summary." Holistic Healing website, November 30, 2000. http://www.holisticmed.com/aspartame/summary.html.

———. "The Bitter Truth about Artificial Sweeteners." Extracted from *Nexus* 2, no. 28 (1995), and *Nexus* 3, no. 1 (1996). http://www.nexusmagazine.com/articles/aspartame.html.

———. Email to Judy Tidwell, About.com. "An Email Response to 'Misinformation about Aspartame' Memorandum," January 4, 2004. http://allergies.about.com/cs/aspartame/a/bluc_mgold.htm.

Gordon, Gregory. "NutraSweet: Questions Swirl." *UPI Investigative Report.* October 12, 1987.

Greene, Bob. *Bob Greene's Total Body Makeover.* New York: Simon & Schuster, 2005.

Gross, Adrian. Aspartame Safety Act of 1985 Hearing. *Congressional Record* (1985): S10834–81040.

Heller, Rachel F., and Richard F. Heller. *Carbohydrate Addicted Kids*. New York: HarperCollins, 1997.

Henkel, John. "Sugar Substitutes: Americans Opt for Sweetness and Lite." *FDA Consumer*, November/December 1999. http://www.fda.gov/fdac/features/1999/699_sugar.html.

Hill, James O., and John C. Peters. *The Step Diet Book*. With Bonnie T. Jortberg. New York: Workman, 2004.

Hill, Napoleon. *Think and Grow Rich*. New York: Fawcett Publications, 1960.

Holistic Healing. "Aspartame Testing on Humans." http://www.holisticmed.com/aspartame/.

———. "What Is Neotame?" http://www.holisticmed.com/neotame/whatis.html.

Hull, Janet Starr. "Chlorine—In Your Pool and Diet Cola." *Healthy Newsletter*, July 2004. http://www.janethull.com/newsletter/0704/chlorine-in-your-pool-and-diet-cola.php.

———. "Splenda Case History." *Healthy Newsletter*, July 2004. http://www.janethull.com/newsletter/0704/splenda-case-history.php.

———. "Splenda—Here We Go Again." *Healthy Newsletter*, July 2004. http://www.janethull.com/newsletter/0704/splenda-here-we-go-again.php.

———. "Splenda: Is it Safe or Not?" *Healthy Newsletter*, December 2003. http://www.sweetpoison.com/newsletter/splenda.

———. *Sweet Poison: How the World's Most Popular Artificial Sweetener Is Killing Us—My Story*. Far Hills, NJ: New Horizon Press, 1999.

Hunter, B. T. "Sucralose." *Consumers' Research Magazine* 73, no. 10 (1990): 8–9.

Innovations Report. "Sweetener Stevioside Is a Safe Sugar Substitute," December 23, 2004. http://www.innovations-report.com/html/reports/medicine_health/report-38242.html.

Institute for Agriculture and Trade Policy. "IATP Files Complaint with U.S. Federal Trade Commission Regarding Splenda Advertising." Press release, January 28, 2005. http://www.iatp.org/iatp/library/admin/uploadedfiles/IATP_Files_Complaint_With_US_Federal_Trade_Com.pdf.

———. "Splenda Uses Misleading Advertising." *IATP News* 9, no. 1 (2005). http://www.iatp.org/iatp/iatpnews/img/0502.html.

Institute of Medicine of the National Academies, Food and Nutrition Board. "Dietary Reference Intakes: Macronutrients." http://www.iom.edu/Object.File/Master/7/300/0.pdf.

Jacobson, Michael. "Artificial Sweetener 'Sunett' Should Not Be Used in Diet Soda." Press release, July 31, 1996. Center for Science in the Public Interest. http://www.cspinet.org/new/ask.html.

———. "Repeal of Saccharine Warning Label Criticized." Center for Science in the Public Interest. http://www.cspinet.org/new/saccharin_labeling.html.

Jacobson, Michael F., Lisa Y. Lefferts, and Anne Witte Garland. *Safe Food: Eating Wisely in a Risky World*. Los Angeles: Living Planet Press, 1991.

Jensen, Bernard. *Foods That Heal*. Garden City Park, NY: Avery, 1993.

Keeney, Keith. "For 87 Million Diet Soft Drink Consumers, Acesulfame Potassium's Soft Drink Approval a Welcome New Choice." Press release, June 30, 1998. Calorie Control Council. http://www.caloriecontrol.org/pr6-30-98.html.

Labare, M.P., and M. Alexander. "Microbial Cometabolism of Sucralose, a Chlorinated Disaccharide, in Environmental Samples." *Applied Microbiology and Biotechnology* 42 (1994): 173–78.

Larimer, Mary E., Rebekka S. Palmer, and G. Alan Marlatt. "Relapse Prevention: An Overview of Marlatt's Cognitive-Behavioral Model." *Alcohol Research and Health* 23, no. 2 (1999): 151–60.

Larson, Joan Mathews. *Depression-Free, Naturally*. New York: Ballantine, 1999.

Lieberman, Shari. *Dare to Lose: 4 Simple Steps to a Better Body*. With Nancy Bruning. New York: Avery, 2002.

Lord, G. H., and P. M. Newberne. "Renal Mineralization—a Ubiquitous Lesion in Chronic Rat Studies." *Food and Chemical Toxicology* 28 (1990): 449–55.

Maher, Timothy J., and Richard J. Wurtman. "Possible Neurologic Effects of Aspartame, a Widely Used Food Additive." *Environmental Health Perspectives* 75 (1987): 53–57. http://ehp.niehs.nih.gov/members/1987/075/75010.PDF.

Marlatt, G. Alan, and Judith R. Gordon, eds. *Relapse Prevention: Maintenance Strategies in the Treatment of Addictive Behaviors*. New York: Guilford Press, 1985.

Mars, Brigitte. *Addiction-Free Naturally: Liberating Yourself from Sugar, Caffeine, Food Addictions, Tobacco, Alcohol, Prescription Drugs*. Rochester, VT: Healing Arts Press, 2001.

Maudlin, R. K. "FDA Approves Sucralose for Expanded Use." *Modern Medicine* 67, no. 10 (1999): 57.

May, James A. *The Miracle of Stevia: Discover the Healing Power of Nature's Herbal Sweetener*. New York: Kensington, 2003.

Mayo Clinic. "Sugar Substitutes: Sweet Taste without all the Calories." http://www.mayoclinic.com/invoke.cfm?objectid=C367D268-8929-4BA8-8DBACAD0320E8099.

McGraw, Phil. *The Ultimate Weight Solution: The 7 Keys to Weight Loss Freedom*. New York: Free Press, 2003.

MedHelp International. "Phenylketonuria." http://www.medhelp.org/lib/pku.htm.

Medical Letter on Drugs and Therapeutics. "Sucralose—a New Artificial Sweetener." 40, no. 1030 (1998): 67–68.

Medline Plus. "Phenylketonuria." http://www.nlm.nih.gov/medlineplus/phenylketonuria.html.

Medline Plus Medical Encyclopedia, s.v. "Sweeteners." http://www.nlm.nih.gov/medlineplus/ency/article/002444.htm.

The Merck Manual of Medical Information—Second Home Edition Online. "Gas and Chemical Exposure." http://www.merck.com/mmhe/sec04/ch049/ch049j.html.

Mercola.com. "The Secret Dangers of Splenda (Sucralose), an Artificial Sweetener." http://www.mercola.com/2000/dec/3/sucralose_dangers.htm.

Metcalfe, Ed. "Sweet Talking." *Ecologist* 30, No. 4 (June, 2000).

Mindell, Earl. *Earl Mindell's Vitamin Bible for the 21st Century*. New York: Warner Books, 1999.

Misner, Scottie. "Sugar Substitutes: Are They Safe?" May 2001. http://ag.arizona.edu/pubs/health/az1229.pdf.

Mission Possible. Press release, May 26, 1998. http://www.aspartame.com/Stevia%20Press%20Release.html.

———. http://www.dorway.com/possible.html.

Moran, Victoria. *Fit from Within: 101 Simple Secrets to Change Your Body and Your Life—Starting Today and Lasting Forever*. New York: Contemporary Books, 2002.

Mullarkey, Barbara Alexander, and Adell V. Newman. "Sweet Delusion: How Safe Is Your Artificial Sweetener." *Informed Consent* 1, no. 4 (1994). http://www.dorway.com/betty/consent.txt.

National Cancer Institute. "Cancer Facts: Artificial Sweeteners." http://www.cancer.gov/cancertopics/factsheet/Risk/artificial-sweeteners.

National Center for Biotechnology Information. "Phenylketonuria," *Genes and Disease*. http://www.ncbi.nlm.nih.gov/books/bv.fcgi?call=bv.View..ShowSection&rid=gnd.section.234.

National Multiple Sclerosis Society. "Stories Linking Aspartame and Multiple Sclerosis Unfounded." http://www.nationalmssociety.org/headlines-aspartame.asp.

National PKU News website. http://www.pkunews.org/.

National Soft Drink Association. "Objections of the National Soft Drink Association to a Final Rule Permitting the Use of Aspartame in Carbonated Beverages and Carbonated Beverage Syrup Bases and a Request for a Hearing on the Objections" (Docket No. 82F-0305, Draft, July 28, 1983) appearing in *Congressional Record* 131, no. 58 (1985): 5507–11. http://www.dorway.com/nsda.html.

Novick, Jeff. "Stevia, the Herbal Sweetener—How Safe Is It Really?" *Chef Jeff's Weekly Health Up-date*, October 23, 2000. http://www.aboutbreathing.com/articles/stevia.htm.

The NutraSweet Company. "Customers and Partners." http://www.nutrasweet.com/custpart/index.asp.

Pescatore, Fred. *The Hamptons Diet*. Hoboken, NJ: John Wiley & Sons, 2004.

PMC Specialties Group, Inc., website. http://www.pmcsg.com/.

PR Newswire. "Five Lawsuits Filed Against Splenda; Johnson & Johnson Under Fire Concerning False Advertising and Misleading Consumers about Splenda." Press release from the Truth about Splenda campaign, January 27, 2005. http://www.prnewswire.com/cgi-bin/stories.pl?ACCT=109&STORY=/www/story/01-27-2005/0002908706&EDATE.

———. "The Sweet Truth about Sugar Substitutes," October 30, 2003.

Rael, Shelley. "Artificial Sweeteners: What's Out There?" *EHPP Nutrition Notes Newsletter* 1, no. 3 (2000). http://ehpp.unm.edu/ListServe3.htm.

Reitz, David Oliver. "The National Soft Drink Association." Dorway.com. http://www.dorway.com/nsda.html.

Richard, David. *Stevia Rebaudiana: Nature's Sweet Secret*. Bloomingdale, IL: Blue Heron Press, 1996.

Roberts, H. J. "Aspartame Disease: An FDA-Approved Epidemic." Mercola.com. http://www.mercola.com/2004/jan/7/aspartame_disease.htm.

———. *Aspartame Disease: An Ignored Epidemic*. West Palm Beach, FL: Sunshine Sentinel Press, 2001.

———. "Aspartame (NutraSweet) Addiction." *Townsend Letter for Doctors and Patients* 198 (2000): 52–57. http://nancymarkle.com/tldaddic.txt.

———. *Aspartame (NutraSweet): Is It Safe?* Philadelphia: Charles Press, 1990.

———. "Section 13—Aspartame Disease." *Useful Insights for Diagnosis, Treatment, Public Health: An Updated Anthology of Original Research*. West Palm Beach, FL: Palm Beach Institute for Medical Research, 2002.

Ross, Julia. *The Mood Cure: The 4-Step Program to Rebalance Your Emotional Chemistry and Redis-cover Your Natural Sense of Well-Being*. New York, Viking, 2002.

Rowett, Christine A. "Smithsonian Revisits Remsen, Fahlberg Debate." *Johns Hopkins University Gazette*, August 22, 1994. http://www.jhu.edu/~gazette/1994/aug2294/remsen.html.

Ruggiero, Roberta. *The Do's and Don'ts of Hypoglycemia: An Everyday Guide to Low Blood Sugar Too Often Misunderstood and Diagnosed*. Hollywood, FL: Frederick Fell, 2003.

Sahelian, Ray, and Donna Gates. *The Stevia Cookbook: Cooking with Nature's Calorie-Free Sweet-ener*. New York: Avery, 1999.

Schardt, David. "Sweet Nothings—Not All Sweeteners Are Equal." *Nutrition Action Health Letter*, May 2004. http://www.cspinet.org/nah/05_04/sweet_nothings.pdf.

Siegel, Bernie. *Peace, Love and Healing*. New York: Harper & Row, 1989.

———. *Prescriptions for Living*. New York: Quill, 1998.

Smith, Kathy. *Kathy Smith's Lift Weights to Lose Weight*. With Robert Miller. New York: Warner Books, 2001.

Somer, Elizabeth. *Food and Mood: The Complete Guide to Eating Well and Feeling Your Best*. New York: Henry Holt, 1999.

Splenda, Inc. "About Splenda." http://splenda.com.

———. "American Diabetes Association and McNeil Nutritionals, Maker of Splenda Brand Products, Announce Sponsorship," January 20, 2004. http://www.splenda.com/page.jhtml?id=splenda/pressctr/ada_sponsor.inc.

———. "Frequently Asked Questions." http://splenda.com/page.jhtml?id=splenda/faqs/faqmain.inc.

———. "Healthcare Professionals Regulatory Approval." http://www.splenda.com/page.jhtml?id=splenda/hcp/regapproval.inc.

———. "Healthcare Professionals Safety of Sucralose." http://www.splenda.com/page.jhtml?id=splenda/hcp/safety.inc.

———. "Healthcare Professionals Splenda Basics." http://www.splenda.com/page.jhtml?id=splenda/hcp/basics.inc.

———. "List of U.S. Products with Splenda Brand Sweetener." http://www.splenda.com/library/assets/splenda/productswithsplenda.pdf.

———. "The Science of Splenda Brand Sweetener." http://www.splendaprofessional.com/page.jhtml;jsessionid=WNE1HTHARV4YYCQPCAOSUYYKB2IIWNSC?id=/splendaprofessional/include/science.inc.

Spoon, Mary. "Is Sweetener Stevia Safe?" *Reno Gazette-Journal,* January 27, 2003. http://www.rgj.com/news/stories/html/2003/01/27/32946.php.

Stark, Christina. "Sugar Substitutes—FDA Consumer Article." *Cornell Cooperative Extension Food and Nutrition,* November/December 1999.

Stellman, S. D., and L. Garfinkel. "Artificial Sweetener Use and One-Year Weight Change Among Women." *Preventive Medicine* 15 (1986): 195–202.

———. "Patterns of Artificial Sweetener Use and Weight Change in an American Cancer Society Prospective Study." *Appetite* 11, suppl. 1 (1998): 85–91.

Stoddard, Mary Nash. *The Deadly Deception: Story of Aspartame.* Dallas, TX: Odenwald Press, 1998.

———. Interview by Ernie Brown. *The Ernie Brown Show.* KRLD Radio (1080AM) Dallas and Texas State Network, February 18, 1997. http://www.aspartamesafety.com/Transcript4.htm.

Stoddard, Mary Nash, and George Leighton. "Aspartame and Flying: The Incredible Untold Story." *Extraordinary Science,* July 1995. http://www.aspartamesafety.com/Article4.htm.

Stoll, Andrew L. *The Omega-3 Connection.* New York: Fireside, 2001.

Sugar Association website. http://www.sugar.org/.

Takayama S., A. G. Renwick, S. L. Johansson, U. P. Thorgeirsson, M. Tsutsumi, D. W. Dalgard, and S. M. Sieber. "Long-Term Toxicity and Carcinogenicity Study of Cyclamate in Nonhuman Primates." *Toxicological Sciences* 53, no. 1 (2000): 33–39.

Truth about Splenda. "The 'Truth about Splenda' Website Launched." Press release, January 10, 2005. http://www.truthaboutsplenda.com/news/01-10-05-website.html.

U.S. Department of Health and Human Services. Centers for Disease Control and Prevention. "Defining Overweight and Obesity." http://www.cdc.gov/nccdphp/dnpa/obesity/defining.htm.

———. "Facts about Phosgene." http://www.bt.cdc.gov/agent/phosgene/basics/facts.asp.

U.S. Food and Drug Administration. Code of Federal Regulations, Chapter 1, Subchapter B, Part 172, Subpart I, Section 172.829. "Neotame," April 1, 2004. http://www.accessdata.fda.gov/scripts/cdrh/cfdocs/cfcfr/CFRSearch.cfm?FR=172.829.

———. "FDA Approves New Non-nutritive Sugar Substitute Neotame," July 5, 2002. http://www.fda.gov/bbs/topics/ANSWERS/2002/ANS01156.html.

———. "Final Rule" for Sucralose, 21 CFR Part 172, Docket No. 87F-0086.

———. "Food Allergies Rare but Risky." *FDA Consumer,* May 1994. http://www.cfsan.fda.gov/~dms/wh-alrg1.html.

———. IA #45-06 "Automatic Detention of Stevia Leaves, Extract of Stevia Leaves, and Food Containing Stevia," May 28, 2003. http://www.fda.gov/ora/fiars/ora_import_ia4506.html.

———. Letter from Arlyn H. Baumgarten to Anthony Costello, President of Optimum Nutrition, Inc., May 7, 2002. http://www.fda.gov/foi/warning_letters/g3288d.htm.

———. "'Nutrition Facts' to Help Consumers Eat Smart," 1994. www.fda.gov/fdac/special/foodlabel/facts.html.

Waldron, J. T. and Cori Brackett. *Sweet Misery: A Poisoned World*. Documentary. Tucson, AZ: Sound and Fury Productions, Inc., 2004.

Walker, Sophie. "J&J Sued Over Splenda Ad Campaign." *Reuters*, January 31, 2005.

Walton, Ralph G. "The Possible Role of Aspartame in Seizure Induction." In *Dietary Phenylalanine and Brain Function*, edited by Richard J. Wurtman and Eva Ritter-Walker. Boston: Birkhauser, 1988.

———. "Survey of Aspartame Studies: Correlation of Outcome and Funding Sources," 1998. http://www.dorway.com/peerrev.html.

Walton, Ralph, Robert Hudak, and Ruth J. Green-Waite. "Adverse Reactions to Aspartame: Double-Blind Challenge in Patients from a Vulnerable Population." *Biological Psychiatry* 34, no. 1 (1993): 13–17.

Warner, Melanie. "Splenda Is Leaving Other Sugar Substitutes with That Empty Feeling." *New York Times*, December 22, 2004.

Weil, Andrew. *Ask Dr. Weil*. New York: Fawcett Columbine, 1998.

———. "Aspartame: Can a Little Bit Hurt?" Weil Website, September 25, 2002. http://www.drweil.com/u/QA/QA106654/.

———. *Natural Health, Natural Medicine: A Comprehensive Manual for Wellness and Self-Care*. New York: Houghton Mifflin, 1998.

Whitaker, Julian. *Dr. Julian Whitaker's Health and Healing* 5, no. 11 (1995).

Wilson, Steve. "Sweet Suspicions." TV broadcast transcript (1984) appearing in *Congressional Record* 131, no. 106 (1985): S10826–S10827.

The WINDS. "Aspartame: Is There Poison in That Can?" http://www.apfn.org/THEWINDS/1999/02/aspartame.html.

World Healthy Organization. "Populations with High Sugar Consumption Are at Increased Risk of Chronic Disease, South African Researchers Report." Press release, August 28, 2003. http://www.who.int/bulletin/releases/2003/PR0803/en/.

Wurtman, Richard. J. "Neurochemical Changes Following High-Dose Aspartame with Dietary Carbohydrates." *New England Journal of Medicine* 309 (1983): 429–30.

Yale-New Haven Hospital. "Eat Any Sugar Alcohol Lately?" www.ynhh.org/online/nutrition/advisor/sugar_alcohol.html.

AFTERWORD: RAYS OF HOPE AND SIGNS OF PROMISE

Ascribe Business and Economics News Service. "Parents, Socially Conscious Food Companies Team Up to Promote Healthy Eating at Home," September 25, 2005. www.highbeam.com/browse/Business-Finance-AScribe+Business+~A~+Economics+News+Service/September-2005-p1-65k.

Brent Zook, Kristal. "We Can't Let the Obesity Epidemic Claim Our Children." *Essence*, April 2005. http://www.findarticles.com/p/articles/mi_m1264/is_12_35/ai_n13596183.

Calhoun School website. http://www.calhoun.org.

CBS News. "Cookie Monster Changes His Tune," April 8, 2005. http://www.cbsnews.com/stories/2005/04/08/entertainment/main686684.shtml.

CNN. "Diabetes Epidemic Continues to Worsen; Body Shape Is Risk Factor; The Role of Diet and Exercise to Control Diabetes; Type 2 Diabetes on the Rise in Kids." House Call with Dr. Sanjay Gupta, November 12, 2005. http://transcripts.cnn.com/TRANSCRIPTS/0511/12/hcsg.01.html.

Cross Roads News. "Sugar-Free Teacher to Share Her Story of Triumph." http://www.johnsonmedia.com/crossroadsnews/getarticle.php3?id=2827.

DeKalb County Schools. "Achieving Academic Excellence Through Nutrition and Exercise. Welcome to the Sugar-Free Zone." http://www.dekalb.k12.ga.us/brownsmill/health.html.

Eat Smart Grow Strong website. http://www.eatsmartgrowstrong.com/Home.aspx.

The Edible Schoolyard website. http://www.EdibleSchoolyard.org.

Ennovy website. http://www.ennovyinc.com.

Greenearth Institute. "Case Study: Appleton Central Alternative Charter High School." http://www.greenearthinstitute.org/nutrition/Documents/ACACaseStudyFinalVersion.doc.

"Harkin Pushes Comprehensive Wellness Initiative to Fight Chronic Disease, Obesity." Senator Tom Harkin's website. http://harkin.senate.gov/news.cfm?id=222816.

Healthy Arkansas website. http://www.arkansas.gov/ha/home.html.

Institute for Integrative Nutrition website. http://www.integrativenutrition.com/.

National Farm to School Program website. http://www.FarmToSchool.org.

National Governors Association. "Healthy America." http://www.nga.org/portal/site/nga/menuitem.5cd31a89efe1f1e122d81fa6501010a0/?vgnextoid=032578e483a25010VgnVCM1000001a01010aRCRD.

National Public Radio. "School Lunch, Chef Bobo Style." http://www.npr.org/templates/story/story.php?storyId=1185900.

National Weight Control Registry website. http://www.nwcr.ws/.

New York City Department of Education. "School Food." www.opt-osfns.org/osfns/.

Rosenthal, Joshua. Comments made at the Instititute for Integrative Nutrition, where Connie studied, and in the IIN catalogue.

Sanders-Butler, Yvonne, and Barbara Alpert. *Healthy Kids, Smart Kids: The Principal-Created, Parent-Tested, Kid-Approved Nutrition Plan for Sound Bodies and Strong Minds.* New York: Penguin, 2005.

Schibsted, Evantheia. "Brain Food." Edutopia website. http://www.edutopia.org/magazine/ed1article.php?id=Art_1421&issue=dec_05.

School Lunch Initiative website. http://www.schoollunchinitiative.org/.

Stitt, Barbara. *Food and Behavior.* Natural Press, 1997.

Surles, Robert. *Chef Bobo's Good Food Cookbook.* Des Moines, IA: Meredith Books, 2004.

Two Angry Moms website. http://www.AngryMoms.org.

University of Arizona Integrative Medicine Program website. http://www.integrativemedicine.arizona.edu/about2.html.

Whole Foods Market website. http://www.wholefoodsmarket.com/company/index.html.

Wild Oats Natural Marketplace website. http://www.wildoats.com.

INDEX

Page numbers in **bold** indicate tables.

TRADEMARK INFORMATION